Human Well-Being Research and Policy Making

Series Editor

M. Joseph Sirgy, Department of Marketing, Virginia Polytechnic Institute and State University, Blacksburg, USA

This series includes policy-focused books on the role of the public and private sectors in advancing quality of life and well-being. It creates a dialogue between well-being scholars and public policy makers. Well-being theory, research and practice are essentially interdisciplinary in nature and embrace contributions from all disciplines within the social sciences. With the exception of leading economists, the policy relevant contributions of social scientists are widely scattered and lack the coherence and integration needed to more effectively inform the actions of policy makers. Contributions in the series focus on one more of the following four aspects of well-being and public policy:

- Discussions of the public policy and well-being focused on particular nations and worldwide regions
- Discussions of the public policy and well-being in specialized sectors of policy making such as health, education, work, social welfare, housing, transportation, use of leisure time
- Discussions of public policy and well-being associated with particular population groups such as women, children and youth, the aged, persons with disabilities, and vulnerable populations
- Special topics in well-being and public policy such as technology and well-being, terrorism and well-being, infrastructure and well-being.

This series was initiated, in part, through funds provided by the Halloran Philanthropies of West Conshohocken, Pennsylvania, USA. The commitment of the Halloran Philanthropies is to “inspire, innovate and accelerate sustainable social interventions that promote human well-being.” The series editors and Springer acknowledge Harry Halloran, Tony Carr and Audrey Selian for their contributions in helping to make the series a reality.

Aurora Adina Colomeischi
Editor

Wellbeing in Schools of Southeastern Europe

Integrating Research and Practice

Springer

Editor
Aurora Adina Colomeischi
Faculty of Psychology and Sciences
of Education
"Ştefan cel Mare" University of Suceava
Suceava, Romania

ISSN 2522-5367 ISSN 2522-5375 (electronic)
Human Well-Being Research and Policy Making
ISBN 978-3-032-10524-0 ISBN 978-3-032-10525-7 (eBook)
https://doi.org/10.1007/978-3-032-10525-7

This Springer imprint is published by the registered company Springer Nature Switzerland AG
The registered company address is: Gewerbestrasse 11, 6330 Cham, Switzerland

To my beloved Tudor, whose unwavering support, strength, and kindness have been a constant source of resilience and wellbeing.

And to my dear son, Codrin, whose curiosity, joy, and light remind me every day of the importance of nurturing wellbeing in every child.

To all the teachers who struggle beyond their powers to fulfill their mission of spreading kindness, beauty, and knowledge into the world.

Contents

Editor and Contributors

About the Editor

Aurora Adina Colomeischi, Ph.D., is an Associate Professor at "Ştefan cel Mare" University of Suceava, having 29 years of experience in education, currently also serving as Dean of the Faculty of Psychology and Educational Sciences. She brings extensive experience in teaching, counseling, and educational research. Her teaching areas are emotional education, psycho-pedagogical counseling, positive psychology, psychology of resilience and teacher training. She initiated and coordinated two master programs, one for teachers in the field of counseling and emotional education and another one for teacher training in resilience.

With a multidisciplinary background as a trained teacher, counselor, and registered psychologist, Dr. Colomeischi's work centers on advancing mental health, resilience, and emotional wellbeing in educational contexts. She has successfully led numerous Erasmus+ projects, developing and implementing innovative curricular frameworks that integrate social-emotional learning (SEL), resilience, and mental health practices into schools and designs teacher training programs based on international experience.

Her scholarly contributions include over 70 publications—spanning topics like emotional education, resilience, social-emotional learning, and teacher wellbeing—and more than 1300 citations of her work. Dr. Colomeischi's research interests focus on children's wellbeing, school resilience, and the application of SEL strategies in education. Her contributions to the field extend beyond academia, as she frequently delivers workshops and training sessions for educators both nationally and internationally, addressing the critical need for resilience and mental health initiatives in schools.

A committed educator and researcher, Dr. Colomeischi champions emotional and psychological wellbeing in schools and universities through both her academic work and leadership roles.

Researcher ID: AEO-7524-2022.

Contributors

Angelica Mariana Andrei Faculty of Psychology and Sciences of Education, "Ştefan cel Mare" University of Suceava, Suceava, Romania

Liliana Bujor Faculty of Psychology and Sciences of Education, "Ştefan cel Mare" University of Suceava, Suceava, Romania

Aurora Adina Colomeischi Faculty of Psychology and Sciences of Education, "Ştefan cel Mare" University of Suceava, Suceava, Romania

Antoci Diana "Ion Creanga" State Pedagogical University of Chisinau, Chişinău, Republic of Moldova

Diana Sinziana Duca Faculty of Psychology and Sciences of Education, "Ştefan cel Mare" University of Suceava, Suceava, Romania

Olena Homoniuk Jan Kochanwski Unversity, Kielce, Poland

Maria Magdalena Iordăchescu Dimitriu Faculty of Psychology and Sciences of Education, "Ştefan cel Mare" University of Suceava, Suceava, Romania

Nadia Koltcheva Department of Cognitive Science and Psychology, New Bulgarian University, Sofia, Bulgaria

Inna Kovalchuk Yuriy Fedkovych Chernivtsi National University, Chernivtsi, Ukraine

Cornelia Ilciuc Faculty of Psychology and Sciences of Education, "Ştefan cel Mare" University of Suceava, Suceava, Romania;
"Al. I. Cuza" University of Iaşi, Iaşi, Romania

Maria Oliinyk Yuriy Fedkovych Chernivtsi National University, Chernivtsi, Ukraine;
Khmelnytski National University, Khmelnitskyi, Ukraine

Maria Poulou Patras University, Patras, Greece

Petruta P. Rusu Faculty of Psychology and Sciences of Education, "Ştefan cel Mare" University of Suceava, Suceava, Romania

Nadia Laura Serdenciuc Faculty of Psychology and Sciences of Education, "Ştefan cel Mare" University of Suceava, Suceava, Romania

Mislitchi Valentina "Ion Creanga" State Pedagogical University of Chisinau, Chişinău, Republic of Moldova

Sanja Tatalović Vorkapić Faculty of Teacher Education, University of Rijeka, Rijeka, Croatia

Chapter 1
Introduction

Aurora Adina Colomeischi

The wellbeing of students and teachers within educational environments has become an increasingly critical area of focus, acknowledged globally as essential for cultivating resilient and inclusive societies. The significance of school wellbeing extends far beyond academic performance, encompassing broader aspects of psychological health, social inclusion, and overall quality of life. Recognizing schools as important environments where children spend significant developmental years, educational policies at the European level have strongly advocated for comprehensive wellbeing initiatives aimed at creating positive and supportive learning climates.

Recent international crises, such as the COVID-19 pandemic and geopolitical disruptions including the invasion of Ukraine, have underscored the vulnerability of educational systems and amplified the urgent need for robust mental health and emotional wellbeing strategies in schools. These events have had profound implications, increasing anxiety, stress, and mental health concerns among students and educators alike, thus highlighting the necessity for systemic interventions and support mechanisms.

In the context of South-Eastern Europe, the challenges related to school wellbeing are notably distinct and complex, exacerbated by historical, socio-economic, and geopolitical factors unique to the region. Issues such as limited access to mental health resources, inadequate professional support for teachers, rural–urban disparities, and the impact of conflict and displacement significantly complicate efforts to foster effective wellbeing practices.

The book proposes a comprehensive approach, both theoretical and practical, to the issue of promoting wellbeing in schools in South Eastern European countries. Having two main parts, the book brings together relevant theoretical and practical

A. A. Colomeischi (✉)
Faculty of Psychology and Sciences of Education, "Ştefan cel Mare" University of Suceava, Suceava, Romania
e-mail: adina.colomeischi@usm.ro
URL: https://www.usv.ro

A. A. Colomeischi (ed.), *Wellbeing in Schools of Southeastern Europe*, Human Well-Being Research and Policy Making, https://doi.org/10.1007/978-3-032-10525-7_1

information to provide a clear, complex, and comprehensive lens for understanding how schools and society have been concerned with ensuring children's wellbeing at school in recent years. The first part includes theoretical and educational policy approaches at European and regional level, focusing on the elements that describe the main actors involved in education (the school as an institution, the school climate, teachers, and the impact they have on the lives of the children they work with, parents and the family), identifying relevant and significant aspects in terms of promoting wellbeing in schools. The second part highlights, through case studies, dimensions relevant to the education systems in six European countries (Bulgaria, Croatia, Greece, Moldavia, Romania, Ukraine).

The first part of this book explores essential dimensions of school wellbeing through interconnected chapters that collectively build a comprehensive understanding of the topic. In the opening chapter, "Wellbeing in European Schools—Policies and Recommendations. Peculiarities for South-Eastern European Region," Angela Andrei and Aurora Adina Colomeischi set the groundwork by discussing European educational policies, emphasizing how they seek to address various dimensions of wellbeing. Special attention is given to the South-Eastern European context, highlighting regional peculiarities, challenges, and actionable recommendations. Following this foundational chapter, the discussions deepened by focusing specifically on "Teachers' Wellbeing and Resilience—Implications for School Wellbeing." This chapter underscores the critical role teachers play as central agents in fostering a healthy school environment. It examines how teachers' wellbeing and resilience directly influence educational outcomes, teacher retention, student engagement, and overall school culture. Expanding the scope further, Diana Sinziana Duca and Maria Magdalena Dimitriu address the broader environmental aspects in their chapter, "School Climate and Wellbeing—Theoretical and Empirical Framework." This chapter offers a comprehensive analysis of how the school climate significantly impacts student and teacher wellbeing. The authors provide both theoretical insights and research results, emphasizing the need for supportive, inclusive, and nurturing school environments. Lastly, Petruta P. Rusu and Cornelia Ilciuc investigate the familial dimension in the chapter "Parental Stress, Family Support, and Students' Wellbeing at School." Recognizing the interconnectedness between home and school environments, this chapter explores how parental stress and family dynamics influence students' emotional and academic wellbeing. The chapter concludes by emphasizing the need to include family stress management and parenting support in interventions aimed at enhancing children's wellbeing both at home and at school.

Together, these chapters create a robust, multidimensional framework for understanding and improving wellbeing within educational contexts, emphasizing the importance of comprehensive, integrative approaches that involve educational policies, students, teachers, school climates, and family partnerships.

The second part of the book enriches the discourse by presenting case studies from various European countries, each one illustrating unique national contexts, policies, and practices. Nadia Koltcheva examines "Children Wellbeing in Bulgaria: Policies,

Practices, and Prospects," exploring current Bulgarian approaches and future opportunities for improving child wellbeing. Sanja Tatalović Vorkapić discusses "Challenges and Opportunities for Enhancing Wellbeing in Croatian Kindergartens and Schools," providing practical insights into Croatian educational practices, critically discussing evidence-based SEL and positive psychology programs implemented in Croatia, which showed significant positive effects on children's and teachers' mental health. Maria Poulou's analysis of "Mental Health and Wellbeing in Schools: The Case of Greece" presents Greek policies and practices, emphasizing effective strategies and areas for further development and concluding with recommendations for holistic, evidence-based approaches that integrate teacher support, student-focused interventions, and policy reforms to create safe, inclusive, and mentally supportive school environments. Further, Antoci Diana and Mislitchi Valentina delve into "Wellbeing in the Educational System of the Republic of Moldova: Conceptualization, Promotion, Assurance," showcasing Moldova's efforts and challenges in embedding wellbeing into their educational system and calling for holistic, evidence-based strategies that integrate psychological, social, and institutional dimensions to sustainably improve wellbeing in Moldovan schools. Aurora Adina Colomeischi goes on with "Wellbeing and Mental Health Promotion at School. The Case of Romania," providing a detailed overview of Romanian initiatives and their impacts, concluding with evidence-based strategies and recommendations for integrating wellbeing systematically across all educational levels. The last chapter is dedicated to the Ukraine case: Mariia Oliinyk, Olena Homoniuk, and Inna Kovalchuk critically explore "To the Problem of Studying the Psychological Health of Students During the War," focusing specifically on Ukrainian educational system, shedding light on the extreme conditions impacting student wellbeing and educational practices in a war context. Together, these chapters provide a comprehensive, multidimensional exploration of school wellbeing, effectively connecting theoretical frameworks, empirical findings, regional peculiarities, and practical case studies, offering valuable insights and actionable recommendations for enhancing wellbeing within educational systems across diverse contexts.

This book is born from a shared vision—a belief that every child, regardless of background or geography, deserves to grow in a school environment that nurtures not only their intellect but also their emotional, social, and psychological development. The authors participated together in different educational projects and initiatives driven by the same belief: that the wellbeing is the foundation upon which thriving learners, empowered teachers, and resilient communities are built. Rooted in the diverse yet interconnected landscapes of South-Eastern Europe, this volume is a significant call to action for educational transformation. It brings together voices from across the region to explore how wellbeing in schools is not merely a desirable goal, but an essential right and a necessary condition for educational equity, inclusion, and excellence. We hope to inspire educators, policymakers, researchers, and communities to reimagine school not just as a place for academic instruction, but as a vibrant space for human flourishing.

Part I

Chapter 2
Wellbeing in European Schools—Policies and Reccomandations. Peculiarities for South-Eastern European Region

Angelica Mariana Andrei and Aurora Adina Colomeischi

2.1 Introduction

The world has undergone unprecedented crises, such as the COVID-19 pandemic and Russia's war of aggression against Ukraine, energy crisis and inflation, in addition to challenges as climate change, biodiversity loss and pollution, increased digitalization and demographic change. Beyond tackling these crises, addressing mental health challenges is crucial to boosting the resilience of individuals and societies.

After the COVID-19 pandemic, mental health problems, in particular anxiety and depression expanded, with many pupils suffering from reduced emotional wellbeing and motivation. Following the Russian invasion of Ukraine, ensuring the inclusion of Ukrainian refugee children in schools, across other European countries makes wellbeing in schools even more relevant.

The wellbeing is considered a key component of mental health in children (Simões et al., 2021), underlining the importance of school interventions that focus both on improving wellbeing, as well as reducing mental health problems.

Therefore, it is crucial to design and implement socio-emotional learning, mental health, wellbeing and bullying prevention programmes in schools for children and young people, including those disadvantaged and marginalized.

A. M. Andrei · A. A. Colomeischi (✉)
Faculty of Psychology and Sciences of Education, "Ştefan cel Mare" University of Suceava, Suceava, Romania
e-mail: adina.colomeischi@usm.ro
URL: https://www.usv.ro

A. M. Andrei
e-mail: angelica.andrei@usm.ro

A. A. Colomeischi (ed.), *Wellbeing in Schools of Southeastern Europe*, Human Well-Being Research and Policy Making, https://doi.org/10.1007/978-3-032-10525-7_2

An Overview upon the Main Educational and Health Policies at the European Level Significant for School Wellbeing

The European policies emphasize the importance of wellbeing in schools and there are recommendations at the European level that address these issues.

The first strategic priority of the Council Resolution on a strategic framework for European co-operation in education and training towards the European Education Area and beyond (2021–2030) (Official Journal of the European Union, 2021) is to improve quality, equity, inclusion and success for all in education and training. The working groups of the European Commission's Education and training 2020 framework are supporting EU countries and the European Commission to make the European Education Area (EEA) a reality. The working groups on schools, namely Pathways to School Success and Learning for Sustainability offer a forum to exchange experiences and practices on addressing common challenges.

The first group supports the implementation and follow-up of the forthcoming Council Recommendation on Pathways to School Success by promoting mutual learning and the exchange of best practices, including on issues related to wellbeing at school as a key component of school success. Moreover, Pathways to School Success aims to promote better educational outcomes for all learners and the well-being of learners and educators at school. This policy document (Official Journal of the European Union, 2022a) recommends by 2025, a further strengthening of an integrated and comprehensive strategy towards school success, comprising prevention, intervention and compensation measures. These measures should be evidence-based and a combination between universal measures with targeted and/or individualized provisions for learners requiring additional attention and support in inclusive settings. This strategy will benefit from a systematic co-operation between actors at different policy levels, sufficient funding and a detailed implementation and evaluation plan.

Another important European policy document issued by the Council of Europe, namely the Framework of competences for democratic culture (Council of Europe, 2018) offers a detailed description of the competences that need to be acquired by learners to become democratically and interculturally competent citizens. Equipping learners with the competences specified by the Framework is crucial to ensure the future health of our culturally diverse democratic societies and the empowerment of all young people who live within them.

A recent Communication from the European Commission (2023) promotes a comprehensive, prevention-oriented and multistakeholder approach to mental health. It stresses the prevention of mental health problems, access to help and reintegration in society as integral components to the right to healthcare. EU funding for mental health (in total, EUR 1.23 billion) is available for research programmes, awareness campaigns, capacity building and transfer of mental health good practices. The impact of these programmes will be monitored by employing reliable, comparable and recent data but also indicators, monitoring and evaluation systems, to ensure follow-up and accountability.

At national, regional and local level, cohesion policy funding, in particular the European Social Fund Plus (ESF+) and the European Regional Development Fund

(ERDF) are available to support equal access to health care (European Commission, 2023). The Technical Support Instrument (TSI) is available to provide technical support to Member States for projects on mental health. For example, EUR 2 million in 2023 and in 2024, further resources from the TSI have been allocated to support capacity building for mental health on a demand driven basis in the Member States.

This comprehensive approach (European Commission, 2023) aims to promote and protect the mental health and psychosocial wellbeing of learners, and their teachers through education actions. The Commission's expert group on supportive learning environments for groups at risk of underachievement and for supporting wellbeing at school have developed guidelines (in 2024) on a systemic, whole-school approach for wellbeing for policymakers at local, regional and national level and for school. These guidelines encompass the topics of mental wellbeing and prevention of bullying, and also address work-related stress of teachers and violence, as well as bullying of teachers as part of a whole-school approach. The documents (European Commission, 2024a, 2024b) provide a deeper understanding of how policymakers, leaders, and teachers should address wellbeing in schools. They offer eleven recommendations with specific action points, indicators of success, tips, inspiring practices, and additional resources. The recommendations emphasize the importance of integrating wellbeing into teacher education, creating national frameworks, monitoring implementation, and funding mental health services and school-based support teams to reduce inequalities in wellbeing outcomes and promote equity and inclusion. These recommendations should be promoted within a whole-school approach that emphasizes embedding wellbeing into the school's culture, curriculum, and environment rather than treating it as a separate initiative. Teachers and students are both mentioned. Teachers must pursue initial training and continuous professional development to model and foster students' wellbeing. Students should have a voice, and their sense of agency, connection, and belonging to the school community should be cultivated.

The European Commission will propose a self-assessment and self-improvement toolkit on wellbeing at school and will put forward recommendations for awareness raising activities at national and EU level.

The European proposal for promoting wellbeing comprises recommendations such as: for physical activities, addressing students' mental health, supporting professional development for teachers, nurturing the inner life of teachers, promoting positive school culture, integrating technology to support wellbeing. These recommendations are briefly discussed below based also on analysis of other European policy documents.

Physical activity and sports have an important role in the promotion of good mental health in the EU. They are promoted in the EU work plan for sport and the European Week of Sport (European Commission, 2023).

Addressing students' mental health and wellbeing through early interventions and whole-school approach programmes to promote mental health by involving all educational actors and community members. Particularly, bullying prevention programmes in schools are powerful ways to support the psychological wellbeing of children and young people. Targeted tools and initiatives are essential to address the specific challenges of children and youth living in rural or remote areas and particularly affected by insufficient mental health support services.

Supporting Professional Development for Teachers

Teachers need support from education authorities to engage in continuing professional development (CPD) and to improve the quality of teaching and learning. Teachers should be stimulated to reflect on their practices and training needs, as well as be motivated and supported to engage by offering quality CPD opportunities, as well as giving them time to participate and providing incentives.

CPD is considered by top-level authorities in almost all European countries to be a teacher's professional duty or one of their statutory obligations (European Commission/EACEA/Eurydice, 2021). Accordingly, TALIS 2018 survey data (OECD, 2019a, 2019b) showed that a high proportion of lower secondary teachers in Europe engage in CPD activities and in the EU, 92.5% of lower secondary teachers had attended at least one type of professional development activity in the 12 months prior to the survey.

Apart from adequate CPD, teachers need a good allocation of time, space and support to work effectively with all learners, including those at risk of exclusion, underachievement and early leaving.

Nurturing the Inner Life of Teachers

The European Council conclusions on 'European teachers and trainers for the future' (Official Journal of the European Union, 2020) considered teachers' wellbeing a key factor for enhancing the attractiveness of the teaching profession. Teachers need a supportive school climate to enhance their personal and professional wellbeing and receive guidance on how to navigate the challenges of their profession while maintaining a healthy work-life balance.

Important aspects related to the wellbeing of teachers, mentioned in the same European policy document (Official Journal of the European Union, 2020) are the following: understanding and managing work expectations; workload and appropriate work environments; available peer and institutional support; relationships with learners, parents, peers and institution leaders; and respect and appreciation given by the wider community.

Promoting a Positive School Culture

All the members of the school community should work together to implement policies and practices to promote a positive school climate, for example to increase prosocial behaviours and decrease antisocial behaviours of students and to build mutually supportive relationships with other educational staff, learners and families.

Integrating Technology to Support Wellbeing

The potential of technology should be valorized to empower schools in enhancing the wellbeing of students, teachers and parents and of the educational community.

Individuals should be supported to engage positively in all digital learning environments with the aim to develop their potential and self-realization (Official Journal of the European Union, 2022b).

Organization for Economic Co-Operation and Development (OECD)'s Research on Wellbeing

The outcomes of the research of the Organization for Economic Co-operation and Development (OECD) on Programme for International Student Assessment (PISA) signaled a decrease in pupils' sense of belonging at school and a prevalence of (cyber)bullying. Regarding students' and teachers' wellbeing, the OECD outcomes of the Programme for International Student Assessment (PISA) of 2015 and 2018 as well as the outcomes of Teacher and Learning International Survey (TALIS) 2018 are examined below.

OECD PISA 2015 (OECD, 2017) investigated students' wellbeing in four main areas of their life: their performance in school, their relationships with peers and teachers, their home life, and how they spend their time outside of school. On average across OECD countries, students reported a level of 7.3 on a life-satisfaction scale ranging from 0 to 10.

In addition, anxiety about schoolwork is one of the sources of stress most often cited by school-age children and adolescents. On average across OECD countries, students who reported the highest levels of anxiety also reported a level of life satisfaction that is 1.2 points lower (on a scale of from 0 to 10) than students who reported the lowest levels of anxiety.

OECD PISA 2018 results (OECD, 2019a, 2019b) showed that students who took part in the 2018 PISA test (OECD, 2019a, 2019b) cited three main aspects of their lives that influence how they feel: how satisfied they are with the way they look, with their relationships with their parents, and with life at school. PISA 2018 results (OECD, 2019a, 2019b) analysed the indicators of school climate (the disciplinary climate, students' sense of belonging at school and teacher support) in relation to other PISA data on important student outcomes (academic achievement, student misbehaviour and students' wellbeing), and to key factors that shape students' learning (teachers' practices and parental involvement). The main findings on the students' wellbeing showed that: on average across OECD countries, 67% of students reported being satisfied with their lives (students who reported between 7 and 10 on the 10-point life-satisfaction scale). Between 2015 and 2018, the share of satisfied students decreased by 5 percentage points.

Teacher and Learning International Survey (TALIS) 2018 (OECD, 2019a, 2019b) investigated how the dimensions of school safety, student–teacher relations and classroom discipline have changed since 2008. For example, regarding the principals' perceptions and awareness of incidents related to school safety, the results showed that, on average across the OECD, schools in 2018 were, for the most part, immune from weekly or daily school safety incidents and, thus, provide students with safe learning environments. However, an issue of concern is related to intimidation or bullying among students, which are significantly higher than for the other school safety incidents, occurring at least weekly in 14% of schools on average across the OECD. Moreover, 3% of schools face issues of intimidation or verbal abuse of teachers or staff at least weekly, with consequences for their wellbeing, stress levels, confidence and, eventually, for their retention in the profession.

Another OECD study (Viac & Fraser, 2020) introduces a comprehensive conceptual framework that defines teachers' wellbeing based on four key components: physical and mental, cognitive, subjective and social. It also brings new perspectives on how working conditions, at both system and school levels, can impact and shape teachers' wellbeing.

To conclude, the OECD studies (PISA of 2015 and 2018) emphasized the importance of assuring the wellbeing of students and teachers in schools based on a comprehensive conceptual framework. OECD PISA 2015 (OECD, 2017) reported anxiety about schoolwork as one of the sources of stress most often cited by school-age children and adolescents associated with a lower level of life satisfaction. OECD PISA 2018 results (OECD, 2019a, 2019b) analysed the indicators of school climate in relation with student outcomes (academic achievement, student misbehaviour and students' wellbeing). TALIS 2018 survey showed an increase of the cases of intimidation or bullying among students.

2.2 Literature Review—Comparative International Studies

A cross-cultural approach in 35 OECD countries (Govorova et al., 2020) aimed to identify the wellbeing components that significantly affect student academic performance and to estimate the magnitude of school effects on the wellbeing of students in OECD countries. The school effect was understood as the ability of schools to increase subjective student wellbeing.

By analyzing responses of 248,620 students from 35 OECD countries (including among the South-Eastern countries, Greece and Turkey) to PISA 2015 questionnaires, the results demonstrated that student wellbeing significantly impacts student performance. Higher cognitive wellbeing is associated with better achievement results, increasing science performance by up to 22 points on the PISA scale. This research highlighted the importance of students' quality of life and happiness and emphasized the comprehensive approach to education where socio-emotional development is integrated in school.

Another international study (Patalay et al., 2017) mapped the current approaches to school mental health provision in ten European countries (including Serbia and Ukraine, among the countries of South-Eastern Europe). An online survey involved 1466 schools in France, Germany, Ireland, Netherlands, Poland, Serbia, Spain, Sweden, UK and Ukraine. These countries were chosen based on their geographical spread, diversity of political and economic systems, and access to the research group and presence of collaborators.

Regarding the schools' approach of mental health support for their students, the outcomes found that on average, schools indicated a greater focus on universal approaches compared with targeted approaches. Schools across the surveyed countries in Europe implemented interventions that are mostly reactive with respect to existing or emerging mental health problems, while they focused less on preventative and promotional approaches. The most frequently used strategies in mental health support included social skills development programmes, behaviour support, and creative activities. Less traditional strategies such as mindfulness practices and the use of designated spaces for wellbeing have been used to a much lesser extent. The types of professionals involved in the mental health provision varied across countries. School location also predicted the extent of available provision, with schools in rural locations reporting significantly lower amounts of provision and lesser extent of professionals delivering support services. The conclusions of this study (Patalay et al., 2017) showed that no country provided the whole range of integrated targeted and universal approaches and support for their students due to lack of staff capacity, availability of professionals, and funding.

A research report on mental health and wellbeing in schools in the European Union (Simões et al., 2021) brings evidence and made recommendations regarding the effective adoption of mental health and wellbeing within a whole-school approach across the EU. It contains a consistent theoretical framework to guide schools to adopt a whole-school approach to promote the mental health and wellbeing of their educational community.

To sum up, the comparative studies included in this analysis showed the importance of assuring school wellbeing for students and teachers and highlighted the role of preventative and comprehensive approaches to education where socio-emotional component is integrated in schools.

Peculiarities and Challenges in the South-Eastern Europe Regarding the School Wellbeing

The South-Eastern European region is characterized by some peculiarities and challenges and we try to point it out showing the necessity of addressing the school wellbeing. Depending on their social, political, economic context, South-Eastern European countries face similar challenges with the other European countries, in their efforts to develop high-quality, democratic, inclusive, and beneficial for everyone education systems.

A particular situation is faced in Ukraine, where the long duration of the war has a strong effect on mental health impacts for adults and children affected by trauma. South-Eastern countries have made consistent efforts to host refugees and support the enrolment of Ukrainian students in their education systems.

Mental health and wellbeing are not considered policy priorities as they are strongly connected to social issues such as poverty, social exclusion and access to education and health services. Mental health and wellbeing policies and practices that are implemented in education, health care, social services or employment sectors are not sufficiently coordinated. Research outcomes indicated the absence of a whole-school approach or preventative and early intervention approaches in schools on mental health and wellbeing as OECD studies (PISA of 2015 and 2018) emphasized the importance of assuring the wellbeing of students and teachers in schools based on a comprehensive conceptual framework.

International comparative studies (European Commission/EACEA/Eurydice, 2021; Taylor et al., 2024) showed high levels of teacher stress, depression, anxiety, and poor physical health observed across countries, including those in the South-Eastern Europe. Moreover, the high level of occupational stress, burnout on the job and workload, perceived by teachers, compared with other professions may lead them to abandon their profession. A study including among others, South-Eastern countries (Patalay et al., 2017) highlighted that schools in rural locations have significantly lower amounts of wellbeing provision and lack of staff capacity, availability of professionals, funding to deliver support services for students.

2.3 Recommendations and Suggestions

Recommendations and suggestions are derived from the previous analysis of European policy documents and literature review.

- Approaching mental health and wellbeing in the context of a rapidly changing society with risk factors for mental health problems (e.g. urbanization, globalization, climate change, rapid advances in technology, shifts in family systems, migration, etc.).
- Adopting an approach that promotes mental health and wellbeing across all policies and prioritizing mental health as it is strongly related to social issues such as poverty, social exclusion and access to education and health services with the aim to reduce mental health inequalities.
- Designing coordinated policies, reforms, and actions in education, health, employment, social work and encouraging interdisciplinary, integrated practices in education, health care, social services, employment, etc.
- Improving working conditions for teachers as the OECD study (Viac & Fraser, 2020) demonstrated that the working conditions, at both system and school levels, can impact and shape teachers' wellbeing.
- Creating a supportive school climate and improving school wellbeing as studies highlighted that a low teacher wellbeing has a negative impact on teaching and pupils, but also the cost of attrition, recruitment, and absenteeism.
- Ensuring a good allocation of time, space and support for teachers to work effectively with all learners, including those at risk.
- Implementing measures (in partnerships with parents, community organizations and health or social services) to reduce bullying in schools as TALIS 2018 survey showed an increase in the cases of intimidation or bullying among students.
- Ensuring initial and continuous teachers' training in the use of technology as research showed that lack of training and low confidence can have negative impacts on wellbeing-related factors such as workload and stress.

- Assuring sufficient funding and building capacity for schools in rural locations reporting significantly lower amounts of wellbeing provision and lesser extent of professionals delivering support services due to lack of staff capacity, availability of professionals, funding, etc.

Competing Interests The authors have no conflicts of interest to declare that are relevant to the content of this chapter.

References

Council of Europe. (2018). *Reference framework of competences for democratic culture. Context, concepts and model* (Vol. 1). Council of Europe Publishing.

European Commission. (2023). *Communication from the Commission to the European Parliament, the Council, the European Economic and Social Committee and the Committee of the Regions on a comprehensive approach to mental health*, 7.6.2023 COM(2023) 298 final.

European Commission/EACEA/Eurydice. (2021). *Teachers in Europe: Careers, development and wellbeing*. Eurydice report. Publications Office of the European Union.

European Commission: Directorate-General for Education, Youth, Sport and Culture. (2024a). *Wellbeing and mental health at school: guidelines for education policymakers*. Publications Office of the European Union. https://data.europa.eu/https://doi.org/10.2766/901169.

European Commission: Directorate-General for Education, Youth, Sport and Culture. (2024b). *Wellbeing and mental health at school: Guidelines for school leaders, teachers and educators*. Publications Office of the European Union. https://data.europa.eu/ https://doi.org/10.2766/760136.

Govorova, E., Benítez, I., & Muñiz, J. (2020). *How schools affect student wellbeing: A cross-cultural approach in 35 OECD countries*, Front. Psychol., 25 March 2020, Sec. Educational Psychology (Vol. 11). https://doi.org/10.3389/fpsyg.2020.00431

OECD. (2017). *PISA 2015 results (Volume III): Students' wellbeing*. OECD Publishing.

OECD. (2019a). *PISA 2018 results (Volume III): What school life means for students' lives*. OECD Publishing.

OECD. (2019b). *TALIS 2018 results (Volume I): Teachers and school leaders as lifelong learners*. OECD Publishing.

Official Journal of the European Union. (2020). *Council conclusions on European teachers and trainers for the future*, 2020/C 193/04.

Official Journal of the European Union. (2021). *Council Resolution on a strategic framework for European cooperation in education and training towards the European Education Area and beyond (2021–2030)*, 2021/C 66/01.

Official Journal of the European Union. (2022a). *Council Recommendation of 28 November 2022 on Pathways to School Success and replacing the Council Recommendation of 28 June 2011 on policies to reduce early school leaving*, 2022/C 469/01

Official Journal of the European Union. (2022b). *Council conclusions on supporting wellbeing in digital education*, 2022/C 469/04

Patalay, P., Gondek, D., Moltrecht, B., Giese, L., Curtin, C., Stanković, M., & Savka, N. (2017). *Mental health provision in schools: Approaches and interventions in 10 European countries*, Published online by Cambridge University Press. https://doi.org/10.1017/gmh.2017.6

Simões, C., Caravita, S., & Cefai, C. (2021). *A systemic, whole-school approach to mental health and wellbeing in schools in the EU. Analytical Report*. European Union.

Taylor, L., Zhou, W., Boyle, L., Funk, S., & De Neve, J-E. (2024). *Wellbeing for school teachers* (Report No. 2). International Baccalaureate Organization.

Viac, C., & Fraser, P. (2020). *Teachers' wellbeing: A framework for data collection and analysis*, OECD Education Working Papers, No. 213. OECD Publishing.

Chapter 3
Teachers' Wellbeing and Resilience—Implications for School Wellbeing

Aurora Adina Colomeischi, Liliana Bujor, and Nadia Laura Serdenciuc

3.1 Arguments for Teachers' Wellbeing

"I have come to a frightening conclusion. I am the decisive element in the classroom. It is my personal approach that creates the climate. It is my daily mood that makes the weather (…)". (Ginott 1976 in Becker et al. 2014).

The wellbeing of teachers is intricately connected to the wellbeing of the world, as evidenced by the staggering number of 90 million teachers in the global working population. Their power of influence extends far beyond the classroom, as the wellbeing of teachers today directly impacts the wellbeing of tomorrow's adults (Biladeau et al. 2022). According to the World Bank Ed-States, there are 9.36 million in pre-primary level, 30.27 million in elementary, 32.12 in secondary and 12.49 in tertiary education. Furthermore, 68.8 million teachers will need to be recruited by 2030 (UNESCO Institute for Statistics, (Kim et al. 2019).

Since 2007, when Lyubomirsky argued the importance of teachers' wellbeing (TWB) in terms of creativity, cognitive performance, and psychological health, as well as adding all the dimensions of social and organizational life, research related to this psychological reality has made considerable progress (Tsuyuguchi 2023). In the same time, searching for a coherent meaning and understanding of this concept, we can find a lot of conceptualizations. European Agency for Safety and Health at Work,

A. A. Colomeischi (✉) · L. Bujor · N. L. Serdenciuc
Faculty of Psychology and Sciences of Education, "Ştefan cel Mare" University of Suceava, Suceava, Romania
e-mail: adina.colomeischi@usm.ro
URL: https://www.usv.ro

L. Bujor
e-mail: liliana.bujor@usm.ro

N. L. Serdenciuc
e-mail: nadia.serdenciuc@usm.ro

A. A. Colomeischi (ed.), *Wellbeing in Schools of Southeastern Europe*, Human Well-Being Research and Policy Making, https://doi.org/10.1007/978-3-032-10525-7_3

in 2013, proposed a definition for occupational wellbeing that includes areas such as physical and mental wellbeing, psychosocial wellbeing, and working environment.

Teacher wellbeing is directly related to the instructional performance, especially with the level of students' wellbeing. There is evidence that the perceived 'emotions' of teachers and students' own emotions are related, a kind of relationship manifesting itself during and also beyond the school lessons. The teacher's power to influence students' emotions can be explained by direct un-conscious crossover processes such as emotional contagion, or consciously through empathy. The model of prosocial classroom (Jennings and Greenberg 2009) considers that teacher wellbeing is the primary factor influencing healthy teacher-student relationships, students' social, emotional, and academic outcomes. The systematic review of 44 qualitative and quantitative studies conducted by Dreer (2023) provides evidence that the teacher-student relationship and the teacher wellbeing have a positive influence on students' learning experiences and outcomes. This suggests that when teachers prioritize their own wellbeing, it can contribute to a more conducive learning environment and better student outcomes. Additionally, Becker et al. (2014) highlight the connection between students' enjoyment/anger and teachers' instructional behavior. This implies that the way teachers interact with their students can impact emotional experience in the classroom.

From an integrative view, based on a literature search that included meta-analysis and the systematic review of over 5000 articles on teachers, it was found that the effect size of the relation between student achievement and teacher effectiveness was smaller compared to the effect size of teacher wellbeing (Bardach et al. 2022).

These findings emphasize the importance of prioritizing teacher wellbeing that has positive influence on teacher-students' relationship and learning environment. To focus on teachers' wellbeing is an investment in humanity, in qualitative terms (values and virtues like human heritage) and in quantitative terms (economic costs concerning all the consequences of mental health problems, these problems being the reverse side of wellbeing).

3.1.1 Some Arguments on Wellbeing from the Burnout Perspective

Two psychological realities in reaching careers—wellbeing and burnout—are interconnected and represent two different sides of the same coin. The level of effectiveness in the teaching profession can greatly influence a teacher's satisfaction and overall wellbeing in their professional life. When teachers feel effective and successful in their role, it can contribute to their motivation, job satisfaction and overall commitment to the profession. On the other hand, the decision to renounce the teaching profession can be influenced by various factors, including job-related challenges and individual circumstances. If a teacher consistently feels ineffective or faces significant obstacles, it may lead to burnout and even to the decision of leaving the profession.

Burnout is a syndrome of emotional exhaustion, depersonalization, and reduced personal accomplishment, as stated by Maslach et al. (1997). It is a particular risk for individuals working with other people. The teaching profession, being a social one, involves prolonged engagement and interactions with students, parents, and staff, which can serve as potential triggers for burnout. 'Teacher burnout' (TB) is related to the emotional demands of teaching, such as managing classroom dynamics, addressing individual students' needs, or dealing with parental expectations. All of these could contribute to emotional exhaustion. Additionally, the depersonalization, like the burnout aspect, may arise when teachers develop an uncaring or detached attitude towards their students or colleagues as a coping mechanism. The feeling of reduced personal accomplishment, characterized by a low sense of competence and work satisfaction, results from factors like high workload, lack of support, and/or limited resources.

The practitioners, policymakers, and researchers have been recognizing the complex interplay between these two psychological realities, with two main questions related to the teaching profession emerging: what are the personal characteristics of effective teachers and what are the personal characteristics of teachers with low burnout tendencies?

In this chapter, our focus will be on shedding light on the teachers' wellbeing and burnout drawing from research, particularly recent meta-analysis. By examining these aspects, our aim is to provide a clearer understanding of the professional reality experienced by teachers. By delving into the findings of recent meta-analyses, we can gain insights into the prevalence of burnout and wellbeing among teachers, the factors that contribute to them, their consequences, and how to sustain strategies and interventions promoting teachers' wellbeing and preventing burnout.

Dimensions and determinants of teachers' wellbeing versus teachers' burnout.

Taken together, wellbeing related to job satisfaction and burnout explain 27% of the variance in teachers' intention to quit, as shown by the data from a meta-analysis that aims to understand burnout and job satisfaction in relation to teacher attrition (Madigan and Kim 2021). Indeed, when it comes to predicting teachers' intention to quit their job, both burnout and job satisfaction play significant roles.

According to the wellbeing conceptualization (Diener et al. 1985, Ryff 1989) from the last research years, studies proposed two dimensions operationalized in two indicators for measuring teachers' wellbeing in schools: positive states (commitment, job satisfaction, engagement) and negative states (stress, burnout, depression, psychosomatic reactions).

The dimensions of TWB and TB need a framework that gives a coherent understanding of these concepts. According to the Job-Demands-Resources model (JD-R), (Schaufeli and Bakker 2004), there are some physical, psychological, social, and organizational aspects of work related to TWB and TB.

The need for coherence in teachers' wellbeing understanding puts the results of research in a four-dimensional framework, consisting of cognitive wellbeing, physical and mental wellbeing, social and subjective wellbeing (Organization for

Economic Cooperation and Development- OECD). In a research review searching for a single comprehensive framework, Viac and Fraser framed the potential outcomes by distinguishing the internal outcomes of teacher wellbeing (i.e., stress, burnout, and motivation to leave the profession) from external outcomes (i.e., classroom processes and student wellbeing). All these dimensions were operationalized through specific scales: (1) cognitive dimension (ability to concentrate on one's job and teacher self-efficacy); (2) subjective dimension (satisfaction with job/teaching profession, moods and emotions regarding job activities, purposefulness, satisfaction with the life, (3) physical and mental dimension (psychosomatic symptoms, number of school days missed due these symptoms), (4) social dimension (social function of relationships with principals, colleagues and students, feeling of trust), (Viac and Fraser 2020).

From a burnout perspective, various concurrent dimensions that contribute to the phenomenon were identified, such as individual factors, organizational factors, and transactional factors. Individual factors include characteristics such as gender, years of experience, coping strategies, and personality traits. Organizational factors refer to aspects within the school or educational institution, like high work demands, the socio-economic status of the school, and the overall organizational culture. Transactional factors involve interactions between individual and organizational factors. This includes how teachers perceive the behaviors of their students and the support from the principal, peers, and administration) (Kim et al. 2019).

The determinants of TWB and TB have practical implications for guiding the intervention programs. However, as there are contradictory conclusions, various factors have been identified as predictors of TWB and TB, including class composition, class size, numbers of years in teaching activity, age, and gender. These factors can have different impacts on TWB and TB and it is important to connect research findings for a comprehensive understanding (Hascher and Waber 2021). A systematic review of longitudinal studies identified four types of determinants of burnout onset in teachers: support, conflict, organizational context, and individual characteristics (Mijakoski et al. 2022). There is some over-lap between the determinants of TWB and TB, which are frequently classified into three factors: workplace environment, job environment, and individual characteristics (Tsuyuguchi 2023).

Workplace environment is about qualitative relationships with colleagues, principals, students, and parents, it is built on values and goals, and offers an organizational trust, in terms of work attitude (Tsuyuguchi 2023). A didactic career is a social profession and the main work instruments are relationships and social networking. This is a scientifically proven truth by the longest psychological research from the history of psychology, Harvard Study (almost 80 years old), and from a research about teacher wellbeing that analyzed studies published between 2000 and 2019 and was conducted in over 40 different countries, covering different continents (e.g., Australia, Belgium, Canada, China, Germany, India, Israel, Norway, Russia, South Africa, Taiwan, United Kingdom, United States), although no causal explanation was found about teacher wellbeing (Hascher and Waber 2021). Waldinger, the actual director of the Harvard study, disseminated the conclusion of all these research years - the quality of relationships has a powerful influence on our physical and psychological health. Positive relationships are relevant to TWB, this being confirmed by the quantitative and qualitative studies analyzed in the last 19 years. Professional learning community strongly mediated between the pay level satisfaction and TWB. Principals can provide a supportive work environment, teachers can encourage collaborative work of the students, and students give the meaning to the teaching profession. A positive teacher-student relationship was found to be supportive for TWB (Hascher and Waber 2021) and teachers' sense of relatedness with students was associated with gains in work enthusiasm one year later (Aldrup et al. 2018). Organizational trust is a proxy indicator of a work environment that integrates trust relationships with principals, colleagues, students, and parents. In a survey about causal effects of TWB on 4399 people working at 76 public high schools in Japan, variables such student trust, colleagues trust, and principal trust were confirmed as determinants of TWB. The lacking effect of the parents' trust can be attributed to the level of schooling, particularly in high school. The colleagues‘ trust is also a moderation variable that increases the level of wellbeing, even in overtime hours situation. More than that, variations in colleagues and principal trust have causal effects on teachers' depressive symptoms. An increase in overtime hours does not directly lead to a decrease in TWB. The factor that directly determines work engagement was the aging of teachers rather that trust relations. Teachers in their 50 s or older tend to significantly decrease work engagement (Tsuyugchi 2023).

Job environment is a second factor with an important role in TWB and TB. It can serve as a proxy index for factors such as autonomy and the sense of self-efficacy. A positive job environment provides individuals with the freedom to make decisions, and a sense of effectiveness. To the contrary, certain factors such as excessive pressure, workload, and long overtime hours can negatively impact TWB and increase burnout (Tsuyuguchi 2023). Creating a supportive and positive job environment and providing resources and support are direct ways of promoting wellbeing and job satisfaction.

A third dimension of teachers' wellbeing/burnout is represented by the individual characteristic. This factor describes the individual characteristics in terms of ability, educational background, or basic personal attributes - age, gender, or number of years in teaching activity. There is no convergent data that could explain wellbeing/ burnout in the teacher career: age, years of teaching, or gender were neither proven to have an impact on wellbeing or not.

In relation to the personality traits (OCEAN model: openness to experience, conscientiousness, extraversion, agreeableness -Wong and Zhang 2014), the ambivalence is not the same. From the teacher personality perspective, using the Big Five framework, research through meta-analyses has indicated certain correlations between the personality traits and burnout. These findings suggest that emotional stability (also known as neuroticism) is the strongest correlate of burnout among teachers. Teachers who score low on emotional stability, meaning they are more prone to experiencing negative emotions and stress, are more likely to experience burnout. Extraversion is the second strongest correlate of burnout. Meta-analysis summarizing findings from multiple occupations reports conscientiousness to be the strongest predictor of job performance (Salgado 2003). Teachers who are more extroverted, being in constant and qualitative social interactions, are more susceptible to not develop burnout. Conscientiousness is a strong correlate, particularly in relation to the depersonalization domain, agreeableness is a moderate correlate, and openness is the weakest correlate of burnout (Kim et al. 2019, Roloff et al. 2022). Results are convergent and show that, for emotional exhaustion and depersonalization, neuroticism is the personality trait with the highest association, while for reduced personal accomplishment, extraversion is more important.

Subjective variables such as interpersonal virtues and character strengths, including optimism and social responsibility, have been found to be positively correlated with TWB, (Hascher and Waber 2021). These variables are part of a multidimensional construct known as psychological capital, which encompasses various resources for TWB that include self-efficacy, hope, optimism, and resilience (Luthans and Youssef-Morgan 2017).

Psychological capital, a construct related to individual characteristics defined from positive psychology perspective, promotes a positive organizational behavior approach with focus on strengths, more exactly on four fundamental characteristics: self-efficacy (having confidence to take on and put in the necessary efforts to succeed at challenging tasks), hope (persevering towards goals and, when necessary, redirecting paths to goals), optimism (making a positive attribution about succeeding now and in the future), and resilience (when beset by problems and adversity, sustaining and bouncing back and even beyond to attain success) (Luthans Yousseff and Avolio, 2007, Luthans and Youssef-Morgan 2017). In the Southeastern part of Europe, in Turkey, the teacher psychological capital increased when teachers helped their students to succeed and to overcome problems, particularly if the teachers were working in low socio-economic schools, and if they had teamwork experiences with the colleagues (Çimen and Özgan 2018). A study on Greek secondary teachers identified a positive correlation between resilience and occupational wellbeing (Brouskeli et al. 2018). Psychological capital of teachers, directly related to wellbeing, can be built by training and experience (Soykan et al. 2019). Psychological characteristics of teachers are considered to be linked to teachers' wellbeing. A meta-analysis literature search, based on the systematic review of 5144 articles, examined the relationship between the teachers' psychological characteristics and teachers' wellbeing in an integrative view, summarizing eight psychological characteristics - self-efficacy, causal attribution, expectations, personality, enthusiasm, emotional intelligence, emotional labor, and mindfulness. Teachers' self-efficacy has consistently been found to be related to wellbeing aspects (Bardach et al. 2022). For leadership, three key skills that influence teachers' wellbeing are: relationship building, contextual competence, and social and emotional competence (Cann et al. 2021).

The teachers' characteristic with the greatest influence on student's academic performance, validated by a meta-analysis of 40 studies published be-tween 2000 and 2019, was the teachers' reflective attitude (López-Martín et al. 2023).

At the leadership level, in a model developed by Cann (2019), the main three leadership habits that interact and influence teachers' wellbeing at high level are: teachers feeling that they are valued - when they are listened to and feel understood (habit 1), meaningful professional development- organization flourishing is about teachers' needs for growth and development (habit 2), and enabling teacher agency in decision making and chances - if leaders include all the teachers in their decisions, this will impacts TWB (habit 3), (Cann et al. 2021).

This variable keeps its significance in the European space. In a survey measuring the wellbeing of the school staff from Finland and Estonia, teachers found trust and working community-related interaction (working atmosphere, appreciation of others, cooperation, information) to be important factors in terms of work satisfaction and occupational wellbeing (Laine et al. 2018). For Romanian teachers (North-West region of Romania), self-efficacy, promotion, positive student behavior, and working conditions influence wellbeing in the teaching profession (Ortan et al. 2021). In Southeastern Europe, specifically in Turkey, a small negative correlation was found between the increasing age and TWB (Özü et al. 2017).

Recently, researchers expressed their interests to examine TWB fluctuation over time. For example, during one school year, teachers registered a decline of vigor (meaning the subjective vitality) and this was related to their level wellbeing (Collie and Martin 2023).

While the whole world's life is sequenced before and after COVID-19, a global representation of TWB and TB must be approached by taking into account the two perspectives: during and after this human experience. The results of studies, published from 2019 to 2021, show that teachers report levels of anxiety (17%), depression (19%), and stress (30%) with some differences between regions and level of schools: in Asia, there has been more anxiety in schools, while stress levels were higher in universities (Ozamiz-Etxebarria et al. 2021).

Consequently, The International Barometer of Education Personnel's Health and Wellbeing was launched in 2021 by the Education and Solidarity Network (ESN), a multi-territory online survey of education staff providing timely data on work conditions and the health and wellbeing of education staff. Six countries were included in this barometer: Québec and Mexico in the Americas, France and the French Community of Belgium/Federation Wallonia-Brussels in Europe, and Morocco and The Gambia in Africa. A total of 8000 teachers answered at a questionnaire, with 100 questions organized into 8 sections: physical and mental health; professional experience; working conditions and environment; organization and school administration; relationships; conditions, information, and support regarding health; experience regarding health; and socio-demographic characteristics. The feeling of safety at school and the autonomy at work are important and potential universal determinants of teachers' wellbeing. In Morocco the student-teacher and the teacher- superior relation-ships were not associated with the teachers' wellbeing. The same perspective was confirmed also in Gambia and Mexico. For all these countries, the physical environment (material conditions, school facilities) is more important (finding compatible with the Maslow' pyramid). An interesting discovery, after several waves of the COVID-19, is that remote working does not appear to be a determinant of teacher wellbeing, because the proportion of teachers working from home was small (except in Belgium, where full-time remote work has been linked to an increased level of stress), according to Billaudeau et al. 2022. In the same pandemic context, a study examined the relationship between the perceived stress of Romanian teachers during the online period of schooling and their wellbeing, with job crafting as a mediator and problem-focused coping as moderator. The results showed that the effect of stress on wellbeing was mediated by job crafting for teachers who scored low on problem-focused coping. In such a special context, where individuals have no means to change the situation, it can be helpful using low problem-focused coping (Ciuhan et al. 2022).

Throughout the arguments explored above, we can observe a continuum between determinants and consequences of teachers' wellbeing/burnout that offer a clear perspective with proximal implications, in the form of a genuine understanding of the teaching profession and a distal implication in developing adaptative interventions. Even during the pandemic period, the teachers' profile kept its content, except in some cases related to cultural differences.

The teaching profession is about qualitative relationships with colleagues, principals, students, and parents in the workplace environment, autonomy in relation with the job environment and self-efficacy as individual characteristics. By considering these determinants, their complexity, and interconnectedness, the intervention programs for improving TWB and preventing TB can be tailored in a realistic way.

3.2 Teachers' Resilience

Gu and Day (2013) presented three reasons to explain why resilience is important for teaching: firstly, teachers as role models for students need to be resilient in order to foster resilience in their students; secondly, teaching is considered a demanding job in the ever-changing world, resilience is a robust factor that explains teachers' commitment and motivation in such times. The third reason is explained by the teaching profession itself, as it is very close to a vocation; only a strong sense of purpose, commitment, and self-efficacy support students' performance.

Friedman (2000) emphasized that educators are charged with fostering not only the academic growth of their students, but also their personal development. In today's educational landscape, teachers find themselves under the weight of parental expectations regarding student achievement, facing constant changes due to educational policies, and being criticized for any perceived shortcomings (Friedman 2000). In addition, teachers are expected to maintain effective relationships with colleagues and supervisors, build teaching teams and provide support for children in need. The high level of emotional labor puts teachers at risk of stress and burnout. Teachers' wellbeing and resilience are essential for their effectiveness in the classroom and for the overall health and wellbeing of pupils.

The main risk factors for teachers, particularly in south-eastern European countries, could be workload, low salaries, and lack of support from government and administration. For example, Romania faced in 2023 one of the biggest strike of teachers, more of one-month, teachers asked for their rights, related to the quality of education and also to their income. They gained some salary increase, also some facilities such as didactic prime (an amount of money for books and mate-rials necessary for teaching). In Ukraine, the salary of teachers is very low, and this leads to the migration of teachers, as workers in Western European countries. Thus, the shortage of teachers adds another vulnerable area within the overall situation in the country. Low income leads to frustration and low life satisfaction, which could affect teachers' role in the relationship with students.

A potential risk factor is workload, which combines academic responsibilities with the cognitive, social, and emotional needs of students, managing parental expectations and fulfilling various administrative tasks. Teachers therefore need to balance all these professional demands and their own psychological capital, to have resilient resources to manage professional life. By recognizing and addressing the various stressors inherent in the teaching profession, schools can create an environment conducive to both effective teaching practice and the flourishing of educators themselves.

A study conducted in the Republic of Moldova (Balode 2018) showed that a significant proportion of teachers exhibit burnout symptoms, including feelings of being overwhelmed due to excessive involvement in their work, driven by a strong desire to perform at a high level. Two other prominent indicators of burnout are a lack of control over teaching outcomes and a lack of recognition for efforts made. Teachers with lower levels of burnout show greater motivation for professional development, effectively manage their basic needs for autonomy, competence, and relatedness within the organizational environment, and perceive a more positive psychosocial climate in their workplace. These teachers tend to remain in the teaching profession longer (with more years of teaching experience) and demonstrate greater resilience to stress and burnout. Dumulescu et al. 2023 identified three significant predictors of resilience among Romanian teachers: fear of negative evaluation, emotion self-regulation strategies and teaching self-efficacy. In a Bulgarian study, the authors (Stoyanova et al. 2023) indicated that teachers' resilience acts as a protective factor against burnout when it comes to the online learning environment. Papazis et al. (2023) analyzed the resilience of Greek teachers during the COVID pandemic and the results indicated that teachers' self-perception of resilience significantly influenced their attitudes towards distance teaching during the pandemic and their stress levels. This study reinforces the crucial role of resilience in coping with challenging situations and provides clear guidance on identifying teachers who may need counselling and professional support to enhance their resilience. We could conclude that schools could act as agents in promoting teachers' resilience by providing them with re-sources for professional development and also by providing a healthy working environment. Therefore, cultivating resilience is paramount for teachers to maintain their unwavering commitment to the educational endeavor, preserve their intrinsic motivation and pursue continuous professional growth (Day and Gu 2013).

A 2021 study (García-Crespo et al. 2021) of students and teachers from European countries, based on data from the international PIRLS 2016 study, which examined the role of families, teachers and student profiles in supporting academic resilience, found that the teaching-related factors that most strongly predicted resilience were effective classroom management and a safe and orderly school environment, both of which could increase the likelihood of resilience by up to 62%. In addition, teaching that focused on understanding and reflection had the potential to increase the likelihood of resilience by up to 61%.

3.3 The Importance of Teachers' Personal and Professional Development

Over the past 20 years, there have been numerous studies focused on enhancing teacher' wellbeing by exploring different models and psychological approaches. These studies have examined various interventions and programs such as Gordon's teacher effectiveness training (TET), Autonomy-supportive intervention program (ASIP), Achiever Resilience Curriculum (ARC) and Social and Emotional Learning (SEL). In terms of psychological approaches, studies investigated psychoeducation, mindfulness, cognitive-behavioral skills, acceptance-based skills, and behavioral stress management skills. Sixteen types of burnout and stress-reduction interventions were identified, including the pandemic period, in Asia, North America, Oceania, Europe, and Africa. The most studied were Mindfulness-Based Interventions alone or in combination with yoga or Cognitive Behavioral Therapy (CBT), followed by Rational Emotive Behavioral Therapy-REBT (Agyapong et al. 2023). The research sheds light on the impact of mindfulness training interventions on teacher wellbeing. A meta-analysis revealed significant positive effects of mindfulness training on various aspects of teacher wellbeing. A large effect of mindfulness on feelings was identified, alongside a moderate effect on stress and anxiety decrease, and a small effect on mindfulness on depression and burnout (Zarate et al. 2019). The conclusion of this analysis was a heterogeneous effectiveness related to the definitions and indicators of wellbeing, burnout, or stress. The long-term effects and the impact of exposure to an intervention remains a direction for further explorations (Hascher and Waber 2021). However, some interesting conclusions can be drawn in order to guide the interventions programs for enhancing personal and professional development. Two systematic reviews, conducted by Von der Emse et al. (2019) and Dreer and Gouase (2021) as cited in Beames et al. (2023), highlight the effective-ness of mindfulness, behavioral, and cognitive-behavioral programs in reducing stress and burnout. These programs have shown positive outcomes in promoting wellbeing and generating changes in thinking and feeling.

The meta-analysis conducted by Beames et al. (2023) examined 88 unique studies on psychological programs and aimed to improve the mental health, professional burnout, and wellbeing of teachers. The findings revealed that the evaluated programs had a significant and large effect on reducing stress levels, and moderate effects in reducing anxiety, depression, professional burnout, and improving overall wellbeing when compared to the control groups.

In the same context of professional development, the learning of specific emotion regulation strategies such as the expression of emotions, has been found to have positive associations with variables like wellbeing and satisfaction (Wang et al. 2019). Additionally, focusing on enhancing teachers' emotional intelligence capacities and cultivating a reflective attitude towards the teaching career through mindfulness interventions, has shown promising results (Bardach et al. 2022).

The effects of Social and Emotional Learning Program (SEL) on teachers' burnout was measured in a meta-analysis of 13 empirical studies. SEL had a significant medium effect size on emotional exhaustion and personal accomplishment, while the analysis did not find statistically significant impacts on depersonalization (Oliveira et al. 2021). A meta-analysis, proposed by Maricuţoiu et al. (2023), explored two perspectives of teachers' wellbeing: hedonic and eudaimonic. The hedonic perspective focuses on teachers' psychological functioning and the overall subjective wellbeing includes factors such job satisfaction, positive emotions, absence of negative emotions, and stress. The eudaimonic perspective emphasizes self-realization and personal growth such as finding meaning and purpose in teaching, experiencing a sense of competence, autonomy, and concordance with personal values. Both perspectives of wellbeing are related and important for differentiated interventions in the teaching development, focusing on the teachers' psychological functioning (hedonic perspective) or on self-realization (eudaimonic perspective), both having implications for students' wellbeing.

Teachers' self-efficacy, which is closely linked to TWB, could be enhanced by providing concrete training opportunities. One effective way is through vicarious experiences, where teachers would have the opportunity to learn and to observe how mentors effectively deal with multiple complex and challenging situations. Additionally, mastery experiences could provide opportunities to practice and experiment using the skills learned by engaging in real-life teaching scenarios (Bardach et al. 2022). By incorporating these concrete methods to enhance the teachers' wellbeing, a positive impact on all the components of the school life can be generated.

In the last years, European educational policies have been giving special attention to and had a new focus on supporting the wellbeing of teachers in the personal and professional development training. The policy agenda of English schools emphasized, in 2018, the importance of focusing on the employees' mental health and on wellbeing (Manning et al. 2020). The Education and Solidarity Network launched, in 2021, the International Barometer of Education Personnel's Health and Wellbeing, mobilizing partners around the world - UNESCO Chair Global Health and Education (Billaudeau et al. 2022).

Being related to the quality of teaching, teachers' wellbeing becomes a concern for the European political structures. Council conclusions on European teachers and trainers for the future (Council of the European Union 2020, p. 15) emphasize that, besides developing their professional competences, sustaining autonomy and involvement in their work, it is also important "to foster their personal and professional wellbeing, motivation and feeling of value". Joining together the three components - wellbeing, motivation, and feeling of value - the aforementioned document configures a behavior oriented affective-attitudinal area responsible for developing coping strategies in order to adequately face different learners' needs. Influencing teachers' job satisfaction and the level of enthusiastic implication in their work, teachers' wellbeing correlates with motivation and learning performances of teaching process beneficiaries (Ibid., p.16). Analyzing the European policy document, we can observe that four paragraphs (out of the fourteen emphasizing some focal points regarding teachers and trainers of the future) make explicit reference to the teachers' wellbeing, delineating some factors of influence (workload, work environments, relationships with students, parents, peers and superiors, respect and appreciation from the part of community members), or a few consequences related to these factors' absence or their negative effects (physical and emotional exhaustion, stress and burnout, affected mental and physical health). Collaboration is viewed as a solution in order to determine teachers' wellbeing: educational policies oriented on building and promoting learning communities, adding the perspective of a "collaborative team culture" that involves teachers, peers, learners, parents and other different stake-holders. While educational institutions are considered responsible for a "participatory leadership", the use of constructive evaluation and the appraisal criteria for teachers, general educational policies have to support the continuous professional development of teachers within the national career frameworks associated with internationalization strategies, improving working conditions and career prospects.

The wellbeing perspective viewed in relation with the educational domain can be approached both as a context of learning and as a goal of personal development in order to help learners construct a better response to the contemporary challenges of a global world. To follow the Global Education 2030 Agenda, UNESCO proposed a strategy regarding education focusing on two key concepts: health and wellbeing (UNESCO 2022). The document emphasizes the role of schools and education systems in building a genuine integrative approach of health and wellbeing. Although the wellbeing of learners is explicitly presented as being a priority of the educational sector, teachers' wellbeing plays an important role in building safe and comprehensive learning environments optimizing health and education outcomes.

European and national policy agendas delineate teachers' wellbeing and their resilience as focal points, recognizing these as influence factors for education quality and learners' performances (European Commission/EACEA/Eurydice 2021, p.141). Examining qualitative data related to national policies and quantitative data from the Teaching and Learning Survey (TALIS) on teacher practices and perceptions, the Eurydice report highlights the role of national regulations in sustaining teaching profession. The suggested dimensions for intervention are teachers' social competences and schools' collaborative culture.

The inner life of teachers has been addressed through various European projects developed to improve educational policies in different European countries. For example, a European Partnership for the Promotion of Mental Health in Schools (PROMEHS), coordinated by the University of Milan Biccoca and involving six other universities and public authorities from six countries, pointed out that a structured intervention for the promotion of mental health could also contribute to developing teachers' potential in terms of social and emotional skills and resilience (Cavioni et al. 2023, Colomeischi 2022, Tatalović Vorkapić et al. 2023, Poulou et al. 2022).

The profession of teachers is demanding and emotionally challenging, with individual resources not being enough in order to achieve qualitative performance. This is why it has to be supported by schools' educational policies or by macrostructural policies as a "pay it forward" form of investment in learners' wellbeing and achievements through teachers' flourishing.

Competing Interests The authors have no conflicts of interest to declare that are relevant to the content of this chapter.

References

Agyapong, B., Brett-MacLean, P., Burback, L., Agyapong, V. I. O., & Wei, Y. (2023). Interventions to reduce stress and burnout among teachers: A scoping review. *International Journal of Environmental Research and Public Health, 20*(9), 5625. https://doi.org/10.3390/ijerph20095625

Aldrup, K., Klusmann, U., Lüdtke, O., Göllner, R., & Trautwein, U. (2018). Stu-dent misbehavior and teacher wellbeing: Testing the mediating role of the teacher-student relationship. *Learning and Instruction, 58*, 126–136. https://doi.org/10.1016/j.learninstruc.2018.05.006

Balode, Neli. (2018). Teachers' resilience to occupational stress and burnout in new approaches in social and humanistic sciences - NASHS 2017, p.78–93, Editura Lumen, Lumen.

Bardach, L., Klassen, R. M., & Perry, N. E. (2022). Teachers' psychological characteristics: Do they matter for teacher effectiveness, teachers' wellbeing, retention, and interpersonal relations? *An Integrative Re-view. Educational Psychology Review, 34*(1), 259–300. https://doi.org/10.1007/s10648-021-09614-9

Beames, J. R., Spanos, S., Roberts, A., McGillivray, L., Li, S., Newby, J. M., O'Dea, B., & Werner-Seidler, A. (2023). Intervention programs target-ing the mental health, professional burnout, and/or wellbeing of school teachers: Systematic review and meta-analyses. *Educational Psychology Review, 35*(1), 26. https://doi.org/10.1007/s10648-023-09720-w

Becker, E. S., Goetz, T., Morger, V., & Ranellucci, J. (2014). The importance of teachers' emotions and instructional behavior for their students' emotions—An experience sampling analysis. *Teaching and Teacher Education, 43*, 15–26. https://doi.org/10.1016/j.tate.2014.05.002

Billaudeau, N., Alexander, S., Magnard, L., Temam, S., & Vercambre, M.-N. (2022). What levers to promote teachers' wellbeing during the COVID-19 pandemic and beyond: Lessons learned from a 2021 online study in six countries. *International Journal of Environmental Re-search and Public Health, 19*(15), 9151. https://doi.org/10.3390/ijerph19159151

Cann, R. F., Riedel-Prabhakar, R., & Powell, D. (2021). A model of positive school leadership to improve teacher wellbeing. *International Journal of Applied Positive Psychology, 6*(2), 195–218. https://doi.org/10.1007/s41042-020-00045-5

Cavioni, V., Grazzani, I., Ornaghi, V., Agliati, A., Gandellini, S., Cefai, C., & Conte, E. (2023). A multi-component curriculum to promote teachers' mental health: Findings from the PROMEHS program. International journal of emotional. *Education, 15*(1), 34–52. www.um.edu.mt/ijee

Ciuhan, G. C., Nicolau, R. G., & Iliescu, D. (2022). Perceived stress and wellbeing in Romanian teachers during the COVID-19 pandemic: The intervening effects of job crafting and problem-focused coping. *Psychology in the Schools, 59*(9), 1844–1855. https://doi.org/10.1002/pits.22728

Collie, R. J., & Martin, A. J. (2023). Teacher wellbeing and sense of relatedness with students: Examining associations over one school term. Teaching and Teacher Education, 132, 104233. doi:https://doi.org/10.1016/j.tate.2023.104233.

Colomeischi, A. A. (2022). Promoting Mental Health at School: Implications for Teachers' Personal Development in Pracana, C, Wang, M (2022). Psychological applications and trends, in science press, Lisbon.

Council of the European Union. (2020) Council conclusions on European teachers and trainers for the future. Official Journal of the European Union. C193, 11–19.

Day, C., & Gu, Q. (2013). Resilient teachers, resilient schools: Building and sustaining quality in testing times (1st ed.). Routledge. doi:https://doi.org/10.4324/9780203578490.

Diener, E., Emmons, R. A., Larsen, R. J., & Griffin, S. (1985). The satisfaction with life scale. *Journal of Personality Assessment, 49*(1), 71–75. https://doi.org/10.1207/s15327752jpa4901_13

Dreer, B. (2023). On the outcomes of teacher wellbeing: A systematic review of research. *Frontiers in Psychology, 14*, 1205179. https://doi.org/10.3389/fpsyg.2023.1205179

Dumulescu, D., Andronache, D., Necula, C. V., & Mara, D. (2023). Teachers resilience: Relationships with fear of negative evaluations and emotion regulation. *Educatia, 21*(25), 386–393.

European Commission/EACEA/Eurydice (2021). Teachers in Europe: Careers, Development and Wellbeing. Eurydice report. Luxembourg: Publications Office of the European Union.

Friedman, I. A. (2000). Burnout in teachers: Shattered dreams of impeccable professional performance. *Journal of Clinical Psychology, 56*(5), 595–606. https://doi.org/10.1002/(SICI)1097-4679(200005)56:5%3C595::AID-JCLP2%3E3.0.CO;2-Q

García-Crespo, F. J., Fernández-Alonso, R., & Muñiz, J. (2021). Academic resilience in European countries: The role of teachers, families, and student pro-files. *PLoS One, 16*(7), e0253409. https://doi.org/10.1371/journal.pone.0253409

Gu, Q., & Day, C. (2013). Challenges to teacher resilience: Conditions count. *British Educational Research Journal, 39*(1), 22–44. https://doi.org/10.1080/01411926.2011.623152

Hascher, T., & Waber, J. (2021). Teacher wellbeing: A systematic review of the research literature from the year 2000–2019. *Educational Research Re-view, 34*, 100411. https://doi.org/10.1016/j.edurev.2021.100411

Jennings, P. A., & Greenberg, M. T. (2009). The prosocial classroom: Teacher social and emotional competence in relation to student and classroom outcomes. *Review of Educational Research, 79*(1), 491–525. https://doi.org/10.3102/0034654308325693

Kim, L. E., Jörg, V., & Klassen, R. M. (2019). A meta-analysis of the effects of teacher personality on teacher effectiveness and burnout. *Educational Psychology Review, 31*(1), 163–195. https://doi.org/10.1007/s10648-018-9458-2

Laine, S., Saaranen, T., Pertel, T., Hansen, S., Lepp, K., Liiv, K., & Tossavainen, K. (2018). Working community-related interaction factors building occupational wellbeing—Learning based intervention in Finnish and Estonian schools (2010–2013). *International Journal of Higher Education, 7*(2), 1. https://doi.org/10.5430/ijhe.v7n2p1

López-Martín, E., Gutiérrez-de-Rozas, B., González-Benito, A. M., & Expósito Casas, E. (2023). Why do teachers matter? A meta-analytic review of how teacher characteristics and competencies affect students' aca-demic achievement. *International Journal of Educational Research, 120*, 102199. https://doi.org/10.1016/j.ijer.2023.102199

Luthans, F., & Youssef-Morgan, C. M. (2017). Psychological capital: An evidence-based positive approach. *Annual Review of Organizational Psychology and Organizational Behavior, 4*(1), 339–366. https://doi.org/10.1146/annurev-orgpsych-032516-113324

Madigan, D. J., & Kim, L. E. (2021). Towards an understanding of teacher attrition: A meta-analysis of burnout, job satisfaction, and teachers' intentions to quit. *Teaching and Teacher Education, 105*, 103425. https://doi.org/10.1016/j.tate.2021.103425

Manning, A., Brock, R., & Towers, E. (2020). Responding to research. JSSE - Journal of Social Science Education, Vol 19 No 2 (2020): Research and impact in social sciences education. doi:https://doi.org/10.4119/JSSE-3312.

Maricuţoiu, L. P., Pap, Z., Ştefancu, E., Mladenovici, V., Valache, D. G., Popescu, B. D., Ilie, M., & Vîrgă, D. (2023). Is teachers' wellbeing associated with students' school experience? A meta-analysis of cross-sectional evidence. *Educational Psychology Review, 35*(1), 1. https://doi.org/10.1007/s10648-023-09721-9

Maslach, C., Jackson, S. E., & Leiter, M. P. (1997). Maslach burnout inventory. Scarecrow Education.

Mijakoski, D., Cheptea, D., Marca, S. C., Shoman, Y., Caglayan, C., Bugge, M. D., Gnesi, M., Godderis, L., Kiran, S., McElvenny, D. M., Mediouni, Z., Mesot, O., Minov, J., Nena, E., Otelea, M., Pranjic, N., Mehlum, I. S., Van Der Molen, H. F., & Canu, I. G. (2022). Determinants of burnout among teachers: A systematic review of longitudinal studies. *Inter-national Journal of Environmental Research and Public Health, 19*(9), 5776. https://doi.org/10.3390/ijerph19095776

Oliveira, S., Roberto, M. S., Veiga-Simão, A. M., & Marques-Pinto, A. (2021). A meta-analysis of the impact of social and emotional learning interventions on teachers' burnout symptoms. *Educational Psychology Review, 33*(4), 1779–1808. https://doi.org/10.1007/s10648-021-09612-x

Ortan, F., Simut, C., & Simut, R. (2021). Self-efficacy, job satisfaction and teacher wellbeing in the K-12 educational system. *International Journal of Environmental Research and Public Health, 18*(23), 12763. https://doi.org/10.3390/ijerph182312763

Ozamiz-Etxebarria, N., Idoiaga Mondragon, N., Bueno-Notivol, J., Pérez-Moreno, M., & Santabárbara, J. (2021). Prevalence of anxiety, depression, and stress among teachers during the COVID-19 pandemic: A rapid systematic review with meta-analysis. *Brain Sciences, 11*(9), 1172. https://doi.org/10.3390/brainsci11091172

Özü, Ö., Zepeda, S., Ilgan, A., Jimenez, A. M., Ata, A., & Akram, M. (2017). Teachers' psychological wellbeing: A comparison among teachers in U.S.A., Turkey and Pakistan. *International Journal of Mental Health Promotion, 19*(3), 144–158. https://doi.org/10.1080/14623730.2017.1326397

Papazis, F., Avramidis, E., & Bacopoulou, F. (2023). Greek teachers' resilience levels during the COVID-19 pandemic lockdown and its association with attitudes towards emergency remote teaching and perceived stress. *Psychology in the Schools, 60*(5), 1459–1476.

Poulou, M. S., Grazzani, I., Cavioni, V., Ornaghi, V. M., Conte, E., Cefai, C., Camilleri, L., & Bartolo, P. (2022). Teachers' and students' changes in social and emotional competences following the implementation of PROMEHS: A Europe- a program for promoting mental health at schools. *Educational Research Applications, 7*, 205. https://doi.org/10.29011/2575-7032.100205

Roloff, J., Kirstges, J., Grund, S., & Klusmann, U. (2022). How strongly is personality associated with burnout among teachers? *A Meta-analysis. Educational Psychology Review, 34*(3), 1613–1650. https://doi.org/10.1007/s10648-022-09672-7

Ryff, C. D. (1989). Happiness is everything, or is it? Explorations on the meaning of psychological wellbeing. *Journal of Personality and Social Psychology, 57*(6), 1069–1081. https://doi.org/10.1037/0022-3514.57.6.1069

Salgado, J. F. (2003). Predicting job performance using FFM and non-FFM personality measures. *Journal of Occupational and Organizational Psychology, 76*(3), 323–346.

Schaufeli, W. B., & Bakker, A. B. (2004). Job demands, job resources, and their relationship with burnout and engagement: A multi-sample study. *Journal of Organizational Behavior: The International Journal of Industrial, Occupational and Organizational Psychology and Behavior, 25*(3), 293–315.

Soykan, A., Gardner, D., & Edwards, T. (2019). Subjective wellbeing in New Zealand teachers: An examination of the role of psychological capital. *Journal of Psychologists and Counsellors in Schools, 29*(2), 130–138. https://doi.org/10.1017/jgc.2019.14

Stoyanova, R., Karabeliova, S., Pandurova, P., Zheckova, N., & Mitev, K. (2023). EFFECT OF RESILIENCE ON BURNOUT IN ONLINE LEARNING ENVIRONMENT. *Strategies for Policy in Science and Education/Strategii na Obrazovatelnata i Nauchnata Politika, 31*(4).

Tatalović Vorkapić, S., Colomeischi, A. A., & Onaghi, V. (2023). PROMEHS teachers' training: The effect of PROMEHS curriculum on teachers' mental health in Croatia and Romania. *Revista Romaneasca Pentru Educatie Multidi-mensionala, 15*(3), 400–418. https://doi.org/10.18662/rrem/15.3/773

Tsuyuguchi, K. (2023). Analysis of the determinants of teacher wellbeing: Focusing on the causal effects of trust relationships. *Teaching and Teacher Education, 132*, 104240. https://doi.org/10.1016/j.tate.2023.104240

UNESCO (2022) UNESCO strategy on education for health and wellbeing. https://unesdoc.unesco.org/ark:/48223/pf0000381728

Viac, C., & Fraser, P. (2020). Teachers' wellbeing: A framework for data collection and analysis.

Wang, H., Hall, N. C., & Taxer, J. L. (2019). Antecedents and consequences of teachers' emotional labor: A systematic review and meta-analytic investigation. *Educational Psychology Review, 31*(3), 663–698. https://doi.org/10.1007/s10648-019-09475-3

Wong, Y. P., & Zhang, L. (2014). Perceived school culture, personality types, and wellbeing among kindergarten teachers in Hong Kong. *Australa-sian Journal of Early Childhood, 39*(2), 100–108. https://doi.org/10.1177/183693911403900213

Zarate, K., Maggin, D. M., & Passmore, A. (2019). Meta-analysis of mindfulness training on teacher Well-being. *Psychology in the Schools, 56*(10), 1700–1715. https://doi.org/10.1002/pits.22308

Chapter 4
School Wellbeing and Educational Climate

Diana Sinziana Duca and Maria Magdalena Iordăchescu Dimitriu

4.1 Theoretical Frameworks

4.1.1 The School Wellbeing of Educational Participants

Improving wellbeing has become a priority for international authorities because of the links between this variable and important aspects of children's development. Defined as a state in which an individual feels good and functions well, wellbeing is a complex concept not limited to the presence of happiness or the absence of illness. It encompasses emotions such as happiness, engagement, interest, commitment, affection, and trust (Huppert 2009).

According to Allardt (1976), wellbeing is a state in which people can satisfy their basic needs. Within the conceptual model of wellbeing proposed by the author, three categories of needs are distinguished: a) having, which expresses impersonal and general material needs; b) loving, which refers to social needs, and c) being, which describes personal development needs. Allardt also developed a classification of subjective and objective indicators of wellbeing based on these three categories of needs. To measure the having dimension, the objective indicators are: standard of living and environmental conditions, and the subjective ones: subjective feelings of dissatisfaction—satisfaction with living conditions. The objective indicators of the loving dimension are relationships with others, while the subjective indicators are one's feelings about social relationships, located on the sadness-happiness axis. The category includes, at the objective level, the measurement of a person's relationship with society and nature; at the subjective level it focuses on one's feelings, on the alienation-personal development axis (Konu & Rimpelä,2002).

D. S. Duca (✉) · M. M. Iordăchescu Dimitriu
Faculty of Psychology and Sciences of Education, "Ştefan cel Mare" University of Suceava, Suceava, Romania
e-mail: diana.duca@usm.ro

A. A. Colomeischi (ed.), *Wellbeing in Schools of Southeastern Europe*, Human Well-Being Research and Policy Making, https://doi.org/10.1007/978-3-032-10525-7_4

Seligman (2011), within the framework of positive psychology, proposes a multidimensional model of wellbeing. According to this perspective, wellbeing is a construct composed of five core elements: positive emotions, engagement, positive relationships, meaning, and accomplishment (PERMA). Positive emotions encompass hedonic aspects such as pleasure, comfort, warmth, and joy. Engagement refers to a state of deep psychological involvement in activities, often described as flow, characterized by intense concentration and absorption. Positive relationships involve feeling socially integrated, cared for, supported by others, and satisfied with one's interpersonal connections. Meaning relates to perceiving one's life as purposeful and experiencing a sense of belonging to something larger than oneself. Accomplishment refers to the pursuit and attainment of goals, as well as feelings of competence, success, and personal achievement.

Similarly, Ryff and Keyes (1995) conceptualize psychological wellbeing as consisting of six dimensions: autonomy, environmental mastery, personal growth, positive relations with others, purpose in life, and self-acceptance. This model emphasizes optimal psychological functioning and long-term personal development rather than momentary emotional states.

Although developed from different theoretical perspectives, the two models share several common elements. Both emphasize the importance of positive relationships, personal growth, purpose or meaning in life, and active engagement with life. Together, they provide complementary frameworks for understanding wellbeing as a complex and multidimensional construct that integrates emotional, psychological, and social components.

4.1.2 Student's Wellbeing

Examining children's environments is necessary to understand better the mechanisms underlying their wellbeing. The school environment influences their wellbeing, as they spend much time there.

Based on Allardt's conceptual model of wellbeing, a model of wellbeing in schools has been developed by Konu and Rimpelä (2002). The health dimension is added to the original three categories of needs described by Allardt. The model illustrates the interaction between wellbeing, teaching, and learning (Fig. 4.1). It also highlights the impact of the family and community environment on children's school life. The four categories into which wellbeing in the school environment has been divided are: conditions (having), social relationships (loving), means for self-fulfillment (being) and health (health). Several factors thus influence wellbeing. The category of school conditions refers both to the environment around and within the school, the subjects, the organization within the school, the timetable, the size of classes, the disciplinary strategies, the safety measures, the lunch provided by the school, the temperature in the school and other such factors. The school climate, group dynamics, teacher-student relationships, family involvement, bullying influence social relationships. Self-fulfillment has many sources in the school environment, such as the value of

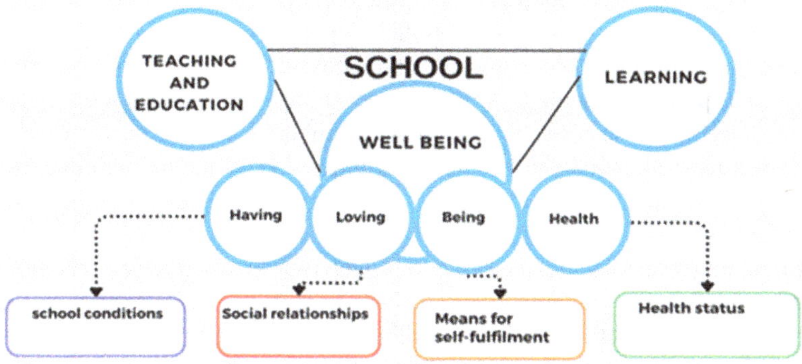

Fig. 4.1 The School Wellbeing Model (adapted by Konu and Rimpelä 2002)

pupils' work, guidance, encouragement, opportunities, promotion of self-esteem, creativity. At the level of health, wellbeing is influenced by psychosomatic symptoms, chronic diseases, other types of illnesses, even the common cold (Fig. 4.1) (Konu and Rimpelä 2002). Noble et al. (2008) define wellbeing more systematically as "a sustained state of positive mood and attitude, resilience, and satisfaction with self, relationships, and school experiences". Drawing on an extensive literature, they summarize seven school-based pathways to student wellbeing: physical and emotional safety; pro-social values; a supportive, inclusive, and caring school community; social and emotional learning; a strengths-based approach; a sense of meaning and purpose; and a healthy lifestyle.

Similarly, Schultz et al. (1987) argues that school wellbeing depends on interpersonal relationships, school improvement practices, systemic analysis, and problem-solving procedures. In his view, the teacher-student relationship is central to pupil wellbeing at school. Therefore, educators must promote cooperative learning, develop social skills, use effective instructional methods, and use positive discipline strategies.

Based on an extensive review of the literature on wellbeing, Soutter et al. (2014) developed a conceptual framework that details indicators of student wellbeing in a school context. The authors presented seven domains that influence this variable, separately and together: having, being, releasing, feeling, thinking, functioning, and striving. These are grouped into three overarching categories: assets, appraisals, and actions.

The first domain includes the dimensions of having, relating and being. Having refers to external resources, tools, and opportunities specific to the educational environment. For example, having access to technological tools, highly qualified teachers, and a safe and pleasant environment. On the other hand, the relational dimension focuses on children's interpersonal relationships. An important aspect of this dimension is the interaction between pupils and their teachers, which must be based on support and friendship to maintain children's wellbeing. In addition, a wellbeing school is characterized by inclusiveness and all pupils, regardless of cultural affiliation, ability, health, and socio-economic status, have access to all school services and are valued as part of the school. Being includes intrapersonal characteristics such as autonomy, self-awareness, resilience, physical wellbeing, and independence. Schools can contribute to students' wellbeing in this dimension by setting high expectations and providing opportunities for students to take on adult-like responsibilities and act autonomously.

The category that included evaluations had two levels: feeling and thinking. Feeling refers to recognizing pupils' different emotions and encouraging appropriate expression and management. Wellbeing schools focus on how pupils feel and teach children how to manage their emotions, integrating this dimension into the whole teaching and learning process, regardless of subject and class. Thinking includes constructive, contemplative, critical and mindful thinking. To support wellbeing, schools must teach students how to learn, develop metacognitive strategies and make informed decisions.

Finally, there are two dimensions of wellbeing: functioning and striving. The functioning dimension can be described by involvement, flow, grit, and determination. Striving concerns how students view and deal with their difficulties. Schools that promote wellbeing need to teach students how to view challenges so that they remain motivated to pursue personal goals and experience eudaimonic wellbeing.

4.2 Teachers Wellbeing

On the other hand, another important category in the context of school wellbeing is teachers. Their wellbeing is one of the key conditions for the effectiveness of the learning process and also for the wellbeing of the students. Most theoretical approaches to this concept are based on the impact of negative emotions due to stress, fatigue, frustration, and relationship problems on wellbeing.

To clarify the components of this variable, Viac and Fraser (2020) developed a framework defining teachers' professional wellbeing around four key dimensions: cognitive, subjective, physical, mental, and social. Cognitive wellbeing refers to teachers' self-efficacy and ability to work effectively by focusing on their work despite the challenges faced. Subjective wellbeing comprises three elements: life evaluation, which focuses on a reflective assessment of personal life; affect, which refers to emotional state; and eudaimonia, which is expressed through a sense of meaning in life. Teachers' physical and mental wellbeing is related to stress and the psychosomatic symptoms it causes. The last dimension, social wellbeing, is influenced by the quality of social interactions between teachers and pupils, colleagues, parents, school staff, school management and the local community.

The policies of education systems play an important role in promoting teachers' professional wellbeing, ensuring the quality of the working environment at the level of job demands and resources. A balance between these two aspects, school characteristics and teacher characteristics, influences the wellbeing experienced in all four dimensions described above. In turn, the dimensions of teacher wellbeing influence, at the internal level, teachers' stress and burnout and their motivation to leave teaching and, at the external level, teaching practices and students' wellbeing. Therefore, to support students' wellbeing, it is necessary first to consider and ensure teachers' wellbeing.

Other authors define teacher wellbeing in terms of the factors that influence it: workload wellbeing, organizational wellbeing, student interaction wellbeing. These summarize the pressure associated with work responsibilities outside the classroom, the school climate dimension, which represents the perception of the school leadership and culture towards teachers, and teachers' interactions with students, including the perception of students' behavior and motivation (Collie et al. 2015). From Yildirim's (2014) perspective, teacher wellbeing is described by job satisfaction, self-efficacy, aspiration, motivation, and authority. For Spilt et al. (2011), an important aspect of teachers' wellbeing, both professional and personal, is the quality of teacher-student relationships. The authors show that mental representations of relationships with disruptive children can lead to negative affect, the frustration experienced can lead to stress, which in turn affects teachers' wellbeing.

These studies indicate a relationship between teacher and pupil wellbeing and school climate. Research on the subject supports this, showing that components of school climate directly and indirectly affect wellbeing in the school environment.

4.3 Conceptual Models of School Climate

School climate is a concept that has been studied over time concerning the aspects of the school that influence the educational process, its outcomes, and the relationships between educational actors. Researchers have noted the lack of a universal definition of school climate in the literature and have examined the variety of perspectives from which this concept has been approached (Cohen et al. 2009, Hoy and Hannum, 1997, Wang and Degol 2016).

For example, Hoy and Hannum (1997) identified two approaches to the subject in the literature. They use metaphor as a way of characterizing school climate. In analyzing the first perspective, school climate is outlined through the notion of the 'personality' of the school, with all its characteristics. The second metaphor is sketched by the term 'health' of the school, including characteristics such as: positive and healthy relationships, the ability to overcome adverse situations and to function harmoniously, to continue to develop. According to the authors, a healthy school is defined by high levels of teacher connectedness, academic engagement, collegial leadership, availability of material resources, principal influence on the school environment, and institutional integrity.

Cohen et al. (2009) provide a succinct definition of school climate, stating that it encompasses individuals' experiences of school life, operationalized in terms of norms, goals, values, interpersonal relationships, educational practices, and organizational structures. In reviewing the literature, the authors noted the lack of a standardized index that captures the essential characteristics of school climate. Therefore, they extracted four dimensions that comprise the variable: safety, instructional process, relationships, and structural environment.

Similarly, Wang and Degol (2016) present a multidimensional model of school climate that helps characterize school climate quality, based on four dimensions similar to those presented above: academic environment, school as community, school safety and institutional environment.

Regarding the dimensions of school climate, Chirkina and Khavenson (2018) noted that researchers most commonly use the following dimensions to operationalize school climate: relationships between individuals within the school; the physical environment, which includes both the school and classroom space; individual factors, particularly the sense of belonging and discipline; and the organizational culture, which is created by expectations, rules, and norms.

Starting from the characteristics of school climate mentioned in previous studies, Aldridge and Ala'I (2013) conducted a study in which they developed a school climate model based on students' perceptions. The model includes dimensions important for various categories of students regarding school effectiveness. Thus, the six aspects of the school climate that were found relevant were teacher support, peer connectedness, school connectedness, affirming diversity, rule clarity, reporting, and seeking help (Aldridge and Ala'I 2013).

4.4 The Interaction Between School Climate and Wellbeing in Students' Perspective

Aldridge and McChesney (2018) conducted a meta-analysis to examine the relationship between school climate, mental health, and the wellbeing of adolescents. Their research identified four components of school climate: social relationships, school safety, school connectedness, and academics. They found that positive peer and teacher relationships based on connectedness, respect and support were associated with increased psychosocial wellbeing, pro-social behavior and lower prevalence of mental health problems and risk behaviors among adolescents. Identical results were also found for positive perceptions of school safety, school connectedness and a learner-centered educational environment. Peer connectedness is associated with positive wellbeing, as evidenced by two longitudinal studies showing that students reported higher levels of positive emotions when they reported feeling well connected to their peers (Schmidt et al. 2019). Thus, peer connectedness positively affects pro-social conduct among peers (Oldfield et al. 2016). Peer connectedness has also been linked to students' hope to cope with academic challenges successfully (Frisby et al. 2020). In this sense, negative perceptions of peer relationships predict higher levels of psychopathology (Suldo et al. 2012).

A positive perception of safety in the school environment, explained by reporting and help-seeking mechanisms, educational policies, the clarity of school rules and the consequences of breaking them, is positively correlated with student wellbeing and negatively correlated with mental health problems (Aldridge and McChesney 2018).

Other authors have focused their studies on other dimensions of school climate and wellbeing. In this context, Rathmann et al. (2018) used teacher control, demands, autonomy, organization, and interaction to operationalize school climate and school satisfaction and school-related helplessness for academic wellbeing. The study's results, which aimed to examine the relationship between school climate and students' mental health, showed a significant relationship between school climate and academic wellbeing dimensions. According to the results, increased teacher control, autonomy and teaching quality are associated with increased school satisfaction, while increased demands are negatively correlated. On the other hand, the second dimension of wellbeing, helplessness, is negatively influenced by teaching quality and classroom autonomy.

Conversely, research shows that a high level of wellbeing is associated with a positive perception of the school climate, especially regarding specific dimensions of interpersonal relationships: teacher-student relationships, peer relationships, and student and teacher involvement (Cocoradă and Orzea 2017).

4.5 The Interaction Between School Climate and Wellbeing in Teachers' Perspective

The impact of teachers' perceptions of school climate on job satisfaction, stress levels and teaching effectiveness was investigated by Collie et al. (2012). The study revealed that perceptions of student behavior and motivation significantly impacted teaching effectiveness and stress. Stress associated with student behavior negatively predicted teacher effectiveness, while stress associated with workload directly predicted job satisfaction. Positive school climate was also associated with teacher wellbeing and mental health, whereas it was negatively associated with emotional distress (Yang et al. 2022).

A recent study showed that perceptions of school climate indirectly affect teachers' enjoyment of teaching through their psychological wellbeing (Zhang et al. 2023). In other words, there is a correlation between teachers' perceptions of school climate and their psychological health. Teacher engagement in decision-making and school development, collaboration with colleagues, and sharing experiences will likely provide emotional support, a pleasant working atmosphere, and perceptions of an inspiring and motivating work climate, improving psychological wellbeing at work. This improved wellbeing contributes to increased enjoyment of teaching, as teachers could immerse themselves in their role with pleasure and depth in a school climate where they feel valued and can hear their opinions (Zhang et al. 2023).

Both quantitative (Cohen et al. 2009, Grazia and Molinari 2021, Wang and Degol 2016) and qualitative research (Hammar Chiriac et al. 2023, Jessiman et al. 2022, Pandia and Purwanti 2019, Walls et al. 2021) have addressed teachers' multidimensional perspectives on school climate. Teachers described a quality school climate regarding safety and peacefulness, characterized by wellbeing, effective teaching and caring teachers, a climate where students and teachers flourish.

In recent qualitative research, Hammar Chiriac et al. (2023) constructed a grounded theory of teachers' views of what affects school climate, based on two levels, internal-external and influenceable-uninfluenceable, and four types of elements: school social processes and values (i.e., internal influential factors), school spaces and support structures (i.e., internal non-influential factors), external relationships (i.e., external influential factors), and external means of control (i.e., external non-influential factors). There was a difference in how teachers talked about internal and external non-influential factors, even though they considered them to be more or less beyond their control. They accepted the external non-influential factors because they were taken for granted as impossible or almost impossible to modify. Instead, teachers discussed the internal non-influential factors more positively. They formulated their strategies for dealing with the conditions of the internal non-influential factors (e.g., through classroom rules or allocating time for breaks).

4.6 Socio-Demographic Factors Related to School Climate and Wellbeing

Research shows that school climate dimensions interact with wellbeing at different levels of schooling. For example, Lester and Cross (2015) found that peer support was the strongest predictor of wellbeing in the last year of primary school, whereas feeling safe in the school environment was the strongest predictor in the first year of secondary school.

Student gender may also influence the impact of teacher-student relationships (a component of school climate). This was demonstrated in a sample of 415 high school students, where a positive correlation between teacher-student relationships and student wellbeing was found only for female subjects (Suldo et al. 2012). In contrast, a systematic review of the literature focusing on the relationship between school climate and students' mental health and wellbeing found that positive relationships with teachers and peers were associated with increased psychosocial wellbeing and decreased mental health problems and risk behaviors, regardless of the gender of the subjects. Positive relationships were operationalized across studies through respect, connectedness, support, positive attitudes towards diversity, and absence of bullying and victimization (Aldridge and McChesney 2018).

Regarding the structural setting, an OECD report covering 35 countries shows that school or class size had little impact on student happiness. Teaching strategy and teacher support are two other dimensions of school climate that the study shows are closely related to student wellbeing, operationalized by the five dimensions: psychological, social, physical, material, and cognitive wellbeing from the PISA theoretical framework (OECD 2019).

Regarding the structural setting, an OECD report covering 35 countries shows that school or class size had little impact on student happiness. Also, teaching strategy and teacher support are two other dimensions of school climate that the study shows are closely related to student wellbeing, operationalized by the five dimensions: psychological, social, physical, material, and cognitive wellbeing from the PISA theoretical framework (OECD 2019).

Regarding differences at the level of teacher wellbeing, research shows a difference in perceptions of colleague support, principal support, work pressure, and less positive attitudes towards innovation according to age, gender, and educational level. For both primary and secondary school teachers, the age of teachers directly impacts their sense of professional wellbeing. This is because as teachers get older, they perceive certain aspects of the school climate differently, experiencing more work pressure and negative attitudes towards innovation for primary teachers, and less peer support and higher workload for secondary teachers (Aelterman et al. 2007).

Studies suggest that the school context can influence students' wellbeing through differences in perceived safety and engagement. In this context, results show that rural students' perceptions of these two dimensions are significantly lower than those of urban students (Nguyen et al. 2021).

4.7 Mediating Variables in the Relationship Between Educational Climate and School Wellbeing—Resilience and Self-Efficacy

4.7.1 Student Resilience

There is growing recognition that resilience is an important characteristic that students can develop. Resilience is facing adversity and achieving goals despite obstacles (Connor and Davidson 2003, Masten 2007). Several studies have examined the impact of school climate in promoting resilience and its impact on the mental health of educational participants. One research study explored how schools can build a climate that promotes resilience in students and found that resilience-building schools are more likely to have supportive relationships, high academic and social expectations, and opportunities for meaningful participation and contribution (Benard, 2004).

Henderson and Milstein (2003) suggest that resilience interventions include increasing connections with pro-social people, having clear and coherent boundaries, and teaching life skills.

Aldridge et al. (2016) examined the association between students' perceptions of school climate and wellbeing through resilience and identity. The study's results reflect several mediating effects of school climate on wellbeing. For example, the results showed that components of school climate, such as positive connections with peers, led to higher levels of resilience and ethnic and moral identity, leading to higher life satisfaction and wellbeing. In light of these findings, schools might consider the importance of promoting solid social networks and improving relationships. Schools could also give students opportunities to broaden their circle of relationships to feel a sense of connectedness with others, which implies a way to target best students' long-term wellbeing (Aldridge et al. 2016).

Another study indicates that school climate is directly and indirectly associated with student life satisfaction through resilience. Significant indirect effects of resilience were reflected in the relationships between dimensions of school climate, such as school connectedness, affirming diversity, and reporting and seeking help, and student life satisfaction (Aldridge et al. 2020).

4.7.2 Teacher Self-Efficacy

One variable of the educational context that has been much analyzed in recent years and that has been linked to both school climate and wellbeing is teacher self-efficacy. Self-efficacy refers to an individual's beliefs about his or her ability to develop and perform the tasks necessary to achieve specific outcomes (Bandura and Wessels, 1997). Tschannen-Moran and Hoy (2001) defined teacher self-efficacy as a multifaceted construct that includes three elements of effectiveness in using instructional strategies, classroom management, and student engagement.

Teacher self-efficacy is associated with many teacher-related outcomes, as suggested by the OECD (Ainley and Carstens 2018). For example, high levels of self-efficacy may contribute to decisions to retain teachers (Ainley and Carstens 2018, McInerney et al. 2018) and may play a preventive role against burnout. Generally, high levels of self-efficacy are conducive to teacher wellbeing and resilience. Teachers' perceptions of school climate significantly predict teachers' self-efficacy, job satisfaction and stress levels (Collie et al. 2012, Wilson et al. 2020).

Zhang et al. (2023) tested a model whereby teacher self-efficacy, school climate, and psychological wellbeing at work could predict the enjoyment of teaching. The results showed that teacher self-efficacy, school climate perceptions and psychological wellbeing directly predicted teaching enjoyment. Teacher self-efficacy indirectly influenced teaching enjoyment through psychological wellbeing. On the other hand, school climate also indirectly influences the enjoyment of teaching through teacher self-efficacy and psychological wellbeing. Conversely, school climate directly predicted teacher self-efficacy and psychological wellbeing.

4.8 Key Policies and Interventions that Promote School Wellbeing by Improving School Climate

A review of school climate shows that there has been a considerable and increasing focus on school climate reform in recent years due to three main determinants (Thapa et al. 2013):

1. A Substantial Body of Evidence Confirms that Contextual Climate Is Important: Group Tendencies, Such as Standards, Expectations, and Belief Structures, Influence Experiences, Personal Learning, and all Aspects of Interpersonal Relationships
2. It Is Increasingly Recognized that School Climate Reform Generally Supports Practical Violence Prevention and Bully Prevention Efforts. Curricula to Prevent Bullying Do Not Work in Isolation but Need to Work through School Climate Reform
3. Growing Interest in Research-Informed pro-Social Education Interventions, Including Character Education, Social-Emotional Learning and Mental Health Promotion. It Means that School Climate Improvement Is a Process that Inevitably Involves Students, Parents/Caregivers and Educators

Several educational policies and interventions have been implemented worldwide to promote wellbeing by improving school climate. School climate refers to a school's general environment, relationships, and culture. A supportive school climate is critical to students' educational achievement, mental health, and wellbeing. Here are some key policies and interventions that have been effective in improving school climate:

- Anti-Bullying Programs

Implement anti-bullying programs and policies that create a safe and inclusive student environment. These interventions include training staff and students to recognize and address bullying behavior. A meta-analysis of the effectiveness of thirty anti-bullying programs in schools found that they decreased bullying by 20–23% in experimental versus control schools. The main program components for reducing bullying were parental education, improved supervision of playgrounds, discipline practices, school meetings, use of videos, parent awareness, working with colleagues, classroom management, and classroom rules (Ttofi and Farrington 2009).

- Social-Emotional Learning (SEL) Programs

Integrating SEL programs into the curriculum to promote emotional intelligence, interpersonal skills, and self-awareness. Providing teachers with training to incorporate SEL strategies into their teaching practices. SEL programmes aim to strengthen teachers' capacity to promote children's social and emotional skills and improve teaching quality. A systematic literature review examined the effectiveness of universal curriculum-based SEL programmes on teacher outcomes (Blewitt et al. 2020). The findings suggest that SEL programmes can improve teaching quality, particularly in providing responsive teacher-child interactions that develop effective classroom management. Other studies demonstrating the effectiveness of SEL programmes have shown changes in improving students' social and emotional skills and pro-social behavior and reducing internalizing and externalizing behavioral problems (Cavioni et al. 2020, Colomeischi et al. 2022).

- Restorative Justice Practices

They are implementing restorative justice practices to address conflicts and disciplinary issues more constructively and empathetically and fostering a sense of responsibility and accountability among students. A systematic review of practices using restorative justice and restorative practices was published by Lodi et al. (2021). The authors state that these practices are increasingly used in schools, improving school climate, discipline, and positive conflict management through measures to prevent suspensions, exclusions, conflicts, and inappropriate behavior (e.g., bullying). Through developing social and emotional skills, restorative justice and restorative practices promote positive peer and student-teacher relationships and pro-social behavior (Lodi et al. 2021).

- Positive Behavior Interventions and Supports (PBIS)

The central premises that guide PBIS are that: (a) students learn how to behave by teaching positive behaviors and reducing problem behaviors, (b) effective schools teach positive behaviors but also regularly monitor these behaviors, (c) emphasis is placed on preventing problems before they occur, (d) support is provided to all students but is differentiated (some students receive more structured and intensive instruction and feedback support, while others receive individualized support), (e) the organization of behavior support must be school-wide, and (f) appropriate behavior support must be provided, while others receive individualized support), (e) the organization of behavior support must be (e) the organization of behavior support must be school-wide, and (f) appropriate behavior support 'practices' are used with fidelity and sustainability when linked to sustained organizational systems support (Horner and Monzalve-Macaya 2018).

- Teacher Professional Development

Professional development for teachers provides ongoing training to improve their classroom management skills and promote positive interactions with students. Teachers are trained in culturally responsive teaching practices to create an inclusive environment. Price (2008) examined K-12 teachers' perceptions of the benefits of professional development activities in improving student-teacher relationships, student-student interactions, and school climate. The study aimed to understand how practical professional development activities can provide teachers with the skills they need to build more positive teacher-student relationships and, in turn, to improve school climate. The results showed a relationship between professional development activities and improved teacher management and teacher-student relationships. The data suggests that K-12 teachers put more effort into building positive teacher-student relationships after participating in professional development activities.

On the other hand, professional development activities offered to improve classroom management were beneficial for improving school climate. The results show that K12 teachers felt schools safer for staff and students after attending professional development activities. For example, teachers felt that professional development activities to improve classroom management either provided them with valuable strategies for managing their classrooms or reinforced strategies they were already using (Price 2008).

- Parent and Community Involvement

Parental involvement in school is essential for children's socio-emotional, developmental, and academic outcomes (Galindo and Sheldon 2012). Parental engagement refers to parents' involvement in their children's education through various actions (volunteering for school activities, communicating with school staff, helping with homework, attending school events, parent-teacher organizations, and parent-teacher meetings) (Stewart 2008). Through close relationships and regular school communication, parents can significantly contribute to their children's academic success and improve the school environment (Arnold et al. 2008).

Berkowitz et al. (2021) note that parental involvement depends on the efforts of the school system to encourage them to get involved. Schools must engage with parents and broaden their understanding and expectations of parental involvement to consider the cultural attributes and social environment that make up their school experience. Finally, state and local governments should support parental involvement by developing and implementing policies to improve parental involvement and school climate (Berkowitz et al. 2021).

- Mental Health Support Services

School may be an appropriate place to implement mental health support services for children and their families. Such services help to reduce several obstacles that many caregivers may face when trying to access mental health services for their children. School-based mental health services provide mental health counseling and support services in schools. These services promote awareness and decrease the stigma associated with mental health problems (Swick and Powers 2018).

- Inclusive Education Policies

Kozibroda et al. (2020) conducted a meta-analysis of research on inclusive education practices and innovations in schools. Until the 2000s, research focused on beliefs and values as a factor influencing the effectiveness of inclusive education strategies. After the 2000s, research focused on issues more specific to the participants in the educational act: school leaders' attitudes, teachers' self-efficacy, parental support, school culture, models of inclusion in schools, and the severity of impairments as a determinant of teachers' attitudes towards inclusion. Overall, inclusive education policies implement strategies that support inclusive education for students with diverse learning needs and ensure that all students feel valued and included in the school community (Kozibroda et al. 2020).

- Student Voice and Participation

Student Voice and Participation provide opportunities for students to have a voice in decision-making processes within the school and to create student-led initiatives and clubs that contribute to a positive school culture. Recent research examines using student voice to improve school climate (Jones and Bubb 2021). The research was carried out in Norway, focusing on allocating resources to developing pupil wellbeing and involving pupils in school improvement. The findings showed some recognition of the centrality of student voice in implementing democracy in schools. Pupils and teachers had positive perceptions of pupil voice. School leaders were also willing to include student voices in school improvement processes. However, the actual use of students' voices was primarily limited to the operation of student councils for various reasons (e.g., lack of alternative structures, time constraints in implementing some decisions, and doubts about competence). Although adults generally feel that student voice is taken into account, students feel that they have much to offer to school improvement if given the opportunity (Jones and Bubb 2021).

- School Leadership and Governance

Strong leadership prioritizes the wellbeing of students and staff by establishing clear policies against discrimination and harassment. Therefore, researchers consider school leadership an essential determinant of school climate (Bellibas and Liu 2018). Studies have shown that the type of leadership principals provide is essential in explaining variations in school climate. For example, Mendel et al. (2002) found that certain leadership styles (collaborative and distributive) had a much more positive effect on school climate than other traditional styles. Some researchers have linked principal leadership to specific dimensions of school climate (e.g., effective communication, teacher support, participatory decision-making, and fair evaluation procedures) (Kelley et al. 2005).

On the other hand, Bryk (2010) suggested that school safety should be the main component of climate that principals should focus on, especially in schools with students of low socio-economic status. Students' sense of safety in and out of school is fundamental to their learning. It is also emphasized that principals should improve professional collaboration between teachers, which can be achieved through teacher respect (Bryk 2010).

When implemented effectively, these policies and interventions create a positive school climate that promotes students' wellbeing and enhances the educational experience. It is important to tailor these strategies to each school community's needs and context.

4.9 Future Directions for Practice and Research Related to the Relationship Between School Climate and the Wellbeing

Some potential directions for research and practice related to the relationship between school climate and the wellbeing of educational participants might be:

- Investigating the *long-term effects of a positive school climate on students' mental health*, academic achievement, and overall life outcomes. Longitudinal studies could provide insights into how early experiences in a supportive environment shape individuals long-term.
- Investigating the *impact of technology on school climate and student wellbeing.* The role of digital tools, online learning platforms and social media in shaping students' overall school climate and emotional health could be an essential focus for future research.
- Examining how *cultural and contextual factors influence perceptions of school climate and wellbeing.* Understand how these factors vary across communities and regions so that interventions and policies can be tailored to context-specific needs.
- Understanding how *educators' mental health affects schools' overall climate* could lead to developing strategies to support teachers and pupils.
- Exploring the impact of *inclusive practices on school climate* by studying the effects of diverse school programs, inclusive policies, and representation in educational materials on students' overall sense of belonging and wellbeing.
- Investigating how effective *resilience-building programs* and coping mechanisms can be implemented in schools. Understanding how students develop emotional resilience and cope effectively with stressors can promote a healthier school climate.
- Developing *mental health prevention interventions.* Research could explore the effectiveness of mindfulness programs, peer support systems, and other proactive approaches to promoting wellbeing and preventing mental health problems.
- Investigating the role of *parental involvement* in shaping school climate. Understanding how parents contribute to or detract from the overall wellbeing of students and the school community can inform strategies to promote positive home-school relationships.
- Evaluation of *policy changes in school climate* may include studying the effects of changes in discipline, standardized testing, or inclusive education on the overall wellbeing of students and teachers.

These potential lines of research highlight the interconnectedness of different factors in shaping wellbeing and climate within educational institutions. Future researchers can explore these areas to provide valuable information for developing effective strategies and policies.

Competing Interests

The authors have no conflicts of interest to declare that are relevant to the content of this chapter.

References

Aelterman, A., Engels, N., Van Petegem, K., &.Pierre Verhaeghe, J. (2007). The Well-being of teachers in Flanders: The importance of a supportive school culture. Educational Studies, 33(3), 285–297. doi:https://doi.org/10.1080/03055690701423085.

Ainley, J., &.Carstens, R. (2018). Teaching and learning international survey (TALIS) 2018 conceptual framework.

Aldridge, J., &.Ala'I, K. (2013). Assessing students' views of school climate: Developing and validating the what's happening in this school? (WHITS) questionnaire. Improving Schools, 16(1), 47–66. doi:https://doi.org/10.1177/1365480212473680.

Aldridge, J. M., Fraser, B. J., Fozdar, F., Ala'i, K., Earnest, J., & Afari, E. (2016). Students perceptions of school climate as determinants of wellbeing, resilience and identity. *Improving Schools, 19*(1), 5–26. https://doi.org/10.1177/1365480215612616

Aldridge, J. M., & McChesney, K. (2018). The relationships between school climate and adolescent mental health and wellbeing: A systematic literature review. International Journal of Educational Research, 88, 121–145. doi:https://doi.org/10.1016/j.ijer.2018.01.012.

Aldridge, J. M., McChesney, K., & Afari, E. (2020). Associations between school climate and student life satisfaction: Resilience and bullying as mediating factors. *Learning Environments Research, 23*, 129–150.

Allardt, E. (1976). Dimensions of welfare in a comparative Scandinavian study. *Acta Sociologica, 19*(3), 227–239.

Arnold, D. H., Zeljo, A., Doctoroff, G. L., & Ortiz, C. (2008). Parent involvement in preschool: Predictors and the relation of involvement to preliteracy development. *School Psychology Review, 37*(1), 74–90.

Bandura, A., & Wessels, S. (1997). *Self-efficacy* (pp. 4–6). Cambridge University Press.

Bellibas, M. S., & Liu, Y. (2018). The effects of principals' perceived instructional and distributed leadership practices on their perceptions of school climate. *International Journal of Leadership in Education, 21*(2), 226–244. https://doi.org/10.1080/13603124.2016.1147608

Benard, B. (2004). Resiliency: What we have learned. *WestEd.*

Berkowitz, R., Astor, R. A., Pineda, D., DePedro, K. T., Weiss, E. L., & Benbenishty, R. (2021). Parental involvement and perceptions of school climate in California. *Urban Education, 56*(3), 393–423.

Blewitt, C., O'Connor, A., Morris, H., Mousa, A., Bergmeier, H., Nolan, A., Jackson, K., Barrett, H., & Skouteris, H. (2020). Do curriculum-based social and emotional learning programs in early childhood education and care strengthen teacher outcomes? A systematic literature review. *International Journal of Environmental Research and Public Health, 17*(3), 1049. https://doi.org/10.3390/ijerph17031049

Bryk, A. S. (2010). Organizing schools for improvement. *Phi Delta Kappan, 91*(7), 23–30. https://doi.org/10.1177/003172171009100705

Cavioni, V., Grazzani, I., & Ornaghi, V. (2020). Mental health promotion in schools: A comprehensive theoretical framework.

Chirkina, T. A., & Khavenson, T. E. (2018). School climate: A history of the concept and approaches to defining and measuring it on PISA questionnaires. Russian Education and Society, 60(2), 133–160. doi:https://doi.org/10.1080/10609393.2018.1451189.

Cocoradă, E., & Orzea, I. (2017). Relationships between Wellbeing, Resilience and School Climate. *Bulletin of the Transilvania University of Braşov, Series VII: Social Sciences and Law, 10*(2-Suppl), 191–200.

Cohen, J., Mccabe, E. M., Michelli, N. M., & Pickeral, T. (2009). School climate: Research, policy, practice, and teacher education. Teachers College Record: The Voice of Scholarship in Education, 111(1), 180–213. doi:https://doi.org/10.1177/016146810911100108.

Collie, R. J., Shapka, J. D., & Perry, N. E. (2012). School climate and social–emotional learning: Predicting teacher stress, job satisfaction, and teaching efficacy. *Journal of Educational Psychology, 104*(4), 1189–1204. https://doi.org/10.1037/a0029356

Collie, R. J., Shapka, J. D., Perry, N. E., & Martin, A. J. (2015). Teacher wellbeing: Exploring its components and a practice-oriented scale. Journal of Psychoeducational Assessment, 33(8), 744–756. doi:https://doi.org/10.1177/0734282915587990.

Colomeischi, A. A., Duca, D. S., Bujor, L., Rusu, P. P., Grazzani, I., & Cavioni, V. (2022). Impact of a school mental health program on children's and adolescents' socio-emotional skills and psychosocial difficulties. *Children, 9*(11), 1661.

Connor, K. M., & Davidson, J. R. (2003). Development of a new resilience scale: The Connor-Davidson resilience scale (CD-RISC). *Depression and Anxiety, 18*(2), 76–82.

Frisby, B. N., Hosek, A. M., & Beck, A. C. (2020). The role of classroom relationships as sources of academic resilience and hope. Communication Quarterly, 68(3), 289–305. doi:https://doi.org/10.1080/01463373.2020.1779099.

Galindo, C., & Sheldon, S. B. (2012). School and home connections and children's kindergarten achievement gains: The mediating role of family involvement. *Early Childhood Research Quarterly, 27*(1), 90–103.

Grazia, V., & Molinari, L. (2021). School climate multidimensionality and measurement: A systematic literature review. *Research Papers in Education, 36*(5), 561–587. https://doi.org/10.1080/02671522.2019.1697735

Hammar Chiriac, E., Forsberg, C., & Thornberg, R. (2023). Teachers' perspectives on factors influencing the school climate: A constructivist grounded theory case study. *Cogent Education, 10*(2), 2245171. https://doi.org/10.1080/2331186X.2023.2245171

Henderson, N., & Milstein, M. M. (2003). *Resiliency in schools: Making it happen for students and educators.* Corwin press.

Horner, R., and Monzalve-Macaya, M. (2018). A framework for building safe and effective school environments: Positive behavioral interventions and supports (PBIS).

Hoy, W. K., & Hannum, J. W. (1997). Middle school climate: An empirical assessment of organizational health and student achievement. Educational Administration Quarterly, 33(3), 290–311. doi:https://doi.org/10.1177/0013161X97033003003.

Huppert, F. A. (2009). Psychological wellbeing: Evidence regarding its causes and consequences. Applied Psychology: Health and Wellbeing, 1(2), 137–164. doi:https://doi.org/10.1111/j.1758-0854.2009.01008.x.

Jessiman, P., Kidger, J., Spencer, L., Geijer-Simpson, E., Kaluzeviciute, G., Burn, A., Leonard, N., & Limmer, M. (2022). School culture and student mental health: A qualitative study in UK secondary schools. *BMC Public Health, 22*(1), 619. https://doi.org/10.1186/s12889-022-13034-x

Jones, M.-A., & Bubb, S. (2021). Student voice to improve schools: Perspectives from students, teachers and leaders in 'perfect' conditions. *Improving Schools, 24*(3), 233–244. https://doi.org/10.1177/1365480219901064

Kelley, R. C., Hornton, B., & Daugherty, R. (2005). Relationships between measures of leadership and school climate. *Education-Indianapolis hen Chula Vista, 126*(1), 1–7.

Konu, A., & Rimpelä, M. (2002). Wellbeing in schools: A conceptual model. Health Promotion International, 17(1), 79–87. doi:https://doi.org/10.1093/heapro/17.1.79.

Kozibroda, L. V., Kruhlyk, O. P., Zhuravlova, L. S., & Chupakhina, S. V. (2020). Practice and innovations of inclusive education at school. *International Journal of Higher Education, 9*(7), 176–186.

Lester, L., & Cross, D. (2015). The relationship between school climate and mental and emotional wellbeing over the transition from primary to secondary school. Psychology of Wellbeing, 5(1), 9. doi:https://doi.org/10.1186/s13612-015-0037-8.

Lodi, E., Perrella, L., Lepri, G. L., Scarpa, M. L., & Patrizi, P. (2021). Use of restorative justice and restorative practices at school: A systematic literature review. *International Journal of Environmental Research and Public Health, 19*(1), 96.

Masten, A. S. (2007). Resilience in developing systems: Progress and promise as the fourth wave rises. *Development and Psychopathology, 19*(3), 921–930.

McInerney, D. M., Korpershoek, H., Wang, H., & Morin, A. J. (2018). Teachers' occupational attributes and their psychological wellbeing, job satisfaction, occupational self-concept and quitting intentions. *Teaching and Teacher Education, 71*, 145–158.

Mendel, C. M., Watson, R. L., & Mac Gregor, C. J. (2002). A study of leadership Behaviors of elementary principals compared with school climate.

Nguyen, A. J., McDaniel, H., Braun, S. S., Chen, L., & Bradshaw, C. P. (2021). Contextualizing the association between school climate and student Well-being: The moderating role of rurality. Journal of School Health, 91(6), 463–472. doi:https://doi.org/10.1111/josh.13026.

Noble, T., Wyatt, T., McGrath, H., Roffey, S., & Rowling, L. (2008). *Scoping Study into Approaches to Student Wellbeing: Final Report.* https://docs.education.gov.au/documents/scoping-study-approaches-student-wellbeing-final-report

OECD. (2019). *PISA 2018 Results (Volume III): What School Life Means for Students' Lives*. OECD. doi:https://doi.org/10.1787/acd78851-en.

Oldfield, J., Humphrey, N., & Hebron, J. (2016). The role of parental and peer attachment relationships and school connectedness in predicting adolescent mental health outcomes. Child and Adolescent Mental Health, 21(1), 21–29. doi:https://doi.org/10.1111/camh.12108.

Pandia, W. S. S., & Purwanti, M. (2019). Teachers' perceptions of school climate in inclusive schools. *Psikohumaniora: Jurnal Penelitian Psikologi, 4*(1), 27. https://doi.org/10.21580/pjpp.v4i1.3357

Price, B. P. (2008). *Teacher perceptions of the impact of professional development and teacher-student relationships on school climate.* Auburn University.

Rathmann, K., Herke, M., Heilmann, K., Kinnunen, J. M., Rimpelä, A., Hurrelmann, K., & Richter, M. (2018). Perceived school climate, academic wellbeing and school-aged children's self-rated health: A mediator analysis. European Journal of Public Health, 28(6), 1012–1018. doi:https://doi.org/10.1093/eurpub/cky089.

Ryff, C. D., & Keyes, C. L. M. (1995). The structure of psychological wellbeing revisited. Journal of Personality and Social Psychology, 69(4), 719–727. doi:https://doi.org/10.1037/0022-3514.69.4.719.

Schmidt, A., Dirk, J., & Schmiedek, F. (2019). The importance of peer relatedness at school for affective Well-being in children: Between- and within-person associations. Social Development, 28(4), 873–892. doi:https://doi.org/10.1111/sode.12379.

Schultz, E. W., Glass, R. M., & Kamholtz, J. D. (1987). School climate: Psychological health and Well-being in school. Journal of School Health, 57(10), 432.

Seligman, M. E. P. (2011). *Flourish: A visionary new understanding of happiness and wellbeing* (1. Free Press hardcover ed). Free Press.

Soutter, A. K., O'Steen, B., & Gilmore, A. (2014). The student wellbeing model: A conceptual framework for the development of student wellbeing indicators. International Journal of Adolescence and Youth, 19(4), 496–520. doi:https://doi.org/10.1080/02673843.2012.754362.

Spilt, J. L., Koomen, H. M. Y., & Thijs, J. T. (2011). Teacher Wellbeing: The Importance of Teacher–Student Relationships. *Educational Psychology Review*, 23(4), 457–477. doi:https://doi.org/10.1007/s10648-011-9170-y.

Stewart, E. B. (2008). School structural characteristics, student effort, peer associations, and parental involvement: The influence of school-and individual-level factors on academic achievement. *Education and Urban Society, 40*(2), 179–204.

Suldo, S. M., McMahan, M. M., Chappel, A. M., & Loker, T. (2012). Relationships between perceived school climate and adolescent mental health across genders. School Mental Health, 4(2), 69–80. doi:https://doi.org/10.1007/s12310-012-9073-1.

Swick, D., & Powers, J. D. (2018). Increasing access to care by delivering mental health services in schools: The school-based support program. *School Community Journal, 28*(1), 129–144.

Thapa, A., Cohen, J., Guffey, S., & Higgins-D'Alessandro, A. (2013). A review of school climate research. *Review of Educational Research, 83*(3), 357–385. https://doi.org/10.3102/0034654313483907

Tschannen-Moran, M., & Hoy, A. W. (2001). Teacher efficacy: Capturing an elusive construct. *Teaching and Teacher Education, 17*(7), 783–805. https://doi.org/10.1016/S0742-051X(01)00036-1

Ttofi, M., & Farrington, D. (2009). What works in preventing bullying: Effective elements of anti-bullying programmes. *Journal of Aggression, Conflict and Peace Research, 1*(1), 13–24.

Viac, C., & Fraser, P. (2020). *Teachers wellbeing: A framework for data collection and analysis* (OECD Education Working Papers 213; OECD Education Working Papers, Vol. 213). doi:https://doi.org/10.1787/c36fc9d3-en.

Walls, J., Ryu, J., Fairchild, L., & Johnson, J. (2021). Contexts of belonging: Toward a multilevel understanding of caring and engagement in schools. *Educational Policy, 35*(5), 748–780. https://doi.org/10.1177/0895904819843590

Wang, M.-T., & Degol, J. L. (2016). School climate: A review of the construct, measurement, and impact on student outcomes. *Educational Psychology Review, 28*(2), 315–352. https://doi.org/10.1007/s10648-015-9319-1

Wilson, C., Marks Woolfson, L., & Durkin, K. (2020). School environment and mastery experience as predictors of teachers' self-efficacy beliefs towards inclusive teaching. *International Journal of Inclusive Education, 24*(2), 218–234.

Yang, C., Chan, M. K., Nickerson, A. B., Jenkins, L., Xie, J. S., & Fredrick, S. S. (2022). Teacher victimization and teachers' subjective wellbeing: Does school climate matter? *Aggressive Behavior, 48*(4), 379–392. https://doi.org/10.1002/ab.22030

Yildirim, K. (2014). Main factors of teachers professional wellbeing. Educational Research and Reviews, 9(6), 153–163. doi:https://doi.org/10.5897/ERR2013.1691.

Zhang, L. J., Fathi, J., & Mohammaddokht, F. (2023). *Predicting teaching enjoyment from teachers' perceived school climate, self-efficacy, and psychological wellbeing at work: EFL teachers.* Perceptual and Motor Skills.

Chapter 5
Parental Stress, Family Support, and Students' Wellbeing at School

Cornelia Ilciuc and Petruta P. Rusu

5.1 Introduction

The **wellbeing of children** is a complex construct including physical, mental, emotional, social, and academic dimensions. Children wellbeing is characterized by the presence of positive emotions (i.e., joy, confidence, engagement), psychological adjustment, cognitive abilities and concentration, self-esteem, autonomy, positive relationships with family and peers, school achievement, quality of school life, stress management and adequate parental income (Pollard & Lee, 2003). A comprehensive study across 11 countries identified the primary determinants of children's wellbeing to include family dynamics (the frequency of activities such as communication, recreational activities in family, learning experiences, safety, access to resources), educational environments (focusing on peer interactions, school safety, and experiences of bullying) and community (neighborhood safety availability of play areas) (Lee & Yoo, 2015). The aforementioned study revealed that variables associated with family life accounted for 40% of the variance observed in children's wellbeing. In comparison, aspects of school life were responsible for explaining 9% of the variance in wellbeing, and community-related variables contributed to 7% of the observed variance.

Family wellbeing is one of the most important predictors of wellbeing and life satisfaction in both children and adults, shaping emotional health and self-esteem (Jebb et al., 2020; Johnson et al., 2021; Lee & Yoo, 2015; Leto et al., 2019).

C. Ilciuc · P. P. Rusu (✉)
Faculty of Psychology and Sciences of Education, "Ştefan cel Mare" University of Suceava, Suceava, Romania
e-mail: petruta.rusu@usm.ro

C. Ilciuc
"Al. I. Cuza" University of Iaşi, Iaşi, Romania
e-mail: cornelia.ilciuc@usm.ro

A. A. Colomeischi (ed.), *Wellbeing in Schools of Southeastern Europe*, Human Well-Being Research and Policy Making, https://doi.org/10.1007/978-3-032-10525-7_5

Parents significantly influence their children's wellbeing through various mechanisms, including genetic predispositions, modeling behaviors, emotional support, and the provision of resources and opportunities. Their involvement in their children's lives impacts emotional development, academic achievement, social skills, and overall health. Positive parental engagement fosters a supportive environment conducive to child development, whereas negative interactions or neglect can adversely affect children's wellbeing. The wellbeing of families is linked to children's academic wellbeing, reflecting a complex interaction of emotional, social, and environmental factors.

School wellbeing is a critical aspect of children's overall subjective wellbeing, linked to various dimensions of their school life. School wellbeing refers to cognitive outcomes, social and emotional wellbeing at school, measured across indicators such as school satisfaction; enjoyment and interest in learning; motivation; homework attitudes; social class integration, attentiveness, self-perception of academic abilities, and teacher relationships (Knuver & Brandsma, 1993; Opdenakker & Van Damme, 2000). In a review of 186 studies measuring children's wellbeing, wellbeing at school was found to be one of the most frequently explored dimensions, alongside social relationships (family, peers) and integration within the community, physical wellbeing, psychological wellbeing, financial stability, and recreational activities (Cho & Yu, 2020). School wellbeing promotes a sense of belonging and competence, critical components of overall child wellbeing. The responsibility for the wellbeing of children in school extends beyond educational professionals to include parents, due to their significant influence on their children's socio-emotional and cognitive development, even within the school setting.

Community wellbeing refers to safety and security, access to quality education and healthcare, social connections, support services for children and families, recreational facilities, such as parks and playgrounds, environmental quality and cultural and educational opportunities (Atkinson et al., 2020; Lee & Yoo, 2015). Community wellbeing significantly affects physical, emotional, social, and cognitive development of children. Existing studies indicated positive associations of neighborhood safety with children's wellbeing. In contrast, children exposed to community violence (witnessing community violence or being a victim of community violence) report more symptoms of depression, hopelessness, anxiety and post-traumatic stress (Ceballo et al., 2003; Lee et al., 2020). Studies investigating community wellbeing should also focus on social inequalities (e.g., socio-economic inequalities), consider different communities a person belongs (such as residential community) and assess wellbeing in different community subgroups and different generations (Atkinson et al., 2020).

As the quality of family relationships and the home environment significantly influence how children feel at school and in the community, the present chapter will focus on two family variables related to children's wellbeing at school: parental stress and family support. Understanding the dynamic relationship between family wellbeing, school wellbeing and community wellbeing in children development is very important for designing prevention and intervention programs and policies to support children. The nature of children's interactions with their parents, along with the degree of parental involvement in their lives, significantly shapes students' perceptions and their strategies for navigating school-related challenges.

5.2 Family Variables Related to Children's Wellbeing

The concept of wellbeing within the school setting is viewed through a multifaceted lens in the ***School Wellbeing Model*** (Konu, 2002). This model categorizes wellbeing into four distinct dimensions: physical health (health status), personal growth and achievements (means for self-fulfillment, or "being"), the educational environment (school conditions, or "having"), and interpersonal connections (social relationships, or "loving"). The School Wellbeing Model suggests that family background significantly shapes school experiences, influencing both the social dynamics and educational outcomes for students. Family support influences a child's social and emotional development, which, in turn, affects their wellbeing at school. Students with strong family bonds may have better social skills and emotional resilience. In addition, children are more likely to be engaged in learning when they feel secure and supported at home.

In a more recent study, Kiuru et al. (2020) have redefined the concept of school wellbeing, focusing on the emotional dimensions manifested through students' satisfaction with school and the stress they experience. School satisfaction encompasses the overall positive perceptions and feelings students have towards their school environment, highlighting the significance of enjoyment and interest in school-related activities (Eccles, 2004; Huebner & Gilman, 2007). Conversely, school stress is characterized by students' perceptions of school demands and expectations as excessively challenging, arising from a disparity between these demands and the students' available resources to meet them (Salmela-Aro & Upadyaya, 2014; Sonmark & Modin, 2017).

Children interact with their parents at home and with teachers and peers at school. These meaningful interactions influence school students' wellbeing (Umberson & Karas Montez, 2010). Hoferichter et al. (2021) investigated the relationship between parental, teacher, and peer support and student wellbeing by assessing physical, psychological wellbeing and self-worth. The results indicated positive associations of perceived teacher support with students' self-worth and physical wellbeing, while peer support was positively linked to psychological wellbeing. Notably, parental support was positively associated with all three dimensions of students' wellbeing.

Over time, researchers have formulated several theoretical models that explain how the characteristics of the family influence the wellbeing of children. ***The Process of Parenting Model*** (Taraban & Shaw, 2018) illustrates the impact of parenting on children's development and wellbeing, highlighting the dynamic interaction between parental characteristics, child traits, and the family's social context. The model incorporates variables related to parental factors, including parents' depression levels, which were linked to diminished positive parenting and a disconnection from children's positive emotions. Furthermore, the parental relationship quality affects children's wellbeing. Parents with higher levels of marital satisfaction tend to collaborate more effectively in child-rearing and education, engage more in family activities, and are more sensitive to their children's needs. Conversely, negative parenting approaches, characterized by frequent punishment and restrictive measures, are associated with adverse emotional behaviors in children, such as irritability, anger, restlessness, sadness, or fear. Additionally, the family's socio-economic status exerts a significant influence on parenting practices and, by extension, on the wellbeing of both parents and children, as well as on family relationships (Taraban & Shaw, 2018).

We will explore in this chapter two important factors that significantly affect the overall wellbeing of children, and particularly their wellbeing in a school context: parental stress and parental support.

5.2.1 Parents's Stress and Children's Wellbeing

Parental stress (e.g., economic stress, work stress, couple relationship stress) has been negatively associated with parenting functioning and children's wellbeing. Parents experiencing high levels of stress may transfer some of that stress to their children. This can affect children's emotional wellbeing and academic performance. Moreover, children's reactions to stress are influenced by their parents' attitudes and coping mechanisms. If parents are stressed, it can influence how children perceive and respond to stressors in their own lives. Furthermore, stress influences parental involvement, as stressed parents may find it challenging to be actively involved in their child's education, attend school events, or provide necessary support. This lack of involvement can impact a student's sense of security and connection to their family.

5.2.2 Economic Stress

Socio-economic status significantly impacts both parental wellbeing and their children's overall and school-related wellbeing. The Integrated Framework of Child Poverty (IFCP) links child poverty and wellbeing, highlighting school-related variables in this association (e.g., the quality of school, school dropout, school violence, interaction between family and school) (Biggeri & Cuesta, 2021).

Masarik and Conger (2017) reviewed eight longitudinal studies from the perspective of the ***Family Stress Model*** (Conger & Conger, 2002; Conger et al., 2010) to understand how parental stress can influence children's physical, socio-emotional and cognitive development. The review indicated that parental stress increases the likelihood of relational conflicts, maladaptive parenting strategies and lower levels of child wellbeing. The authors formulated an explanatory model with economic stress as a pivotal stressor, noting that its manifestations—low-income job, loss, or significant unexpected expenses—increase psychological distress, hostility, depressive states, and anxiety across various nationalities and marital statuses. Psychological distress, in turn, negatively affects both spousal and parent-child relationships. Specifically, it is associated with escalated conflict frequency and severity, lower levels of partner support, and co-parenting. Moreover, parental psychological distress negatively impacts children, leading to diminished parental support, harsher disciplinary practices, excessive control and punitive measures, and reduced quality time spent together. Such adverse parenting behaviors are linked to an increased likelihood of neglect and abuse, further exacerbating children's and adolescents' adjustment challenges, and significantly undermining their wellbeing at school.

Compared to other EU countries, family income is lower in countries from Eastern Europe (Győrffy, 2022; Popescu et al., 2019; Tesliuc et al., 2014). A large number of eastern-European families experience financial difficulties and the stress caused by them. Economic pressure differs depending on the environmental characteristics. Families living in rural areas are more affected than those living in urban areas (Herman, 2012). The life of both parents and children can be affected by economic hardship in many ways. The Family Stress Model proposed by Conger and colleagues indirectly relates economic difficulties to child outcomes through marital conflict, parents' emotional states, and parenting strategies (Conger et al., 1990, 1994, 2010; Masarik & Conger, 2017). Parents' feelings of frustration or helplessness determined by the lack of financial resources can have a negative impact on the child's development and wellbeing through the parents' use of inappropriate parenting strategies. On the other hand, marital conflict and dissatisfaction related to economic hardship can also influence parenting behaviors. Consequently, unfavorable economic circumstances, the stress caused by them, marital conflict, and over controlling parenting affect the emotional, social, and cognitive development of children and, thus, their wellbeing.

Men and women of lower socio-economic status place a high value on children and parenthood (Edin & Nelson, 2013), yet they face more challenges in child-rearing compared to their higher-income counterparts (Cooper, 2014). Current societal standards for parenting, which include maintaining a more than comfortable living environment and serving healthy, home-prepared meals, exert additional pressure on low-income mothers, making them susceptible to depression (Bowen et al., 2019).

Research indicated that students from wealthier families enjoy greater financial resources and parental support compared to their peers from less affluent backgrounds (Finkelstein et al., 2007; Veiga, 2016) leading to higher motivation for achievement and school wellbeing. Furthermore, children from more privileged backgrounds often exhibit greater self-esteem, self-efficacy, optimism, autonomy, and advanced social skills (Artuch-Garde et al., 2017; Holopainen et al., 2020; Martin, 2013; Zolkoski & Bullock, 2012). In addition, more educated parents typically engage more in school activities, such as attending conferences and teacher meetings, than less educated parents (Kelty & Wakabayashi, 2020). This disparity is attributed to higher socio-economic parents providing their children with more resources (such as money and knowledge), highlighting the importance of education, and setting higher educational expectations than parents with fewer financial resources and lower educational levels

(Alves et al., 2017; Simpkins et al., 2012). School dropout is also influenced by family economic and social resources (Biggeri & Cuesta, 2021).

5.2.3 *Work Stress*

Work-related stress depletes parents' resources (such as energy, cognitive capacity, and attention), resulting in reduced involvement in their children's lives. Studies in the work-family domain have demonstrated that occupational stress factors (including high demands, excessive workload, and a lack of support at work) lead to diminished parental engagement and a decrease in positive family interactions, as these stressors exhaust parents' energy and mental resources (Repetti & Wang, 2017). Thus, parents who experience high stress levels at work are prone to irritation and frustration. These negative emotions influence their behavior within the family by enabling anger, withdrawal, or avoidance of involvement in family activities such as playing with children and helping them do their homework. Parents' lack of involvement in children's lives affects their overall wellbeing, including the wellbeing at school, because family support is one of the decisive factors in forming a positive attitude towards life and school and cultivating interest and pleasure in educational activities.

The challenge of balancing work and family responsibilities is increasingly confronting employees (Nomaguchi, 2009) particularly when they are also parents. This phenomenon known as Work-family conflict (WFC) primarily affects the wellbeing of the individuals who experience it, but also of their family members. Parental WFC indirectly diminishes children's wellbeing by negatively influencing parenting behaviors and reducing the support children receive from their parents (Hess & Pollmann-Schult, 2020). Parents who prioritize their work roles over family commitments are likely to spend less quality time with their children, be less available to meet their children's needs, exhibit more irritability, engage in stricter disciplinary practices, and demonstrate less affection in their interactions with their children (Cooklin et al., 2016). Consequently, parental WFC indirectly impacts child wellbeing through the depletion of parents' emotional, cognitive, and physical resources, which leads them to adopt negative behaviors and provide less support to their children.

5.3 Stress Related to Couple Relationship

Considering that children live within the family, together with their parents, the dynamics and couple relationship quality between parents have an essential role in the children's wellbeing. According to Belsky (1984), the relationship between marital quality and child outcomes can be explained by the fact that parents' perception of marital quality affects parenting behaviors and their psychological adjustment. Thus, marital dissatisfaction can result in increased parental distress and deteriorated parent-child relations, which may lead to affecting the children's wellbeing and the emergence of emotional problems. Fishman and Meyers (2000) found a negative association between parents' level of marital satisfaction and children's psychological distress. Moreover, mothers who experienced higher levels of marital satisfaction reported greater involvement, which, in turn, was associated with lower levels of child distress. However, this mediated pathway did not remain significant in the case of fathers.

Conversely, conflict between parents is a distinct aspect of couple dynamics that can significantly influence the broader spectrum of family life, including its effects on children. Erel and Burman (1995) found that children of all ages are impacted by interparental conflict, though it more severely affects younger children because they are more vulnerable than older ones. Hess (2022) in a longitudinal analysis, found a significant correlation between the frequency of conflicts between parents and the decline in children's social wellbeing, with this relationship being strongly influenced by parenting practices. Specifically, regular disputes between parents result in poorer communication and reduced emotional warmth towards children, which adversely impacts their social wellbeing. Additionally, Jaycox and Repetti (1993) pointed out that children from families experiencing marital conflicts tend to have a lower sense of competence compared to their counterparts, which can undermine their wellbeing and academic performance at school.

Family stability plays a crucial role in the wellbeing of children. Research indicates that children from divorced families often exhibit lower levels of wellbeing compared to those from intact families (Amato, 2001; Amato & Keith, 1991). Størksen et al. (2006) conducted a longitudinal study on the impact of parental divorce on the wellbeing of teenagers. The results showed that parental separation significantly influences adolescents' wellbeing, with girls particularly showing a higher propensity for anxiety and depression symptoms over time compared to boys.

5.4 The Importance of Dyadic Coping in Stress Buffering

Within the studies on stress and parenting, dyadic coping (i.e., support or assistance provided to and received from the partner in coping with stress; joint problem-solving in times of stress), co-parenting and parenting support to their children have been found to be important resources in buffering the effect of stress on dysfunctional parenting and family functioning (Rusu et al., 2016, 2019; Zemp et al., 2016b). Children whose parents display higher levels of dyadic coping have better social skills and fewer externalizing and internalizing problems (Zemp et al., 2016a). Future studies should investigate the role of dyadic coping in promoting children's school wellbeing, as dyadic coping might positively affect children's motivation, self-esteem, enjoyment, and interest associated with school.

5.4.1 Family Support

Parents directly or indirectly influence the socio-emotional and cognitive development of their children and their wellbeing in general, but also at school by offering support or by depriving children of this resource. Children can perceive parental support in multiple ways, including parents' behavior, parental style, emotional warmth of parents, and their involvement in children's education.

Research studies indicate that parental support is positively associated with children's wellbeing (Francis et al., 2021; Gecas & Schwalbe, 1986; Lan et al., 2019). Furthermore, a supportive relationship with parents is a protective factor that may help successful educational transitions (Waters et al., 2014). In contrast, deprivation of parental support has been significantly associated with children's mental and physical problems. Studies show that children who perceive a low level of parental support tend to develop internalizing and externalizing problems (Barber & Harmon, 2002), distress (Costa et al., 2015), and impaired psychological functioning (Inguglia et al., 2018).

On the other hand, parents are the first and most important factors influencing their children's self-esteem, which plays a pivotal role in children's assessment of school demands against their own perceived capabilities. These appraisals significantly influence the wellbeing of the child (Yang et al., 2019). Children's self-esteem tends to grow when they live in an enabling family environment and benefit from positive parenting behaviors. A longitudinal study on children between the ages of 10 and 16 showed that parental warmth, low maternal depression, economic security, monitoring, and the father's presence determine the growth of children's self-esteem (Krauss et al., 2020). On the other hand, studies showed that child neglect (not adequately meeting the child's physical, emotional, and mental needs) significantly affects self-esteem (Ayhan & Beyazit, 2021; Sciarrino et al., 2018). Child neglect can take various forms, such as depriving the child of support, ignoring him, not showing love towards the child, treating him with disrespect, and not fulfilling the needs related to education or health (Lewin & Herron, 2007; Straus & Kantor, 2005).

Positive parenting has an essential role in the development of children's emotional, social, and cognitive skills important to manage situations in the school environment. Positive parenting involves parents' sensitivity to children's needs, emotional warmth, parents' reactivity to children's emotions, thoughts, and intentions, emotional support, empathy, acceptance, secure attachment, open communication with the child and active listening, cognitive stimulation and the child's involvement in activities that favor the development of cognitive processes, the existence of daily routines (e.g., doing homework, reading stories, playing with the child, family meals), encouraging the child, supporting his autonomy (Grusec et al., 2014; Landry et al., 2006; Prime et al., 2023; Taraban & Shaw, 2018). Positive parenting supports the child's self-esteem, and self-efficacy which in turn helps the child to manage the challenges effectively in the school context and experience a high level of wellbeing.

Parenting style has a considerable impact on children's wellbeing. The results of the study conducted by Gul et al. (2021) showed that children whose parents adopt a positive (authoritative) parental style experience a significantly higher level of wellbeing than children whose parents have a negative parental style (authoritarian and permissive). The difference is also maintained when evaluating the relationships between parenting styles and dimensions of wellbeing: autonomy, self-acceptance, the ability to manage external resources, establishing a goal in life, personal growth, and positive relationships with others.

Parents' behavior also influences children's executive functions, parents help children to concentrate, think before acting, resist temptations, operate with information, and face unexpected changes in the school context. Executive functions include working memory (retaining and operating with information), inhibitory control (children's ability to control their thoughts, emotions, and behavior, selective attention, self-control), and cognitive flexibility (acceptance of mistakes, ability to look at things from different perspectives). Valcan et al. (2018) conducted a meta-analysis investigating the relationship between parents' behaviors and children's executive functions. They took into account the positive behaviors of the parents (e.g., warmth, sensitivity), negative behaviors (detachment, control), and cognitive behaviors (supporting the child's autonomy and cognitive stimulation). The results indicated positive correlations between parents' positive and cognitive behaviors and children's executive functions. In addition, Koşkulu-Sancar et al. (2023) showed that positive parenting (emotional support, parental warmth, parental responsiveness, and attachment security) was positively associated with children's executive functions, while negative parenting (inconsistency, parents' negative emotions) was negatively related to the development of children's executive functions.

5.4.2 Emotional Support

A supportive family environment provides emotional stability and a sense of security for children. Families that engage in open communication, express love, and provide encouragement contribute positively to a child's mental wellbeing. Parental emotional support is crucial for children's subjective wellbeing. A recent study demonstrated that increased parental emotional support was positively associated with greater subjective wellbeing of adolescents (Berger et al., 2024).

According to Arrindell and Van der Ende (1984), emotional support is one of the three dimensions of parental style, along with rejection and control attempts. Emotional support implies a responsive parental behavior adapted to the child's needs (Simões et al., 2011). This concept indicates that the quality of the parent-child relationship's emotional side is determined by how the parent expresses himself physically and verbally (Rohner et al., 2005).

Self-perceptions of competence influence motivational processes and students' wellbeing at school and explain different academic results in students with similar cognitive abilities. Côté and Bouffard (2011) showed that emotional support from parents is related to children's under-evaluation of scholastic competence. Students who undervalue themselves reported less parental emotional support and more criticism and disapproval from their parents. This illusion of scholastic incompetence negatively affects students' adaptation and functioning at school. This phenomenon determines several consequences on how the children affected perceive and experience the school activity. These children tend to be less curious and interested in school subjects but are more anxious about evaluation (Harter, 1985; Phillips & Zimmerman, 1990). Likewise, low self-esteem children experience less pleasure and satisfaction in school (Miserandino, 1996). Given the critical role of children's self-perceived competence in their school wellbeing and the pivotal role of parents in shaping these self-perceptions through emotional support, it is imperative for parents to exert effort in this area. By expressing satisfaction with their children's achievements, showing acceptance, encouraging them, and communicating confidence in their abilities, parents can significantly bolster their children's perception of their own competence (Galand & Vanlede, 2004; Nurra & Pansu, 2009).

5.4.3 Involvement in Education

Family support is also reflected in the level of parental involvement in a child's education. The concept of "parental involvement" includes both parent-school communication and the general attitude of the parents towards the school (its value, the attitude towards teachers and peers of their children). Parents who actively participate in their children's academic activities and school events create a positive and supportive learning environment.

The support parents can offer to promote the wellbeing of their children at school involves both *school-based involvement* and *home-based involvement* (Wang & Sheikh-Khalil, 2014). Home-based involvement includes helping children with homework and projects, initiating conversations related to school life and school performance, and conveying the importance of learning to the child. School-based involvement refers to parents' participation in school activities, such as events, conferences, and teacher consultations. Numerous studies prove that parental home-based involvement is essential to students' wellbeing, motivation associated with school, and academic achievement (Spera, 2006; Wang & Sheikh-Khalil, 2014; Wilder, 2014). These relationships can be explained by the fact that parents' involvement in activities and discussions related to school increases the child's perception of the value of school, positive attitudes, and motivation towards school (Pomerantz et al., 2007). The more the child perceives parental warmth, the greater the benefits of parents' involvement will be (Chung et al., 2020; Khaleque, 2013; Rohner et al., 2005).

The degree to which parents are involved in school-related aspects is also influenced by *academic socialization*, which Hill and Tyson (2009) consider a dimension of parental involvement. This concept primarily includes the parents' perception of the usefulness and value of school, which they pass on to their child. This belief influences students' positive or negative attitude towards school. Academic socialization also includes the management of the time that the child allocates to school and personal activities, the promotion of high educational aspirations, the presentation of learning strategies that could help the child, and the parent's involvement in the planning and organization of educational activities.

5.5 Differences Between Mothers and Fathers Regarding the Support Offered to Children

Both mothers and fathers play vital roles in the development and wellbeing of a child, yet research suggests variances in how each parent engages and behaves in their child's life (Canavarro & Pereira, 2007; Craig & Mullan, 2011). Some scholars consider that these differences can be determined by different factors such as socioeconomic status, values about gender and family, and differences regarding paid work.

A study that involved participants from four countries (Australia, Denmark, Italy, and France) showed that parents' gender significantly influenced the extent to which they were involved in child care activities (Craig & Mullan, 2011). These activities were categorized into two types: physical care and activities involving direct interaction with the child (such as feeding, hugging, soothing, and accompanying to school and extracurricular activities), and talk-based care (including conversations, listening, educational support, storytelling, and playing games). Despite Denmark being the most gender-egalitarian among the studied nations, mothers were still found to be more engaged in child-rearing activities than fathers. However, the extent of these differences varied across the countries surveyed, suggesting that the effectiveness of policies aimed at promoting father involvement or equitable parenting is heavily dependent on the cultural and social context.

Research indicates that mothers and fathers typically engage in different parenting approaches and offer varying levels of support to their children (Conrade & Ho, 2001). Studies have found that mothers generally provide more affection and emotional support compared to fathers, with children receiving higher levels of emotional support from their mothers (Canavarro & Pereira, 2007; McKinney & Renk, 2008).

Additionally, it has been observed that mothers are more active in school-related activities. Communication between schools and families often occurs mainly through mothers, who tend to be more involved in their children's academic lives (Lannert & Szekszárdi, 2015). Fletcher and Silberberg (2006) studied father involvement in primary schools in Australia and discovered that, while mothers participate more in school activities, fathers show a preference for engaging in outdoor and sports activities with their children.

5.6 Family and Bullying in School

Bullying in the school environment is increasingly common worldwide, but also in countries from South Eastern Europe. According to official statistics, over one-third of Romanian students face some form of bullying (UNESCO, 2019). This phenomenon is one of the factors that significantly affects the wellbeing of children, overall and at school (Bradshaw et al., 2017; Sivaraman et al., 2019; Varela et al., 2021; Xu & Fang, 2021). The manifestation of bullying behaviors in the school environment damages the wellbeing of students at school, regardless of children becoming victims or perpetrators.

5.6.1 Parenting Behaviors and the Manifestation of Bullying in School

Studies show that one of the aspects that predispose children to adopt such aggressive behaviors is inappropriate parenting. A study demonstrates a significant correlation between specific parenting behaviors that involve upbringing and discipline methods and bullying behaviors among students. The way children are raised by their families significantly impacts their likelihood of engaging in bullying within the school setting (Papanikolaou et al., 2011). Students are more prone to participate in bullying activities when parents apply disciplinary measures without providing explanations. Furthermore, a connection exists between bullying behavior and parents' reluctance to help with school-related problems.

5.6.2 Protective Role of Family

Research suggests that the way parents raise their children impacts the development of their social skills, emotional regulation, and the ability to form friendships. These factors collectively influence a child's susceptibility to becoming a victim of bullying. Parenting that supports the development of children's social abilities and peer relationships—termed 'facilitative parenting'—plays a crucial role in whether children are bullied by their peers (Healy et al., 2015). The study highlighted that, in comparison to their non-bullied counterparts, bullied children often have weaker relationships with peers and exhibit higher levels of reactive aggression in response to hypothetical peer provocation scenarios.

Warm and non-dominating parenting styles foster social skills in children, potentially reducing their likelihood of being bullied. Such parenting can also mitigate the emotional impacts of bullying by assisting children in managing their responses to challenging circumstances. Research indicates that parents of bullied children often exhibit less warmth and are more controlling or demanding (Ladd & Ladd,

1998). Conversely, social skills—crucial for shielding children from bullying—are associated with consistent parental affection and minimal controlling behaviors over time (McDowell et al., 2003). Warm and supportive parenting can also alleviate the emotional effects of bullying and social exclusion (Graziano et al., 2010). Bowes et al. (2010) highlight that a positive family environment and maternal affection can counteract the adverse emotional and behavioral effects of bullying, underscoring the significance of family dynamics in supporting bullied children. However, parents under considerable stress may engage more in negative interactions with their children than positive ones, adversely affecting the child's wellbeing.

5.7 Implications. Prevention, and Intervention Programs for Parents

The wellbeing of children in school settings is significantly linked to the dynamics within their families, including their interactions with both parents and the level of parental engagement in their daily lives. In light of this, it is essential for educational stakeholders to prioritize enhancing connections between schools and families. Schools should aim to improve communication with parents by employing tools like digital school platforms, organizing consistent meetings, and facilitating activities that include both students and their parents. Additionally, it is crucial to provide services tailored to address contemporary parental challenges, such as stress management, through counseling, prevention and intervention initiatives, and parent-focused seminars.

Children's wellbeing at school significantly benefits from parental support. Improvements in this support can result from initiatives by various stakeholders, such as offering financial assistance to families dealing with economic hardships and improving parental access to resources such as programs, conferences, and workshops. These measures are designed to enlighten parents about the significance of their engagement in their children's educational experiences, assist them in juggling professional and parental responsibilities, and equip them with effective stress management techniques.

In recent years, numerous meta-analyses have been conducted to evaluate the success of various programs targeted at parents. These studies have explored the impact of such programs on enhancing the parent-child bond and children's overall wellbeing, as well as their effectiveness in diminishing levels of anxiety and depression among parents (Eira Nunes et al., 2021; Yap et al., 2016). A recent meta-analysis investigated the efficacy of 23 co-parenting programs (Eira Nunes et al., 2021). The results support a significant effect of these programs on the quality of co-parenting, parents' wellbeing, and couple relationships. The authors of the study identified four strategies that support co-parenting through the analyzed programs: (a) psychoeducation on co-parenting, the importance of parents' involvement and children's support; (b) skills training in co-parenting (communication, parenting, coping, and problem-solving); (c) elaboration of a co-parenting plan that aims to organize tasks and responsibilities related to childcare more clearly; and (d) group-guided discussions. These prevention and intervention programs for parents can be effective tools that decision-makers can implement to support parents and promote the wellbeing of parents and their children. However, we have noticed that most programs for parents have been implemented and validated in the USA and Western Europe. We also note the need to test more interventions in countries from Southeast Europe.

The stress experienced by parents can have adverse effects on their interactions with their partners and children, thereby influencing family harmony and the well-being of all members, both at home and in school settings. Interventions focused on couples, either standalone or combined with parenting programs, have proven to be effective in promoting the wellbeing of children. The Couples Coping Enhancement Training (CCET, Bodenmann & Shantinath, 2004) is one such program designed to assist couples in managing stress more effectively. Research indicates that CCET can enhance communication skills, mutual coping mechanisms, satisfaction in relationships, and decrease conflicts between partners (Bodenmann et al., 2014; Schaer et al., 2008) with these benefits persisting six months post-intervention. Strengthening dyadic coping skills can be an essential part of the intervention for couples in other Southeastern countries facing a significant level of stress. The positive outcomes of CCET, such as improved relationship dynamics and constructive parenting, help mitigate the negative effects of external stress on family interactions (Zemp et al., 2016a, 2016b). Consequently, this leads to better parental behavior and involvement, which supports children's wellbeing, enhancing their experiences both at home and in school.

Acknowledgements This work was supported by a grant of the Ministry of Research, Innovation and Digitization, CNCS – UEFISCDI, project number PN-III-P1-1.1-TE-2021-1203, within PNCDI III.

Competing Interests This study was funded by a grant of the Ministry of Research, Innovation and Digitization, CNCS – UEFISCDI, project number PN-III-P1-1.1-TE-2021-1203, within PNCDI III.

References

Alves, A. F., Gomes, C. M. A., Martins, A., & da Silva Almeida, L. (2017). Cognitive performance and academic achievement: How do family and school converge? *European Journal of Education and Psychology, 10*(2), 49–56.

Amato, P. R. (2001). Children of divorce in the 1990s: An update of the Amato and Keith (1991) meta-analysis. *Journal of Family Psychology, 15*(3), 355.

Amato, P. R., & Keith, B. (1991). Parental divorce and the wellbeing of children: A meta-analysis. *Psychological Bulletin, 110*(1), 26–46. https://doi.org/10.1037/0033-2909.110.1.26

Arrindell, W. A., & Van Der Ende, J. (1984). Replicability and invariance of dimensions of parental rearing behaviour: Further Dutch experiences with the EMBU. *Personality and Individual Differences, 5*(6), 671–682. https://doi.org/10.1016/0191-8869(84)90115-6

Artuch-Garde, R., González-Torres, M. D. C., De La Fuente, J., Vera, M. M., Fernández-Cabezas, M., & López-García, M. (2017). Relationship between resilience and self-regulation: A study of Spanish youth at risk of social exclusion. *Frontiers in Psychology, 8*, 612. https://doi.org/10.3389/fpsyg.2017.00612

Atkinson, S., Bagnall, A.-M., Corcoran, R., South, J., & Curtis, S. (2020). Being well together: Individual subjective and community wellbeing. *Journal of Happiness Studies, 21*(5), 1903–1921. https://doi.org/10.1007/s10902-019-00146-2

Ayhan, A. B., & Beyazit, U. (2021). The associations between loneliness and self-esteem in children and neglectful behaviors of their parents. *Child Indicators Research, 14*(5), 1863–1879. https://doi.org/10.1007/s12187-021-09818-z

Barber, B., & Harmon, E. (2002). Violating the self: Parental psychological control and youth problem behavior. *Intrusive Parenting: How Psychological Control Affects Children and Adolescents*, 53–96.

Belsky, J. (1984). The determinants of parenting: A process model. *Child Development, 55*(1), 83–96. https://doi.org/10.2307/1129836

Berger, L. M., Panico, L., Sheridan, A., and Thévenon, O. (2024). *Parental emotional support and adolescent wellbeing: A cross-national examination of socio-economic and gender gaps based on PISA 2018 surveys*. OECD. https://doi.org/10.1787/2b7a2ac6-en

Biggeri, M., & Cuesta, J. A. (2021). An integrated framework for child poverty and wellbeing measurement: Reconciling theories. *Child Indicators Research, 14*(2), 821–846. https://doi.org/10.1007/s12187-020-09774-0

Bodenmann, G., Hilpert, P., Nussbeck, F. W., & Bradbury, T. N. (2014). Enhancement of couples' communication and dyadic coping by a self-directed approach: A randomized controlled trial. *Journal of Consulting and Clinical Psychology, 82*(4), 580–591. https://doi.org/10.1037/a0036356

Bodenmann, G., & Shantinath, S. D. (2004). The Couples Coping Enhancement Training (CCET): A new approach to prevention of marital distress based upon stress and coping*. *Family Relations, 53*(5), 477–484. https://doi.org/10.1111/j.0197-6664.2004.00056.x

Bowen, S., Brenton, J., & Elliott, S. (2019). *Pressure cooker: Why home cooking won't solve our problems and what we can do about it*. Oxford University Press.

Bowes, L., Maughan, B., Caspi, A., Moffitt, T. E., & Arseneault, L. (2010). Families promote emotional and behavioural resilience to bullying: Evidence of an environmental effect. *Journal of Child Psychology and Psychiatry, 51*(7), 809–817. https://doi.org/10.1111/j.1469-7610.2010.02216.x

Bradshaw, J., Crous, G., Rees, G., & Turner, N. (2017). Comparing children's experiences of schools-based bullying across countries. *Children and Youth Services Review, 80*, 171–180. https://doi.org/10.1016/j.childyouth.2017.06.060

Canavarro, M. C., & Pereira, A. I. (2007). A percepção dos filhos sobre os estilos educativos parentais: A versão portuguesa do EMBU-C. *Revista Iberoamericana de Diagnóstico y Evaluación-e Avaliação Psicológica, 2*(24), 193–210.

Ceballo, R., Ramirez, C., Hearn, K. D., & Maltese, K. L. (2003). Community violence and children's psychological wellbeing: Does parental monitoring matter? *Journal of Clinical Child and Adolescent Psychology, 32*(4), 586–592. https://doi.org/10.1207/S15374424JCCP3204_11

Cho, E.Y.-N., & Yu, F.-Y. (2020). A review of measurement tools for child wellbeing. *Children and Youth Services Review, 119*, Article 105576. https://doi.org/10.1016/j.childyouth.2020.105576

Chung, G., Phillips, J., Jensen, T. M., & Lanier, P. (2020). Parental involvement and adolescents' academic achievement: Latent profiles of mother and father warmth as a moderating influence. *Family Process, 59*(2), 772–788.

Conger, R. D., & Conger, K. J. (2002). Resilience in midwestern families: Selected findings from the first decade of a prospective, longitudinal study. *Journal of Marriage and Family, 64*(2), 361–373. https://doi.org/10.1111/j.1741-3737.2002.00361.x

Conger, R. D., Conger, K. J., & Martin, M. J. (2010). Socioeconomic status, family processes,and individual development. *Journal of Marriage and Family, 72*(3), 685–704. https://doi.org/10.1111/j.1741-3737.2010.00725.x

Conger, R. D., Elder Jr, G. H., Lorenz, F. O., Conger, K. J., Simons, R. L., Whitbeck, L. B., Huck, S., & Melby, J. N. (1990). Linking economic hardship to marital quality and instability. *Journal of Marriage and the Family*, 643–656.

Conger, R. D., Ge, X., Elder, G. H., Lorenz, F. O., & Simons, R. L. (1994). Economic stress, coercive family process, and developmental problems of adolescents. *Child Development, 65*(2), 541. https://doi.org/10.2307/1131401

Conrade, G., & Ho, R. (2001). Differential parenting styles for fathers and mothers: Differential treatment for sons and daughters. *Australian Journal of Psychology, 53*(1), 29–35. https://doi.org/10.1080/00049530108255119

Cooklin, A. R., Westrupp, E. M., Strazdins, L., Giallo, R., Martin, A., & Nicholson, J. M. (2016). Fathers at work: Work-family conflict, work-family enrichment and parenting in an Australian cohort. *Journal of Family Issues, 37*(11), 1611–1635. https://doi.org/10.1177/0192513X14553054

Cooper, M. (2014). *Cut adrift: Families in insecure times*. University of California press.

Costa, S., Soenens, B., Gugliandolo, M. C., Cuzzocrea, F., & Larcan, R. (2015). The mediating role of experiences of need satisfaction in associations between parental psychological control and internalizing problems: A study among Italian college students. *Journal of Child and Family Studies, 24*(4), 1106–1116. https://doi.org/10.1007/s10826-014-9919-2

Côté, S., & Bouffard, T. (2011). Role of parental emotional support in illusion of scholastic incompetence. *European Review of Applied Psychology, 61*(3), 137–145. https://doi.org/10.1016/j.erap.2011.05.003

Craig, L., & Mullan, K. (2011). How mothers and fathers share childcare: A cross-national time-use comparison. *American Sociological Review, 76*, 834–861. https://doi.org/10.1177/0003122411427673

Eccles, J. S. (2004). Schools, academic motivation, and stage-environment fit. In R. M. Lerner & L. Steinberg (Eds.), *Handbook of adolescent psychology* (1st ed., pp. 125–153). Wiley. https://doi.org/10.1002/9780471726746.ch5

Edin, K., & Nelson, T. J. (2013). *Doing the best I can: Fatherhood in the inner city*. University of California Press.

Eira Nunes, C., De Roten, Y., El Ghaziri, N., Favez, N., & Darwiche, J. (2021). Co-parenting programs: A systematic review and meta-analysis. *Family Relations, 70*(3), 759–776. https://doi.org/10.1111/fare.12438

Erel, O., & Burman, B. (1995). Interrelatedness of marital relations and parent-child relations: A meta-analytic review. *Psychological Bulletin, 118*(1), 108.

Finkelstein, D. M., Kubzansky, L. D., Capitman, J., & Goodman, E. (2007). Socioeconomic differences in adolescent stress: The role of psychological resources. *Journal of Adolescent Health, 40*(2), 127–134. https://doi.org/10.1016/j.jadohealth.2006.10.006

Fishman, E. A., & Meyers, S. A. (2000). Marital satisfaction and child adjustment: Direct and mediated pathways. *Contemporary Family Therapy, 22*(4), 437–452. https://doi.org/10.1023/A:1007848901640

Fletcher, R., & Silberberg, S. (2006). Involvement of fathers in primary school activities. *Australian Journal of Education, 50*(1), 29–39. https://doi.org/10.1177/000494410605000103

Francis, A., Pai, M. S., & Badagabettu, S. (2021). Psychological wellbeing and perceived parenting style among adolescents. *Comprehensive Child and Adolescent Nursing, 44*(2), 134–143. https://doi.org/10.1080/24694193.2020.1743796

Galand, B., & Vanlede, M. (2004). Le sentiment d'efficacité personnelle dans la formation: Quel rôle joue-t-il? D'où vient-il? Comment intervenir? *Savoirs, 5*, 91–116.

Gecas, V., & Schwalbe, M. L. (1986). Parental behavior and adolescent self-esteem. *Journal of Marriage and the Family, 48*(1), 37. https://doi.org/10.2307/352226

Graziano, P. A., Keane, S. P., & Calkins, S. D. (2010). Maternal behaviour and children's early emotion regulation skills differentially predict development of children's reactive control and later effortful control. *Infant and Child Development, 19*(4), 333–353. https://doi.org/10.1002/icd.670

Grusec, J. E., Saritaş, D., & Daniel, E. (2014). The nature of effective parenting: Some current perspectives. *Wellbeing: A Complete Reference Guide*, 1–21.

Gul, N., Khan, H., & Niwaz, A. (2021). Parenting styles out comes on psychological wellbeing of children. *Rawal Medical Journal, 46*(3), 652–652.

Győrffy, D. (2022). The middle-income trap in Central and Eastern Europe in the 2010s: Institutions and divergent growth models. *Comparative European Politics, 20*(1), 90–113. https://doi.org/10.1057/s41295-021-00264-3

Harter, S. (1985). Competence as a dimension of self-evaluation: Toward a comprehensive model of self-worth. *The Development of the Self, 2*, 55–121.

Healy, K. L., Sanders, M. R., & Iyer, A. (2015). Parenting practices, children's peer relationships and being bullied at school. *Journal of Child and Family Studies, 24*(1), 127–140. https://doi.org/10.1007/s10826-013-9820-4

Herman, E. (2012). Rural employment in the context of Romanian regional development. *Annals of the Constantin Brancusi University of Targu Jiu, Economy Series, 3*, 131–140.

Hess, S. (2022). Effects of inter-parental conflict on children's social wellbeing and the mediation role of parenting behavior. *Applied Research in Quality of Life, 17*(4), 2059–2085. https://doi.org/10.1007/s11482-021-10022-y

Hess, S., & Pollmann-Schult, M. (2020). Associations between mothers' work-family conflict and children's psychological wellbeing: The mediating role of mothers' parenting behavior. *Journal of Child and Family Studies, 29*(6), 1561–1571. https://doi.org/10.1007/s10826-019-01669-1

Hill, N. E., & Tyson, D. F. (2009). Parental involvement in middle school: A meta-analytic assessment of the strategies that promote achievement. *Developmental Psychology, 45*(3), 740–763. https://doi.org/10.1037/a0015362

Hoferichter, F., Kulakow, S., & Hufenbach, M. C. (2021). Support from parents, peers, and teachers is differently associated with middle school students' wellbeing. *Frontiers in Psychology, 12*. https://doi.org/10.3389/fpsyg.2021.758226

Holopainen, L., Waltzer, K., Hoang, N., & Lappalainen, K. (2020). The relationship between students' self-esteem, schoolwork difficulties and subjective school wellbeing in Finnish upper-secondary education. *International Journal of Educational Research, 104*, Article 101688. https://doi.org/10.1016/j.ijer.2020.101688

Huebner, E. S., & Gilman, R. (2007). Students who like and dislike school. *Applied Research in Quality of Life, 1*(2), 139–150. https://doi.org/10.1007/s11482-006-9001-3

Inguglia, C., Liga, F., Lo Coco, A., Musso, P., & Ingoglia, S. (2018). Satisfaction and frustration of autonomy and relatedness needs: Associations with parenting dimensions and psychological functioning. *Motivation and Emotion, 42*(5), 691–705. https://doi.org/10.1007/s11031-018-9702-6

Jaycox, L. H., & Repetti, R. L. (1993). Conflict in families and the psychological adjustment of preadolescent children. *Journal of Family Psychology, 7*(3), 344–355. https://doi.org/10.1037/0893-3200.7.3.344

Jebb, A. T., Morrison, M., Tay, L., & Diener, E. (2020). Subjective wellbeing around the world: Trends and predictors across the life span. *Psychological Science, 31*(3), 293–305. https://doi.org/10.1177/0956797619898826

Johnson, M. D., Galambos, N. L., & Krahn, H. J. (2021). Family context, life transitions, and subjective wellbeing from age 18 to 50 years. *Developmental Psychology, 57*(11), 1968–1980. https://doi.org/10.1037/dev0001243

Kelty, N. E., & Wakabayashi, T. (2020). Family engagement in schools: Parent, educator, and community perspectives. *SAGE Open, 10*(4), 2158244020973024. https://doi.org/10.1177/2158244020973024

Khaleque, A. (2013). Perceived parental warmth, and children's psychological adjustment, and personality dispositions: A meta-analysis. *Journal of Child and Family Studies, 22*(2), 297–306. https://doi.org/10.1007/s10826-012-9579-z

Kiuru, N., Wang, M.-T., Salmela-Aro, K., Kannas, L., Ahonen, T., & Hirvonen, R. (2020). Associations between adolescents' interpersonal relationships, school wellbeing, and academic achievement during educational transitions. *Journal of Youth and Adolescence, 49*(5), 1057–1072. https://doi.org/10.1007/s10964-019-01184-y

Knuver, A. W. M., & Brandsma, H. P. (1993). Cognitive and affective outcomes in school effectiveness research. *School Effectiveness and School Improvement, 4*(3), 189–204. https://doi.org/10.1080/0924345930040302

Konu, A. (2002). Factor structure of the school wellbeing model. *Health Education Research, 17*(6), 732–742. https://doi.org/10.1093/her/17.6.732

Koşkulu-Sancar, S., van de Weijer-Bergsma, E., Mulder, H., & Blom, E. (2023). Examining the role of parents and teachers in executive function development in early and middle childhood: A systematic review. *Developmental Review, 67*, Article 101063. https://doi.org/10.1016/j.dr.2022.101063

Krauss, S., Orth, U., & Robins, R. W. (2020). Family environment and self-esteem development: A longitudinal study from age 10 to 16. *Journal of Personality and Social Psychology, 119*(2), 457–478. https://doi.org/10.1037/pspp0000263

Ladd, G. W., & Ladd, B. K. (1998). Parenting behaviors and parent–child relationships: Correlates of peer victimization in kindergarten? *Developmental Psychology, 34*(6), 1450–1458. https://doi.org/10.1037/0012-1649.34.6.1450

Landry, S. H., Smith, K. E., & Swank, P. R. (2006). Responsive parenting: Establishing early foundations for social, communication, and independent problem-solving skills. *Developmental Psychology, 42*(4), 627–642. https://doi.org/10.1037/0012-1649.42.4.627

Lannert, J., & Szekszárdi, J. (2015). Miért nem érti egymást szülő és pedagógus? *Iskolakultúra, 25*(1), 15–34. https://doi.org/10.17543/ISKKULT.2015.1.15

Lan, X., Ma, C., & Radin, R. (2019). Parental autonomy support and psychological wellbeing in Tibetan and Han emerging adults: A serial multiple mediation model. *Frontiers in Psychology, 10*, 621. https://doi.org/10.3389/fpsyg.2019.00621

Lee, B. J., & Yoo, M. S. (2015). Family, school, and community correlates of children's subjective wellbeing: An international comparative study. *Child Indicators Research, 8*(1), 151–175. https://doi.org/10.1007/s12187-014-9285-z

Lee, H., Kim, Y., & Terry, J. (2020). Adverse childhood experiences (ACEs) on mental disorders in young adulthood: Latent classes and community violence exposure. *Preventive Medicine, 134*, Article 106039. https://doi.org/10.1016/j.ypmed.2020.106039

Leto, I. V., Petrenko, E. N., & Slobodskaya, H. R. (2019). Life satisfaction in Russian primary schoolchildren: Links with personality and family environment. *Journal of Happiness Studies, 20*(6), 1893–1912. https://doi.org/10.1007/s10902-018-0036-6

Lewin, D., & Herron, H. (2007). Signs, symptoms and risk factors: Health visitors' perspectives of child neglect. *Child Abuse Review, 16*(2), 93–107. https://doi.org/10.1002/car.949

Martin, A. J. (2013). Academic buoyancy and academic resilience: Exploring 'everyday' and 'classic' resilience in the face of academic adversity. *School Psychology International, 34*(5), 488–500. https://doi.org/10.1177/0143034312472759

Masarik, A. S., & Conger, R. D. (2017). Stress and child development: A review of the Family Stress Model. *Current Opinion in Psychology, 13*, 85–90. https://doi.org/10.1016/j.copsyc.2016.05.008

McDowell, D. J., Parke, R. D., & Wang, S. J. (2003). Differences between mothers' and fathers' advice-giving style and content: Relations with social competence and psychological functioning in middle childhood. *Merrill-Palmer Quarterly, 49*(1), 55–76.

McKinney, C., & Renk, K. (2008). Differential parenting between mothers and fathers: Implications for late adolescents. *Journal of Family Issues, 29*(6), 806–827. https://doi.org/10.1177/0192513X07311222

Miserandino, M. (1996). Children who do well in school: Individual differences in perceived competence and autonomy in above-average children. *Journal of Educational Psychology, 88*(2), 203.

Nomaguchi, K. M. (2009). Change in work-family conflict among employed parents between 1977 and 1997. *Journal of Marriage and Family, 71*(1), 15–32. https://doi.org/10.1111/j.1741-3737.2008.00577.x

Nurra, C., & Pansu, P. (2009). The impact of significant others' actual appraisals on children's self-perceptions: What about Cooley's assumption for children? *European Journal of Psychology of Education, 24*, 247–262.

Opdenakker, M.-C., & Van Damme, J. (2000). Effects of schools, teaching staff and classes on achievement and wellbeing in secondary education: Similarities and differences between school outcomes. *School Effectiveness and School Improvement, 11*(2), 165–196. https://doi.org/10.1076/0924-3453(200006)11:2;1-Q;FT165

Papanikolaou, M., Chatzikosma, T., & Kleio, K. (2011). Bullying at school: The role of family. *Procedia - Social and Behavioral Sciences, 29*, 433–442. https://doi.org/10.1016/j.sbspro.2011.11.260

Phillips, D. A., & Zimmerman, M. (1990). The developmental course of perceived competence and incompetence among competent children. In R. J. Sternberg & J. Kolligian, Jr. (Eds.), *Competence considered* (pp. 41–66). Yale University Press.

Pollard, E. L., & Lee, P. D. (2003). Child wellbeing: A systematic review of the literature. *Social Indicators Research, 61*(1), 59–78. https://doi.org/10.1023/A:1021284215801

Pomerantz, E. M., Moorman, E. A., & Litwack, S. D. (2007). The how, whom, and why of parents' involvement in children's academic lives: More is not always better. *Review of Educational Research, 77*(3), 373–410. https://doi.org/10.3102/003465430305567

Popescu, A., Toma Adrian, D., & Stoian, E. (2019). Changes, trends and relationships between average income and consumption expenditures per household in Romania in the period 2007–2017. *Scientific Papers Series Management, Economic Engineering in Agriculture and Rural Development, 19*(2), 363–374.

Prime, H., Andrews, K., Markwell, A., Gonzalez, A., Janus, M., Tricco, A. C., Bennett, T., & Atkinson, L. (2023). Positive parenting and early childhood cognition: A systematic review and meta-analysis of randomized controlled trials. *Clinical Child and Family Psychology Review*, 1–39.

Repetti, R., & Wang, S. (2017). Effects of job stress on family relationships. *Current Opinion in Psychology, 13*, 15–18. https://doi.org/10.1016/j.copsyc.2016.03.010

Rohner, R. P., Khaleque, A., & Cournoyer, D. E. (2005). Parental acceptance-rejection: Theory, methods, cross-cultural evidence, and implications. *Ethos, 33*(3), 299–334. https://doi.org/10.1525/eth.2005.33.3.299

Rusu, P. P., Bodenmann, G., & Kayser, K. (2019). Cognitive emotion regulation and positive dyadic outcomes in married couples. *Journal of Social and Personal Relationships, 36*(1), 359–376. https://doi.org/10.1177/0265407517751664

Rusu, P. P., Hilpert, P., Turliuc, M. N., & Bodenmann, G. (2016). Dyadic coping in an Eastern European context: Validity and measurement invariance of the Romanian version of dyadic coping inventory. *Measurement and Evaluation in Counseling and Development, 49*(4), 274–285. https://doi.org/10.1177/0748175616664009

Salmela-Aro, K., & Upadyaya, K. (2014). School burnout and engagement in the context of demands–resources model. *British Journal of Educational Psychology, 84*(1), 137–151.

Schaer, M., Bodenmann, G., & Klink, T. (2008). Balancing work and relationship: Couples Coping Enhancement Training (CCET) in the workplace. *Applied Psychology, 57*(s1), 71–89. https://doi.org/10.1111/j.1464-0597.2008.00355.x

Sciarrino, N. A., Hernandez, T. E., & Davidtz, J. (2018). *Understanding child neglect: Biopsychosocial perspectives*. Springer.

Simões, S., Farate, C., & Pocinho, M. (2011). Estilos educativos parentais e comportamentos de vinculação das crianças em idade escolar. *Interações: Sociedade e as Novas Modernidades, 20.*

Simpkins, S. D., Fredricks, J. A., & Eccles, J. S. (2012). Charting the Eccles' expectancy-value model from mothers' beliefs in childhood to youths' activities in adolescence. *Developmental Psychology, 48*(4), 1019–1032. https://doi.org/10.1037/a0027468

Sivaraman, B., Nye, E., & Bowes, L. (2019). School-based anti-bullying interventions for adolescents in low- and middle-income countries: A systematic review. *Aggression and Violent Behavior, 45*, 154–162. https://doi.org/10.1016/j.avb.2018.07.007

Sonmark, K., & Modin, B. (2017). Psychosocial work environment in school and students' somatic health complaints: An analysis of buffering resources. *Scandinavian Journal of Public Health, 45*(1), 64–72. https://doi.org/10.1177/1403494816677116

Spera, C. (2006). Adolescents' perceptions of parental goals, practices, and styles in relation to their motivation and achievement. *The Journal of Early Adolescence, 26*(4), 456–490. https://doi.org/10.1177/0272431606291940

Størksen, I., Røysamb, E., Holmen, T. L., & Tambs, K. (2006). Adolescent adjustment and wellbeing: Effects of parental divorce and distress. *Scandinavian Journal of Psychology, 47*(1), 75–84. https://doi.org/10.1111/j.1467-9450.2006.00494.x

Straus, M. A., & Kantor, G. K. (2005). Definition and measurement of neglectful behavior: Some principles and guidelines. *Child Abuse and Neglect, 29*(1), 19–29. https://doi.org/10.1016/j.chiabu.2004.08.005

Taraban, L., & Shaw, D. S. (2018). Parenting in context: Revisiting Belsky's classic process of parenting model in early childhood. *Developmental Review, 48*, 55–81. https://doi.org/10.1016/j.dr.2018.03.006

Tesliuc, E., Pop, L., Grosh, M., & Yemtsov, R. (2014). *Income support for the poorest: A review of experience in Eastern Europe and Central Asia.* World Bank Publications.

Umberson, D., & Karas Montez, J. (2010). Social relationships and health: A flashpoint for health policy. *Journal of Health and Social Behavior, 51*(1_suppl), S54–S66. https://doi.org/10.1177/0022146510383501

UNESCO, I. (2019). *Behind the numbers: Ending school violence and bullying.* UNESCO Digital Library.

Valcan, D. S., Davis, H., & Pino-Pasternak, D. (2018). Parental behaviours predicting early childhood executive functions: A meta-analysis. *Educational Psychology Review, 30*(3), 607–649. https://doi.org/10.1007/s10648-017-9411-9

Varela, J. J., Sánchez, P. A., González, C., Oriol, X., Valenzuela, P., & Cabrera, T. (2021). Subjective wellbeing, bullying, and school climate among chilean adolescents over time. *School Mental Health, 13*(3), 616–630. https://doi.org/10.1007/s12310-021-09442-w

Veiga, F. H. (2016). Assessing student engagement in school: Development and validation of a four-dimensional scale. *Procedia - Social and Behavioral Sciences, 217*, 813–819. https://doi.org/10.1016/j.sbspro.2016.02.153

Wang, M. T., & Sheikh-Khalil, S. (2014). Does parental involvement matter for student achievement and mental health in high school? *Child Development, 85*(2), 610–625. https://doi.org/10.1111/cdev.12153

Waters, S., Lester, L., & Cross, D. (2014). How does support from peers compare with support from adults as students transition to secondary school? *Journal of Adolescent Health, 54*(5), 543–549. https://doi.org/10.1016/j.jadohealth.2013.10.012

Wilder, S. (2014). Effects of parental involvement on academic achievement: A meta-synthesis. *Educational Review, 66*(3), 377–397. https://doi.org/10.1080/00131911.2013.780009

Xu, Z., & Fang, C. (2021). The relationship between school bullying and subjective wellbeing: The mediating effect of school belonging. *Frontiers in Psychology, 12*, Article 725542. https://doi.org/10.3389/fpsyg.2021.725542

Yang, Q., Tian, L., Huebner, E. S., & Zhu, X. (2019). Relations among academic achievement, self-esteem, and subjective wellbeing in school among elementary school students: A longitudinal mediation model. *School Psychology, 34*(3), 328–340. https://doi.org/10.1037/spq0000292

Yap, M. B. H., Morgan, A. J., Cairns, K., Jorm, A. F., Hetrick, S. E., & Merry, S. (2016). Parents in prevention: A meta-analysis of randomized controlled trials of parenting interventions to prevent internalizing problems in children from birth to age 18. *Clinical Psychology Review, 50*, 138–158. https://doi.org/10.1016/j.cpr.2016.10.003

Zemp, M., Bodenmann, G., Backes, S., Sutter-Stickel, D., & Revenson, T. A. (2016a). The importance of parents' dyadic coping for children. *Family Relations, 65*(2), 275–286. https://doi.org/10.1111/fare.12189

Zemp, M., Milek, A., Cummings, E. M., Cina, A., & Bodenmann, G. (2016b). How couple- and parenting-focused programs affect child behavioral problems: A randomized controlled trial. *Journal of Child and Family Studies, 25*(3), 798–810. https://doi.org/10.1007/s10826-015-0260-1

Zolkoski, S. M., & Bullock, L. M. (2012). Resilience in children and youth: A review. *Children and Youth Services Review, 34*(12), 2295–2303. https://doi.org/10.1016/j.childyouth.2012.08.009

Part II

Chapter 6
Children's Wellbeing in Education in Bulgaria: Policies, Practices, and Prospects

Nadia Koltcheva

> If your plan is for one year plant rice. If your plan is for ten years plant trees. If your plan is for one hundred years educate children.
>
> Confucius

Children are the treasure of each parent and the capital of each society. The way we care for and nurture them, the way they develop both physically and mentally, the way they feel and thrive, defines their wellbeing. Each child's wellbeing defines his/her functioning, development, personality growth, quality of life, and success in life. At a societal level, each individual's wellbeing defines the quality of the human capital that the society has.

The concept of wellbeing has gained increasing attention in the last few years, with many organizations and governments recognizing its importance for promoting healthy and fulfilling lives for individuals and communities. As such, efforts to promote wellbeing are often integrated into various policy areas, such as healthcare, education, and social policy.

Wellbeing is a broad concept that refers to an individual's overall state of health, happiness, and satisfaction with his/her life. It encompasses physical, mental, emotional, and social aspects of an individual's experience and is considered an important aspect of overall health and happiness.

Child wellbeing is defined in many different ways. Different approaches exist. Helseth and Haraldstad (2014) state that: "The literature on child wellbeing is largely concerned with the changing concept of wellbeing and the movement from a child-saving to a child-development approach, or from child welfare to child wellbeing" (Ben-Arieh, 2010, in Helseth & Haraldstad, 2014, p. 747).

N. Koltcheva (✉)
Department of Cognitive Science and Psychology, New Bulgarian University, Sofia, Bulgaria
e-mail: nkoltcheva@nbu.bg

A. A. Colomeischi (ed.), *Wellbeing in Schools of Southeastern Europe*, Human Well-Being Research and Policy Making, https://doi.org/10.1007/978-3-032-10525-7_6

Depending on the perspective (practitioners, researchers, policymakers), the definition may have a different focus and encompass different characteristics and indicators: "The child indicator movement stems from the social indicators movement and is concerned with describing the condition of children, monitoring child outcomes, setting goals, and informing and shaping public policy" (Helseth & Haraldstad, 2014, p. 747).

According to Helseth and Haraldstad (2014), there have been major shifts in child indicators. They define the most significant shifts (Aldgate, 2010; Ben-Arieh, 2010, in Helseth & Haraldstad, 2014) as:

(1) from looking at survival to focusing on child wellbeing,
(2) from focusing primarily on negative outcomes to including positive outcomes,
(3) from focusing on a child's future wellbeing to valuing their current wellbeing, and
(4) from an adult perspective to a child perspective, including children's rights and viewing children as shapers of their own lives who influence their wellbeing by participation.

In a broad sense, wellbeing describes the determinants of a good life for children, the promoters of growth and development, and factors that enhance a child's feelings of happiness and satisfaction with life. Wellbeing can be influenced by a range of factors, including personal relationships, work, community involvement, physical health, and access to resources such as healthcare, education, and financial security. Therefore, it is important, when assessing wellbeing, to aim for a holistic approach and to take into account both the objective circumstances and the person's subjective experiences and perceptions, as well as his/her environment and life situation.

The UNICEF definition of child wellbeing has a broad view of wellbeing and is often used as a reference (UNICEF, 2007):

> The true measure of a nation's standing is how well it attends to its children – their health and safety, their material security, their education and socialization, and their sense of being loved, valued, and included in the families and societies in which they are born.
>
> UNICEF (2007, p. 1)

The UNICEF definition is based on the whole-child approach and adopts an ecological perspective on child wellbeing (UNICEF Innocenti, 2020a). It aligns with Urie Bronfenbrenner's bioecological model of human development (Bronfenbrenner & Morris, 2006). This theoretical perspective presents a systemic view of human development, going beyond the idea that developmental processes occur only within the individual or in his/her immediate environment. Instead, it emphasizes their interrelationship and mutual influence.

> Human development takes place through processes of progressively more complex reciprocal interaction between an active, evolving biopsychological human organism and the persons, objects, and symbols in its immediate external environment. To be effective, the interaction must occur on a fairly regular basis over extended periods of time.
>
> Bronfenbrenner and Morris (2006, p. 797)

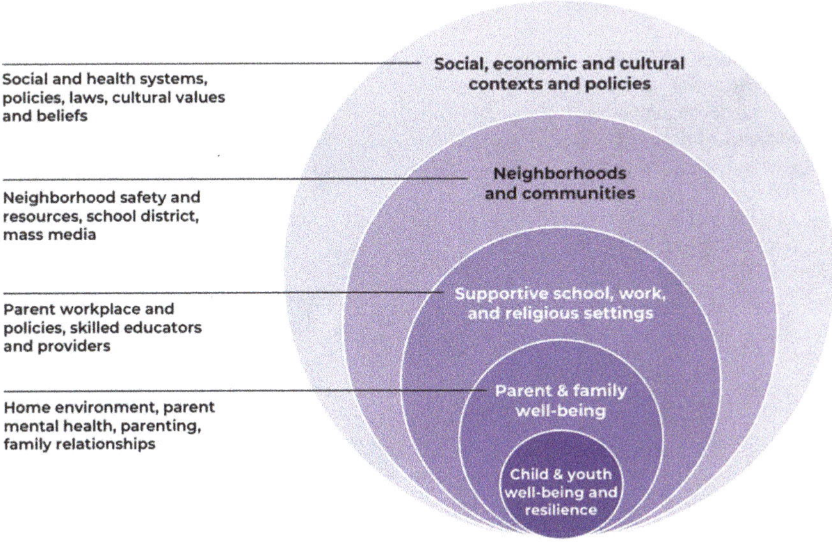

Fig. 6.1 The Center for Child and Family Wellbeing's version of Bronfenbrenner's Bioecological model regarding child and youth wellbeing and resilience. *Source* Center for Child and Family Wellbeing (2023). The Bioecological Model. Retrieved from https://ccfwb.uw.edu/about-us/the-bioecological-model/

According to Bronfenbrenner (1979), the development of the individual always occurs within a context of direct and indirect social influences—starting with the family and extending through various systems to society as a whole. He suggests that an individual's development is influenced by relationships with parents, teachers, peers, partners, and others, as well as by the norms, rules, values, and policies of relevant institutions and organizations within the socio-economic and political context.

Bronfenbrenner (1979) proposed a model of four systems embedded within each other: microsystem, mesosystem, exosystem, and macrosystem, and later added chronosystem to represent the influence of time. This developmental perspective takes into account both biological and environmental factors influencing human development.

The Centre for Child and Family Wellbeing (CCFW), affiliated with the Psychology Department at the University of Washington, translates Bronfenbrenner's bioecological model into a framework for child and youth wellbeing and resilience. The "bioecological" or "whole-child" model is a systemic and holistic framework for human development, and CCFW recognizes it as the core of their approach (Fig. 6.1).

Concerning the concept of wellbeing, UNICEF Innocenti (2020a) also adopts Bronfenbrenner's model and develops a multi-level approach to wellbeing. It sets a broad framework for considering the influence of various factors. The model distinguishes between outcomes that are both objective (e.g., educational achievement) and subjective (e.g., the child's point of view, life satisfaction, feelings). These outcomes

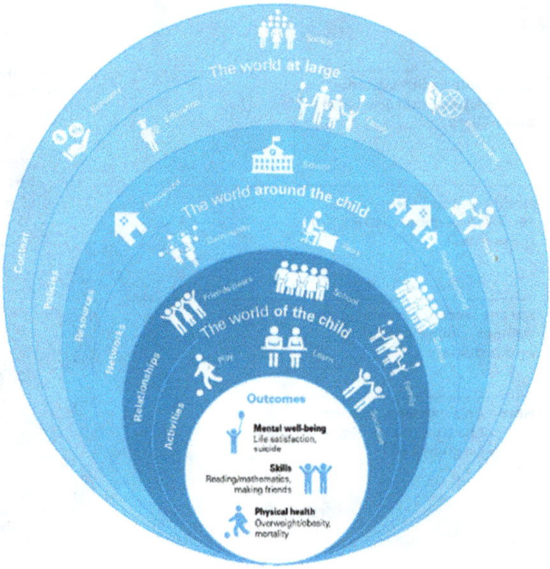

Fig. 6.2 UNICEF's multi-level approach to wellbeing. *Source* UNICEF Innocenti. Worlds of Influence: Understanding What Shapes Child Wellbeing in Rich Countries. Innocenti Report Card 16. UNICEF Office of Research – Innocenti, Florence, 2020a

are organized into three levels: (1) the world of the child, (2) the world around the child, and (3) the world at large (Fig. 6.2).

The world of the child encompasses elements that a child encounters directly, such as his/her activities and relationships (e.g., with parents, teachers, peers). The world around the child comprises resources (e.g., the family's economic status, the quality of the neighbourhood) and networks (e.g., connections among people around the child). The world at large includes policies (e.g., national programs, social policies, education, healthcare) and context (e.g., economic, social, and environmental factors).

UNICEF's approach is multidimensional and includes a wide variety of factors. It provides a strong foundation for cross-country comparisons and for monitoring progress over time. However, similar to previous international reports, less attention is given to children's subjective wellbeing (Bradshaw et al., 2010).

In the current chapter, we focus on children's wellbeing at school. While we mention some indicators that reveal the broader picture, the focus is on the educational system, existing policies, the current state of practices, and the wellbeing of different agents—specifically children, teachers, and parents.

Table 6.1 Children in Bulgaria by age groups

Age group	Total	Males	Females
0	56,526	28,880	27,646
1–4	229,534	117,908	111,626
5–9	304,395	156,208	148,187
10–14	322,964	165,924	157,040
15–19	301,621	155,885	145,736
Total	1,215,040	624,805	590,235

Data National Statistical Institute, Republic of Bulgaria (2023a)

6.1 Republic of Bulgaria

Bulgaria is a Southeast European country and has been a member state of the European Union (EU) since 2007. It is the sixteenth-largest country in Europe and is located on the Balkan Peninsula. Bulgaria is classified as an upper-middle-income country.

According to the National Statistical Institute, the population of Bulgaria in 2022 was 6,447,710 people (National Statistical Institute, 2023a). Data from the 2021 national census show that 84.57% of the population are Bulgarians, 8.40% are Bulgarian Turks, 4.41% are Romani, 1.31% identify with another ethnicity, and 1.31% did not declare their ethnicity. Therefore, the majority groups of children in the Bulgarian educational system are Bulgarians, Bulgarian Turks, and those of Roma origin (National Statistical Institute, 2023b). As of 2022, the total number of children in Bulgaria aged 0–19 was 1,215,040 (624,805 males and 590,235 females), which represents 18.84% of the total population (see Table 6.1).

The wellbeing of children in Bulgaria is a topic of increasing concern, with a range of social, economic, and environmental factors affecting their health and development. In recent decades, Bulgaria has made significant progress in improving children's lives—one notable aspect being the adaptation of its legal framework to the Convention on the Rights of the Child. Despite efforts to improve living standards and support systems, many children in Bulgaria still face challenges in areas such as education, nutrition, and access to healthcare.

6.2 Bulgarian Educational System

The management of the educational system in Bulgaria is organized into four levels: national, regional, municipal, and school. The system is centralized and operates under the supervision and guidance of the Ministry of Education and Science. This Ministry serves as the central public authority responsible for overseeing all levels of education, including kindergarten, school, and university.

Regional Departments of Education (RDEs) function as territorial units under the authority of the Ministry and manage and supervise the education system at the regional level. These departments correspond with the country's territorial and administrative structure.

Each school in Bulgaria functions as a distinct legal entity. Notably, in recent years, school autonomy—both in terms of management and finances—has significantly expanded. This autonomy includes aspects of school governance and specific elements of instructional organization. Schools are required to adhere to State educational standards and a curriculum framework for all subjects, as outlined in Ordinance No. 5 of 03.06.2016 on preschool education and Ordinance No. 5 of 30.11.2015 on general education.

In Bulgaria, there is a distinction in the management and status of education and childcare for children aged 0 to 6 or 7 years. The country operates a so-called "split system" regarding early and preschool education. Children aged 10 months to 3 years may attend nurseries. These nurseries are not included in the formal educational system. Attendance is voluntary and based on parents' needs and decisions, with the main focus placed on young children's care. Nurseries fall under the jurisdiction of the Ministry of Health and are administered by local authorities.

Children aged 3 to 6 or 7 years (who typically start first grade at age 6 or 7) are typically enrolled in kindergartens. Kindergartens are considered educational institutions, and children start attending them at the age of 3. Since 2021, according to amendments to the Preschool and School Education Act (promulgated in the State Gazette, issue 79 (13 October 2015), effective since 01 August 2016, and amended in the State Gazette, issue 11 (02 February 2023), preschool education has been mandatory for children aged 4 years (Ordinance № 5/2016, updated 2022). Until the beginning of the 2023–2024 academic year, municipalities are obliged to create the necessary conditions for implementing compulsory preschool education for children from the age of 4. Education and training in kindergartens are organized and provided in accordance with the Preschool Education State Standards (Ordinance № 5/2016, updated 2022). Preschool education is organized into four age groups (Fig. 6.3):

(1) I Group—3- to 4-year-olds,
(2) II Group—4- to 5-year-olds,
(3) III Group—5- to 6-year-olds,
(4) IV Group—6- to 7-year-olds.

Children start school at the age of 7, or at the age of 6 according to the parents' decision and the child's level of physical and mental development. School education is mandatory up to the age of 16. According to the level, school education is divided into primary and secondary, and according to the content of preparation, it is divided into general and vocational education. Within school education, there are several levels (Fig. 6.3):

ISCED	Age	Grade/Class		Level of education		Institution	Education programme		
8	25-28			Tertiary education	3rd cycle	Higher Education Institution	PhD programmes - 3-4 years		
7	24			Tertiary education	2nd cycle	Higher Education Institution	Integrated Bachelor's and Master;s programmes - 5-6 years	Master's programmes 1-2 years	
	23								
6	22			Tertiary education	1st cycle	Higher Education Institution		Bachelor's programmes - 4 years	
	21								
	20								
	19								
5	19			Tertiary education \ not mandatory to access ISCED 6			Professional Bachelor's programmmes - 3 years		
4	19			Post-secondary non-tertiary education (not mandatory to access tertiary education)			Non-tertiary VET education - 1 year		
3	18	XII class		Secondary education	stage two	School	general secondary education - 2 years	combining general and VET education - 2 years	combining general and VET education - 5 years
	17	XI class							
2	16	X class	compulsory		stage one	School	general secondary education - 3 years		
	15	IX class							
	14	VIII class							
2	13	VII class	compulsory	Basic education/Primary education	stage two	School	Basic education / Primary education (single structure)		
	12	VI class							
	11	V class							
1	10	IV grade	compulsory		stage one	School			
	9	III grade							
	8	II grade							
	7	I grade							
02	6	IV group	beginning of compulsory attendance	Preschool education		Kindergarten	Preschool education / Pre-primary education		
	5	III group							
	4	II group							
	3	I group							
01	2					Nursery	Early childhood educational development		
	10 months								

Fig. 6.3 Overview of the Bulgarian educational system

(1) Basic education / Primary education

   a. Elementary school (primary school)—grades 1–4
   b. Lower secondary—grades 5–7

(2) Secondary education

   a. First secondary stage—grades 8–10
   b. Second secondary stage—grades 11–12

Mandatory education in Bulgaria comprises three stages: preschool education (pre-primary education), basic education (primary education), and secondary education. Compulsory education in Bulgaria is free of charge. According to official data from the National Statistical Institute, over 210,000 children attend kindergartens, and around 550,000 children attend schools (National Statistical Institute, 2023c, 2023d) (Table 6.2).

The coverage of children in preschool education for the academic year 2022/2023 is 87.3% (National Statistical Institute, Report, 2022). The coverage of students in primary education (grades 1–4) for the same academic year is 92.7%, and for students in lower and upper secondary education (grades 5–7 and 8–12), it is 91% (Kateliev et al., 2023). Most children in Bulgaria attend kindergartens and schools. The data show a stable trend of attendance in both kindergartens and schools (Table 6.3). Moreover, the percentage of children attending has risen in the academic year 2022/2023.

Table 6.2 Children enrolled in kindergartens and students enrolled in schools in Bulgaria for several consecutive years, from the academic year 2018/2019 until 2022/2023

	Age/Class	2018/2019	2019/2020	2020/2021	2021/2022	2022/2023
Kindergarten	Under 3 years	8485	8614	7550	7612	8438
	3 years	47,375	47,923	45,808	45,496	46,412
	4 years	51,890	50,523	50,731	50,830	50,350
	5 years	55,174	56,914	55,581	56,494	55,941
	6 years	54,939	53,274	55,126	53,733	54,666
	7 years	790	572	704	646	634
	above 7 years	114	47	166	36	40
	Total	218,767	217,867	215,666	214,847	216,481
School	I–IV class	256,618	248,157	237,556	233,369	232,549
	V–VII class	190,033	191,572	194,412	194,914	189,580
	VIII–XII class	134,616	132,775	133,055	128,547	127,797
	Total	581,267	572,504	565,023	556,830	549,926

Source National Statistical Institute, Republic of Bulgaria (2023c, 2023d)

Table 6.3 Group net enrolment rates by levels of education in Bulgaria for several consecutive years from academic year 2018/2019 until 2022/2023

Level of Education	2018/ 2019	2019/ 2020	2020/ 2021	2021/ 2022	2022/ 2023
Preschool educational	78.4	78.7	78.1	79.1	87.3
Primary education (I–IV grade)	88.4	86.2	84.8	83.6	92.7
Lower and upper secondary education (V–VII и VIII–XII grade)	82.5	82.3	84.4	84.6	91.0

Source National Statistical Institute, Republic of Bulgaria (Kateliev et al., 2023)

94.91% of children in kindergartens (205,476 out of 216,481; data from the National Statistical Institute, 2023e) spend the entire day at the institution. Most children in schools, especially those at the elementary level, also spend a significant portion of the day in school or engaged in school-related activities. On the other hand, school is an important part of children's lives. How are kindergartens and schools ensuring children's physical and mental development and wellbeing? How do children feel at kindergarten or school?

6.3 Wellbeing at School—National, Regional, and School Policies

The wellbeing of children at kindergarten or school is an important aspect of their overall functioning and development, with significant impacts on their academic success and future prospects. Several national and state-level policies govern children's education in Bulgaria. These include the development of a comprehensive education system that provides students with access to quality education.

In 2016, a new law regarding the legal framework pertaining to the provision of preschool and school education in Bulgaria was enacted—the Preschool and School Education Act (State Gazette, issue 11 (02 February 2023)). It addresses the structure, functions, organization, management, and financing of the preschool and school education system in the country. This law regulates the State educational standards within the preschool and school education system. These standards are mandatory and define compulsory requirements for achieving educational outcomes within this framework, along with the conditions and processes for their attainment. The Act also outlines the rights and obligations of the different parties within the educational process—children, students, teachers, principals, and other pedagogical professionals, as well as parents.

Based on the general requirements of the Preschool and School Education Act (State Gazette, issue 11 (02 February 2023)), there are numerous supplementary legal documents regulating different aspects of the Bulgarian educational system. State educational standards are set as mandatory requirements for preschool and school education, as well as the conditions and processes for their achievement. Part of the State educational standards in the educational system are: requirements for preschool (Ordinance No. 5 of 03.06.2016) and school (general) education (Ordinance No. 5 of 30.11.2015); on the civic, health, environmental and intercultural education (Ordinance No. 13 of 21.09.2016); on inclusive education (Ordinance, SG issue 86 of 27.10.2017); on the state requirements for acquiring the professional qualification of a teacher (Ordinance, SG, issue 89 of 11.11.2016); on quality management in the institutions (Ordinance No. 16 of 08.12.2016); on organization of activities in school education (Ordinance No. 10 of 01.09.2016); on the physical environment and information and library provision of kindergartens, schools and personal development support centres (Ordinance No. 24 of September 10, 2020); etc.).

Many endeavours have been made in recent years to improve the Bulgarian educational system. However, we need to admit that due to the unstable political situation in the country over the last couple of years, many planned reforms were not executed, promised reforms were not fulfilled, or there were delays in implementing key policies. Experts from the National Children's Network, analysing different areas of children's development and wellbeing in the country, are rather critical regarding education in their report Notebook 2023. What is the Country's Average Success in Child Care? (National Children's Network, 2023). Their statement reads: "Despite the prescribed norms, the procedures from the normative base are followed formally, leaving the possibilities of the schools, the formal compliance of the regulatory requirements, and the lack of tracking the effectiveness of the measures" (National Children's Network, 2023, p. 87). Good school management and the promotion of teacher effectiveness in Bulgarian schools are seriously advocated as commitments of the Ministry of Education and Science within the goals and activities of the Strategic Framework for the Development of Education, Training and Learning in the Republic of Bulgaria (2021–2030). However, the Action Plan for 2024 for the Strategic Framework is delayed and is still in the process of being finalized.

At the regional level, local authorities might offer measures and/or develop programs aimed at addressing the specific needs of children in their communities. These programs often focus on providing additional resources for kindergartens or schools and addressing local issues depending on the specific profile of the population (for example, there are regions with predominantly Roma or Bulgarian Turkish populations). According to a UNICEF Bulgaria report (2018), "Forty-five percent of Roma children do not attend preschool, and 15% of them do not attend school." This situation requires additional measures to be undertaken.

All schools and kindergartens in Bulgaria, including private ones, must follow state regulations and rules. On the other hand, they have the freedom to experiment and implement extra activities for children, as well as to take part in projects that promote and implement good practices.

6.4 Curricula and Frameworks for Promoting Wellbeing

In Bulgaria, a new law for preschool and school education was adopted in 2016—the Preschool and School Education Act (State Gazette, issue 11 (02 February 2023)). This framework introduced substantial changes to the entire school system and initiated substantial transformations within the educational landscape. The goal was a comprehensive overhaul of the educational system, school dynamics, curriculum and syllabus, and teachers' continuous professional development. This transformative process embraces a novel educational paradigm with far-reaching implications, fostering the intellectual, emotional, social, moral, and physical growth of every child.

The main objectives reflecting the policy of preschool and school education in Bulgaria are outlined in Article 5 of the Preschool and School Education Act (State Gazette, issue 11 (02 February 2023)). Twelve key goals are defined. The first emphasizes the holistic development of the child, supporting "intellectual, emotional, social, spiritual, moral and physical development and support to every child and every pupil in accordance with their age, needs, abilities, and interests." Other aims relate to the "acquisition of competencies" for successful personality development and professional career, active civic life in modern communities, applying principles of sustainable development, understanding and applying principles of democracy, rule of law, human rights, and freedoms, active and responsible citizenship, understanding global processes, trends, and interrelationships, understanding and applying the principles, rules, responsibilities, and rights deriving from European Union membership.

Additionally, objectives include the acquisition of knowledge about national, European, and global cultural values and traditions, and the shaping of tolerance and respect towards ethnic, national, cultural, linguistic, and religious identities, as well as the rights of children, pupils, and people with disabilities. These objectives are operationalized through State educational standards for preschool and school education, which define the expected key competencies students should acquire at each educational level. As mentioned earlier (see Wellbeing at school—national, regional, and school policies), there are two separate ordinances regarding State educational standards—for preschool education: Ordinance No. 5 of 03.06.2016 and for school education: Ordinance No. 5 of 30.11.2015.

The preschool curriculum in Bulgaria covers several key educational areas aimed at holistic child development (Bulgarian language and literature, mathematics, surrounding world, fine arts, music, design and technology, physical culture). Teachers in each kindergarten develop their own academic program for the school year (September 15 to May 31), based on these requirements. The program consists of pedagogical situations—mainly in the form of games—organized weekly according to age groups. Teachers select appropriate pedagogical technologies tailored to the children's characteristics and topics. Kindergartens follow the Ministry-approved programs and teaching aids that meet State educational standards.

The subjects in general education are integrated within the following educational and cultural areas: Bulgarian Language and literature, foreign languages, mathematics, informatics and information technology, social sciences, civil education and religion, natural sciences and ecology, home economics and technology, physical education, and sports. School education aims to provide a general educational minimum as per the State educational standards. Basic education equips students with foundational knowledge and skills, encourages independent and critical thinking, creativity, and active participation. In elementary education (grades 1 to 4), a single teacher typically instructs all subjects. In larger schools, specialized teachers handle subjects like foreign languages, art, music, physical education, and sports. From grades 5 to 8, subject-specific teachers with qualifications in their fields deliver instruction.

The curriculum specifies learning content, expected knowledge, skills, attitudes, new concepts, distribution of lessons throughout the year, and interdisciplinary connections. However, curricula primarily focus on knowledge acquisition rather than skills, and almost none explicitly address children's social and emotional skills—a critical element for wellbeing and mental health.

In 2022, the Ministry of Education and Science initiated a comprehensive review of curricula for grades 1 to 10. The updated curricula will be introduced progressively. The official goal is to reduce unnecessary factual content (Georgieva, 2023). However, Prof. Penov, Minister of Education, cautions against rushing fundamental changes and favours gradual reform, focusing first on subjects with serious proposals for change. Educational experts in Bulgaria have voiced strong criticism regarding this approach. Asenka Hristova, educational expert at the Institute for Research in Education, warns:

> This is a risky approach in a reality where more and more countries are making fundamental changes to their educational models and curricula to address the fact that the world is no longer 'rewarding' students for what they know, but for what they can do with what they know. The current dilemma worldwide is that knowledge and skills easiest to form are also those most quickly and easily automated. Therefore, many education systems are rapidly reorienting from teaching knowledge to applying knowledge, stimulating emo-tional intelligence, and developing a wide palette of skills.
>
> On the contrary, fundamental changes must be hastened, lest it becomes hopelessly too late and many young people without the necessary skills will remain on the fringes of society, technological progress will not translate into economic growth, and Bulgaria, instead of catching up, will fall behind in wellbeing. But it must be known well what and how to be done.
>
> Asenka Hristova, educational expert
>
> Institute for Research in Education (Georgieva, 2023)

There is a clear need for fundamental change, driven by a shift to a competency-based philosophy. Simple adjustments to learning materials or topic relocation within the curriculum framework will not significantly improve outcomes for students.

6.5 Wellbeing for Students

The majority of preschool and school-age children attend educational institutions. Moreover, they spend a large part of their day at kindergarten or school. Educational institutions are key places for children to learn and acquire knowledge. If children could learn everything at home, kindergartens and schools would not have been invented and would not play such a vital role in society. These institutions foster socialization and help children acquire critical life skills, where children can be taught to be citizens. In 2001, the National Conference of State Legislators in the United States of America passed a resolution calling for social and emotional learning (SEL) in schools:

> Legislators have an obligation to help our children acquire the skills they need to become productive and contributing members of our society. As part of this responsibility, we must encourage our schools to ensure that children are well-trained in academic subjects and also given the social-emotional skills that build character and lay the foundation of good citizenship. Scholastic achievement must go hand-in-hand with the acquisition of traits such as honesty, cooperation, fairness, respect for others, kindness, trustworthiness, the ability to resolve conflict, and the insight to understand why such character traits are important.
>
> Resolution on Character Education and Social and Emotional Learning from the National Conference of State Legislatures,
>
> August 2001 (CASEL, 2005, p. 1)

Kindergartens and schools are essential places where wellbeing can be promoted via curricular and extracurricular activities. As mentioned above, in Bulgaria there is a specific ordinance dedicated to civic, health, environmental, and intercultural education (Ordinance № 13/21.09.2016, amended on 01.09.2023). These types of education are "interconnected and form an interdisciplinary complex aimed at acquiring social, civil, and intercultural competencies and health-related competencies and maintaining a sustainable environment" (Ordinance № 13/21.09.2016, Article 3(1)). These types of education should take place in both kindergartens and schools as part of the overall learning process. In kindergartens, they should be integrated into the curriculum across educational areas, in additional pedagogical interactions, or as an independent educational direction when innovative or author programs are applied. In schools, such education can be applied in three ways: (1) During regular class hours, including through student self-government; (2) In activities of interest within a full-day school schedule; (3) Within general support activities for personal development, according to the state educational standard for inclusive education.

According to the ordinance, these educational activities should be carried out throughout all types of school training. However, in practice, the options are limited. Class time usually amounts to one academic hour per week, during which teachers and organizational staff perform various activities with students. The time allocated is very limited. The second option, activities of interest, applies only to elementary school children attending school full-time. The third option applies only to children with special educational needs who attend general support activities. There is a mandatory number of academic hours allocated for such topics, but the amount is surprisingly low—varying between 17 academic hours per academic year (e.g., grades 2 and 3) up to 29h (e.g., grade 10) (Ordinance № 13/21.09.2016).

Extracurricular activities can be a good supplement to kindergarten and school curricula. Usually, there are no supplementary extracurricular activities at kindergartens and schools free of charge for the children. There are rules and regulations for extracurricular activities in kindergartens and schools (for example, Sofia-city municipality—kindergartens: Regulation, Decision No. 135; Regulation, Decision No. 136). There is no standard list that every institution applies. Depending on the educational institution's management and the principal's initiative, there are different types of offers for extracurricular activities in each institution. These activities also vary between academic years. Usually, they are provided by external organizations. These types of activities could be sports (football, basketball, swimming, taekwondo, etc.), foreign language (usually English), arts (drawing, folk dances, Latino dances, etc.), and others. These activities could contribute to children's physical health and skills development. Unfortunately, parents have to choose the type of activity(s) for children to attend and also pay extra fees. Children whose parents cannot afford the fees do not attend. On the other hand, it is important to mention that among the extracurricular activities offered, there are rarely activities targeting the development of children's personality, social, and/or emotional skills. Extracurricular activities could be very good options for group activities that stimulate children's curiosity and interests, and develop skills and qualities such as cooperation, empathy, and tolerance. They could provide shared experiences and interests and build strong friendships. Peer social support is a strong buffer in children's functioning.

On the other hand, "we must mention that a process of promotion and recognition of SES in Bulgaria has started. … However, it is mostly a bottom-up process. On an organizational level, some kindergartens adapt and/or develop and experiment with such practices. Usually, those are initiatives undertaken by any of the following—the kindergarten's pedagogical team, the kindergarten's principal, the kindergarten's psychologist (if such specialist is employed), individual teachers, etc. Such initiative can also be initiated within the framework of projects, in which the kindergarten is a partner" (Koltcheva & Coelho, 2022). There are also many non-governmental organizations applying projects in kindergartens and schools. The aim is to improve children's mental development, functioning, and wellbeing via the implementation of various project activities. Some good examples are projects for the development of language and social and emotional skills for preschool and elementary school children (Trust for Social Achievement, Lachezar Tsotsorkov Foundation), work with Roma minority children (Health and Social Development Foundation (HESED)), child abuse prevention and treatment (Animus Association), etc., or initiatives by university researchers ("Play with Fory") (Koltcheva et al., 2022). "Together in Class," a non-governmental organization, also implements projects in schools for improving children's learning and skills—Learning Together 2021: Overcoming the educational challenges caused by the pandemic, Learning Together 2023: Enhancing self-regulated learning and social-emotional skills (Together in Class, 2021, 2023). The team of prepodavame.bg promotes numerous resources and good practices for teachers, principals, and educational experts in Bulgaria. They also promote a new trend in teaching children social and emotional skills via topics in regular subjects at school (Prepodavame.bg, 2023). In addition, private business organizations offer various activities and programs for children's development (for example, design thinking—Educational Program "Design Champions;" emotional skills—"Mission: Captains of Emotions;" STEAM and social and emotional skills—Lego Education).

Many initiatives and activities are ongoing. However, as N. Koltcheva (2022) wrote, "Their biggest shortcomings, however, are that usually all these offers are very general; rarely is it clear what exactly are the skills that children will develop; if it is a program, there is no clarity about its content; usually there is no information on how the skills will be developed; what is the approach/techniques/methods that will be applied; what is the qualification of the people who will work with the children; no proof of effectiveness, standards of implementation, etc. They follow different approaches, and this is understandable, but rarely is it clear which one is used." The initiatives depend on project availability, the initiatives of teachers, principals, and external finance sources. This makes such initiatives not sustainable, and also, they lack clear capacity and effectiveness.

In Bulgaria, there is a state document according to which children's skills for ensuring their wellbeing must be developed. A state document provides a general framework and guidance. However, there is no assurance on how these guidelines and regulations are applied in each school. Are they at the level of children's skills development and personal development, or are they just additional information children need to be introduced to? It is a matter of school policies and decisions as well as the availability of resources and possibilities. This is a potential threat of inequality between children rather than an option for their personality development and thriving. There are obligatory allocated academic hours, but their number is very low. Skills development needs time and consistency.

We must also mention that there are more than 20 national programs for the development of education in kindergartens and schools. They were approved by the Council of Ministers in 2022 (National programs, 2022). According to the report on the national education development programs for 2022 (published on 04/20/2023 by the Ministry of Education and Science), 201,960,616 levs were spent on these programs. It is a brief document but reports the benefits achieved from all of the programs applied. Conditions are provided for the implementation of innovative pedagogical practices and innovative practices for carrying out activities with children and families in and outside the kindergarten and for promoting children's physical activity within the National program "It's good in kindergarten." Many kindergartens and schools in the country benefited from technical equipment (e.g., laptops, interactive boards, media projectors), software, internet connectivity, etc., to improve the quality of education (National program "Information and communication technologies (ICT) in the system of preschool and school education"). Unfortunately, there is a lack of information as to what extent these investments met the needs of each kindergarten and school. It remains unclear whether the availability of these equipment has improved educational quality or children's outcomes.

The National program "Together for Every Child" has a module for supporting teams for implementation for children who dropped out or are at risk of dropping out of the education system, but also modules for involving parents in kindergarten and school life. The National program "Supporting Municipalities for Educational Desegregation" focuses on assistance in ensuring conditions for equal access to quality education, providing transportation for children, and providing support via appointed educational mediators. There is a National program "Support for Personal Development of Children and Students," but it focuses only on children with special educational needs and does not target the wellbeing and development of all children. The national programs "IT Skills and Career Training" and "Together in Arts and Sports" target, respectively, the development of digital competencies and children's personal development via arts and sports.

Another good practice towards promoting children's wellbeing in kindergartens and schools is the conjoined initiative between the Ministry of Agriculture, the Ministry of Education and Science, and the Ministry of Health: The National Strategy for the Implementation of a Scheme for Offering Fruits, Vegetables, Milk and Dairy Products in Kindergartens, Schools, and Centres for Special Educational Support in The Republic of Bulgaria from 2023/2024 to the End of 2028/2029 Academic Year (Approved: 30.03.2023). Based on the strategy, a regulation on the terms and conditions for the implementation of fruit and vegetable and milk and dairy products schemes in educational institutions was written. They concern two schemes—"School Fruit" and "School Milk" (adopted by PMS No. 251 of 27.09.2016, promulgated State Gazette No. 77, (04 October 2016), changed with Decision No. 8272 of the Supreme Court of the Republic of Bulgaria—No. 59 (16 July 2021), in force from 16 July 2021). These measures aim at providing healthy nutrition to children. For elementary school children (1st–4th grades), free breakfast is provided as well. They are supported via the National Program for the Development of School Education and Preschool Education and Training. The food distributed at schools is intended also as an additional incentive for children at risk of dropping out. It is also a social measure, especially in regions with predominantly Roma populations and families with low socio-economic status.

A very weak point here is the reporting of the effectiveness of all programs and interventions in preschool and school education. Usually, the reports are based mostly on the calculation of the number of beneficiaries covered and the number of activities undertaken, and this approach does not allow critical analyses of their effectiveness, finding good solutions, and making improvements (National Children's Network, 2023).

6.6 Parents' Involvement in School Life

Parents play a crucial role in children's development. Strong parent–child relationships are fundamental to children's development and wellbeing. Parents' involvement in school life is an important aspect of children's wellbeing, but it can also be a significant challenge. According to Article 208 (1) of the Preschool and School Education Act, "The cooperation and interaction between parents and kindergartens or schools shall take place through individual consultations, parents' meetings, training, as well as every time when a specific situation or the behaviour of the child or pupils warrants it" (State Gazette, issue 11 (02 February 2023), p. 68).

More important issues include how this cooperation and interaction take place, how effective they are, what their quality is, whether they manage to ensure children's wellbeing, etc. In the same law, formal ways of including parents in school life can be found. These are the public oversight boards and the boards of trustees. The main activities and tasks of the kindergarten or school public council are to (Preschool and School Education Act, Article 269 (1)):

- Approve the strategy for the development of the kindergarten or school and accept the principal's annual report;
- Participate in the work of the kindergarten or school pedagogical council;
- Propose policies and measures to improve the quality of the educational process;
- Give an opinion on the allocation of the kindergarten or school budget;
- Consult on the kindergarten or school curriculum;
- Participate in the committees that evaluate the activities of the kindergarten or school principal;
- Notify the competent authorities when, in carrying out its activity, it finds violations of the normative acts and regulations;
- Participate in the development and adoption of the Code of Ethics of the kindergarten or school community;
- Participate in the attestation of the kindergarten or school principal;
- Participate in the competition for a new kindergarten or school principal;
- etc.

The boards of trustees are independent voluntary associations that assist the activities of the educational institution. They might be established by an initiative of the kindergarten or school principal and spend their income for the benefit of the kindergarten or school. Boards of trustees focus primarily on supporting kindergartens and schools by helping to raise and manage additional financial and material resources efficiently (Preschool and School Education Act, Article 309 (1)). They assist in maintaining the institution's facilities and contribute to organizing essential services like food and transportation, as well as addressing various social issues. Furthermore, they promote programs that tackle children's problems and encourage interest-based activities, recreation, tourism, and sports. The boards also play a key role in organizing and supporting parents' training related to children's upbringing and development, fostering community involvement, and alerting authorities if any irregularities arise within the kindergarten or school.

The Preschool and School Education Act (State Gazette, issue 11, (02 February 2023)) gives greater powers to the Public Council compared to the Board of Trustees. It guarantees its possibility to propose activities and/or policies for improving the educational process and school life in general. The Public Council has not only a controlling but also a purposeful function. The Minister of Education and Science issued a Regulation on the creation, structure, and activity of public councils for kindergartens and schools (State Gazette, issue 75 (27 September 2016, amended 09 May 2023, actualized 01 June 2023)).

According to the report on national education development programs for 2022 (published on 04.20.2023 by the Ministry of Education and Science), the National program "Together Again" has interesting modules targeting cooperation between educational institutions and parents—Module 2: "Good Practices for Interaction with Parents of Children and Students in Compulsory Preschool and School Age" and Module 3: "Get Involved and Change—The Parent, an Active Partner in School Life." Unfortunately, Module 2 targets mainly the parents of children and students who have left the educational system or are at risk of dropping out of kindergarten and school. There is no information regarding the effectiveness of Module 3 due to ongoing activities at the time the report was issued. The expectation was that organized meetings with parents could improve communication between parent-teacher-student to build trust, respect, and tolerance among them and to involve parents in school life.

There are also some good informal practices applied in kindergartens. Some examples are:

- Teacher for one day—invitation of parents to teach children at the kindergarten;
- Morning fairy tale—invitation of parents to read fairy tales to children at the kindergarten;
- Workshops with parents before national or traditional holidays—parents might be invited to the kindergarten to take part in workshops where, together with the children, they make different objects and decorations for holidays such as Christmas, Easter, Baba Marta, etc., or workshops dedicated to key topics (healthy food, safety on the road, etc.);

- Mothers' Day—mothers are invited to participate in workshops with the children at the kindergarten;
- Fathers' Day—fathers are invited to participate in workshops with the children at the kindergarten;
- Professions—invitation of parents to the kindergarten to present their profession to the children;
- Others.

Regular invitations of parents to schools might be rarer than in kindergartens. Such examples of events can be specific celebrations or organized holiday bazaars at the school (for Christmas, for fundraising campaigns, etc.). All informal activities depend on initiatives ongoing at the kindergarten or school, as well as on the initiatives of principals and teachers.

Many activities are ongoing both formally and informally. However, most of them are locally dependent. On the one hand, this is understandable and connected with the kindergarten or school autonomy and ethos. On the other hand, there is no information regarding the quality of the promoted and implemented activities and their effectiveness. There is limited evidence regarding the effectiveness of such initiatives in improving parent-school relationships, how satisfied the parents are, or to what degree their involvement in school life has improved. That is why we strongly recommend that all measures, initiatives, and actions undertaken be systematically assessed, monitored, and followed up. There might be very efficient measures and initiatives implemented, but when no appropriate information is collected, no inferences regarding their effectiveness and added value can be made. Educational professionals can analyse and improve their practices only if they can assess the actions undertaken. Otherwise, improvement may rely on a prolonged process of trial and error. Such an approach may not justify the resources invested.

6.7 Wellbeing of Teachers

The wellbeing at the workplace is linked to personal wellbeing and quality of life, as well as the quality of work performance. There is no doubt that teachers' work performance is closely tied to teacher-student relationships and the children's wellbeing.

In Bulgaria, for the academic year 2022/2023, 75,219 pedagogical staff were employed—19,747 in kindergartens and 55,472 in schools (Kateliev et al., 2023). Unfortunately, the age distribution of teachers in Bulgaria highlights a pressing need for generational renewal. Most of the teachers are 45–50 years of age and up (Table 6.4).

The Ministry of Education and Science has made many efforts in the last few years to make the profession more appealing to young specialists. Besides, there has been a significant improvement in pedagogical staff payment. Due to this increase in teachers' salaries in recent years, the minimum (starting) salary for teachers in

Table 6.4 Pedagogical Staff in Preschool and School Education in Bulgaria by age

Age group	Preschool education	School education	Total
Under 25	556	1,042	1,598
Up 25 to 29	1,256	2,702	3,958
Up 30 to 34	2,057	4,182	6,239
Up 35 to 39	2,497	4,882	7,379
Up 40 to 44	2,982	6,133	9,115
Up 45 to 49	2,957	8,978	11,935
Up 50 to 54	2,455	9,895	12,350
Up 55 to 59	2,650	9,876	12,526
60 and over	2,337	7,782	10,119
Total	19,747	55,472	75,219

Source National Statistical Institute, Republic of Bulgaria (2023f, 2023g)

2022 is higher than the district average salary in 23 out of 28 districts in the country (Ivanov, 2023). This rapid increase in salaries has significantly raised the number of students in pedagogy disciplines at universities. P. Ivanov (2023) calculated that over the past six years, this increase is 42%. Besides many of the enrolled students, many professionals from other fields have also been drawn to teaching. Probably, such measures may help address the issues with the shortage of teachers and the large number of teachers in the country who will retire in the next few years. However, these are not guaranteed to be effective solutions, nor do they ensure a supply of well-prepared, motivated, and qualified teachers who can provide high-quality education for children.

The National program "Motivated Teachers and Qualification" includes modules such as "Training of Newcoming Specialists to the School Education System for Acquiring the Professional Qualification 'Teacher' and Preparation for Their Inclusion in the Educational Process in Schools with a Shortage of Specialists" and "Upgrading Training of Specialists with Higher Education and Qualification 'Teacher' without Previous Professional Experience as Teachers for Their Inclusion in the Educational Process in Schools Working with Predominantly Children from Vulnerable Groups."

In Bulgaria, as in educational systems in many other countries, most teachers are women—85.4% (Table 6.5). Almost all teachers at schools have bachelor's or master's educational qualification degrees (95.5%, 52,949). A higher education degree (Master, Bachelor, or Specialist) is a requirement for a teaching position. Ordinance No. 15 of 22.07.2019 (State Gazette, issue 61 (02 August 2019)), amended and supplemented State Gazette, issue 52 (05 July 2022), besides the requirements for education, defines the functions of the different types of pedagogical staff at kindergartens and schools. Their functions are related to education, upbringing, socialization, and support for the personal development of children at kindergartens and schools. Teachers, whether in kindergartens or schools, have many responsibilities

Table 6.5 Pedagogical Staff in School Education in Bulgaria by level and gender

Educational level	Total
Total	55,472
Primary (I–IV grade)	22,709
Lower secondary (V–VII grade)	19,829
Upper secondary (VIII–XII grade)	12,934
Male	8,077
Primary (I–IV grade)	1,373
Lower secondary (V–VII grade)	4,033
Upper secondary (VIII–XII grade)	2,671
Female	47,395
Primary (I–IV grade)	21,336
Lower secondary (V–VII grade)	15,796
Upper secondary (VIII–XII grade)	10,263

Source National Statistical Institute, Republic of Bulgaria (2023h)

such as planning, organizing, and conducting the educational process; monitoring the progress of children; cooperating and participating in supporting children's personal development; controlling and encouraging children's participation in the educational process; responsibility for children's life and health; participation in the selection of appropriate textbooks and teaching aids, taking into account the specifics of the group or class, etc. It is essential that teachers receive adequate support in order to manage all the required functions.

The educational degree is mandatory, but continuous professional development is needed afterward. It is an ongoing process of improving teachers' knowledge and skills, introducing them to new methods and teaching aids, and acquiring competencies for more effective work performance. Such qualifications can be obtained in higher educational institutions or training organizations, which have training programs licensed by the Ministry of Education and Science and are registered in the information register. The type of qualification might be introductory (support for newly appointed teachers) or continuous (for all pedagogical staff). We must also mention that all pedagogical specialists are obliged to improve their qualifications according to Article 47 in Ordinance No. 15 of 22.07.2019 (State Gazette, issue 61 (02 August 2019), amended and supplemented State Gazette, issue 52 (05 July 2022)).

Besides the regulated qualification options, additional opportunities are offered by approved national programs. The National program "Motivated Teachers and Qualification" includes a module titled "Continuing Qualification for Teachers, Principals and Other Pedagogical Professionals, Research, Forums and Conferences." According to the Ministry's report (Report of the National Education Development Programs for 2022), trainings were conducted on topics such as preparation for the development of tests; practical skills for overcoming aggression and violence in schools; models of communication with parents; leadership skills; motivation;

teamwork; and managing professional stress in educational institution management. The National program "Prevention and Rehabilitation of Pedagogical Specialists" has initiatives focused on protecting and improving pedagogical specialists' health status and providing conditions for rehabilitation.

The qualification options are clearly defined in legal documents. However, there is a lack of information regarding the effectiveness and quality of the training that teachers participate in. On the other hand, are free to choose the training topics themselves. Are the chosen topics the most appropriate ones? Are the conditions at the kindergarten or school suitable for implementing the acquired knowledge and skills? Will there be support from kindergarten or school management for this implementation? Sometimes teachers may choose popular topics without considering how to apply them in their practice.

Experts from the National Children's Network (2023) express some skepticism regarding the existing qualification options and the extent to which they guarantee the quality of education provided. According to them, "At the national level, there are still no policies and mechanisms for mentoring new teachers, who in most cases enter the profession with ideas very different from the school reality. The situation analysis prepared by World Bank experts as part of the Roadmap states that in 2019, 2,573 teachers with up to 5 years of experience left their jobs. For comparison, the number of teachers with 6 to 10 years of experience who left is significantly smaller—698 (p.107)" (National Children's Network, 2023, p. 88). This highlights the urgent need for a system of support, mentoring, and extra training for newly appointed teachers.

P. Ivanov (2023) cites data from a World Bank report showing that of the newly appointed teachers in 2016, only 10% remained teaching in schools after their third year on the job. He stresses the necessity of capacity building for support and training of newly appointed teachers during their first years. This is absolutely essential. Various mechanisms can help achieve this: school mentors could be trained to provide support to novice teachers; Regional Departments of Education could offer more support and methodological assistance; and school management could provide support for newcomers as well as all teachers. Social support is a powerful buffer that improves teachers' subjective wellbeing at the workplace, their motivation, work performance, and satisfaction.

Promoting the effectiveness of teachers in Bulgarian schools is a commitment of the Ministry of Education and Science, as reflected in the goals and activities of the Strategic Framework for the Development of Education, Training, and Learning in the Republic of Bulgaria (2021–2030).

6.8 School Ethos and School Environment

School ethos refers to the shared values, norms, and culture that shape relationships and daily practices within the school. The school environment sets the overall framework for the functioning of the entire school system. On one hand, it is formally defined by numerous laws, legal regulations, and standards. On the other hand, the school climate extends far beyond formal rules. It includes informal norms, management policies, leadership styles, the interplay of individual personalities, people's attitudes and beliefs, and human relationships. These features strongly influence the wellbeing of all involved—school management, teachers, students, and parents.

According to Shriver and Weissberg (1996), the principles of social and emotional learning can serve as an organizing framework for coordinating all school activities related to students' learning, prevention, health, and development. A learning environment that is safe, caring, well-managed, and participatory is one of the main prerequisites for ensuring students' better academic performance and success in life (CASEL, 2005). By establishing such an environment, principals and teachers can improve academic outcomes and help reduce students' engagement in risky behaviours.

Teaching children a range of social and emotional competencies may lead to decreases in risky behaviours, support positive student development, strengthen attachment to school, and promote academic success. The school environment plays a vital role in promoting child wellbeing, focusing not only on the physical and emotional safety of students but also on fostering a supportive and inclusive school culture.

One of the national programs addressing this area is the National Program "Providing a Modern, Safe, and Accessible Educational Environment." However, according to the 2022 report of the National Education Development Programs (published 20 April 2023, by the Ministry of Education and Science), the program's actions are primarily focused on ensuring accessible architecture for people with special educational needs in public schools, maintaining effective access controls to school buildings, improving security through technical means, and enhancing incident control.

Although physical safety is essential, it represents only one aspect of the overall school environment. There is hope that at the local level, there is a clearer understanding of the importance of the school environment for students' mental and physical health, achievements, functioning, and overall wellbeing. The importance of strong school leadership is also emphasized as part of the Strategic Framework for the Development of Education, Training, and Learning in the Republic of Bulgaria (2021–2030).

6.9 Research Results and Good Practices (Studies on the Wellbeing of Students and Teachers)

Wellbeing has increasingly become a key focus in recent decades, recognized as vital to human functioning across all ages, for both children and adults. Numerous international organizations, including UNICEF, OECD, WHO, and Gallup, have conducted surveys and published reports highlighting this issue.

In 2020, the UNICEF Innocenti Research Office released a global report on children's wellbeing covering 41 countries (UNICEF Innocenti, 2020a). The report emphasized that good mental wellbeing, mental health, and a positive attitude are critical components of a high quality of life. Despite this, many children in wealthy countries struggle with mental wellbeing. In 12 of the 41 countries surveyed, fewer than 75% of 15-year-olds reported high life satisfaction. Suicide ranks among the leading causes of death for 15- to 19-year-olds. Other health indicators are concerning: one in 15 babies in rich countries is born underweight, poses survival risks, and in 10 countries, one-third of children are overweight or obese. Alarmingly, many children under 15 lack basic academic and social skills, with two out of five children not acquiring essential reading and math competencies by age 15. Social and emotional skills development and interpersonal relationships are critical, yet many 15-year-olds feel insecure about their ability to make friends, which experts regard as a significant challenge, even in affluent nations.

A crucial part of human wellbeing, both generally and especially for young children and students, depends significantly on relationships with others. Significant others in children's lives include their parents (both mothers and fathers) and their teachers. According to the report (UNICEF Innocenti, 2020a), Bulgaria is in the middle when it comes to ranking in terms of children's mental wellbeing—18 out of 38. Mental wellbeing encompasses the broader sense of positive functioning (various components including emotions such as feeling happy, satisfaction with life, and a sense of flourishing). Research also confirms that adolescents' subjective wellbeing is associated with higher levels of warm and loving relationships with their parents. A 2020 study among Bulgarian adolescents aged 14–18 shows that their subjective wellbeing moderately correlates with the perception they have of their relationships with their parents. The more rejecting they perceive their mothers ($r = -0.551$, $p < 0.001$) and fathers ($r = -0.404$, $p < 0.001$), the lower their level of subjective wellbeing (Koltcheva, 2021). The perceived acceptance and feelings of warmth and affection by both parents positively correlate with the youth's subjective wellbeing (mother—$r = 0.455$, $p < 0.001$; father—$r = 0.384$, $p = 0.013$). According to the Programme for International Student Assessment (PISA), data from 2018, in Bulgaria 73% of the 15-year-olds declare high life satisfaction (UNICEF Innocenti, 2020a). Adolescents' positive attitudes towards life are also related to their perceptions of the relationships with their parents. The more accepted the parents are perceived to be by youth, the more positive the youth's attitude towards life (mother—$r = 0.408$, $p < 0.001$; father—$r = 0.258$, $p = 0.013$) and conversely—when parents are perceived rejected, the youth's positive attitude towards life gets lower (mother—$r = -0.486$, $p < 0.001$; father—$r = -0.320$, $p = 0.002$) (Koltcheva, 2021). Khan et al. (2011) also found a positive correlation between perceived parental acceptance in young people and their life satisfaction. According to Rohner (2021), the perceived relationships with others, especially with parents, are a key factor in the overall mental development and level of psychological adjustment of the individual, especially during childhood and adolescence. This statement has been confirmed in numerous studies in different countries. Putnick and colleagues (Putnick et al., 2014) collected and compared data on 1,247 families from nine different cultures

(China, Colombia, Italy, Jordan, Kenya, the Philippines, Sweden, Thailand, and the United States). They tested a developmental model that included five indicators of children's adjustment (internalizing behaviour, externalizing behaviour, school achievement, prosocial behaviour, and social competence). In this three-year study, they found out that perceived parental rejection (by both the mother and the father) uniquely predicted: (1) increased parent-reported child internalizing and externalizing behaviour problems; (2) poorer child performance in school; (3) decreased children's prosocial behaviour; (4) lower children's social competence. This research provides evidence for the same effects of children's perceived rejection across countries, namely children's perception of paternal and/or maternal acceptance–rejection have approximately the same effects on their adjustment and behaviour. Evidence regarding this provides also Rothenberg and colleagues (Rothenberg et al., 2019, 2020, 2021a, 2021b). They analysed data from 1,315 children and their parents (mothers and fathers) from 12 ethnic groups in nine countries (China, Colombia, Italy, Jordan, Kenya, the Philippines, Sweden, Thailand, and the United States of America) collected annually over five years, from ages 8 to 13. Their results indicate that the effects of parental warmth and control on children's externalizing and internalizing behaviours are consistent across children's development, cultural environment, and both mothers' and fathers' attitudes. They conclude that "parental warmth appears to function as a protective factor similarly across many cultures, preventing the emergence and development of adolescent externalizing and internalizing symptoms, while the effects of behavioural control vary across cultures" (Rothenberg et al., 2020, p. 1). Rothenberg and colleagues (2021b) report in their longitudinal study that all four forms of maternal and paternal perceived rejection (coldness/lack of affection, hostility/aggression, indifference/neglect, and undifferentiated rejection) were independently associated with externalizing and internalizing behaviour problems in children aged 7–14 years. They conclude that the effects of perceived parental acceptance–rejection are similar panculturally. Savova and Koltcheva (2018) conducted a similar study in Bulgaria with 8–11-year-old children and their parents using the same assessment measures as in Rothenberg's and colleagues' and Putnick and colleagues' research studies—Rohner's Parental Acceptance-Rejection/Control Questionnaire, Children (PARQ/C, Child), Mother version and Father version, and Achenbach's Child Behaviour Checklist for Ages 6–18 (CBCL 6–18). The results showed significant correlations between internalizing (mother—$r = 0.427$, $p = 0.002$; father—$r = 0.411$, $p = 0.002$) and externalizing (mother—$r = 0.591$, $p < 0.001$; father—$r = 0.578$, $p < 0.001$) children's behaviour problems and their perceived rejection by both the mother and the father. Parent-child relationships are an important factor regarding children's wellbeing. Parental warmth, affection, and attitude are a powerful buffer for many negative behavioural manifestations in children. Such findings are also of great applied value as the basis for guidelines, training programs, and counselling.

Positive relationships between adolescents and their parents are connected with youths' higher levels of mental wellbeing and low levels of delinquent behaviours (Hair et al., 2008). Numerous findings are derived from the World Health Organization's Health Behaviour among School-Aged Children (HBSC) study. The HBSC study is a large school-based survey on 11-, 13-, and 15-year-old youths. The data are used at national, regional, and international levels to gain insights into adolescent health and wellbeing, understand social determinants of health, and inform policy and practice to improve young people's lives. The HBSC study started in 1983–1984 in a few countries, but it has since grown to include 50 countries and regions across Europe and North America. According to data from 45 countries in Europe and Canada (227,441 students), adolescents' mental wellbeing has declined over time (Inchley et al., 2020). Girls are at greater risk of poor mental wellbeing outcomes than boys. One in four adolescents report feeling nervous, feeling irritable, or having difficulties getting to sleep every week. There was a small increase in multiple health complaints across all age and gender groups between the 2014 and 2018 waves. There are significant differences in mental wellbeing across countries. This proves that cultural, political, and economic factors can play a role in promoting good mental wellbeing. Adolescents from high socio-economic status families report higher levels of life satisfaction and excellent health and lower levels of multiple health complaints. Kotzeva and Dimitrova (2022) tracked Bulgarian youths' wellbeing and health over a 13-year period (2006–2018) using data from three waves (2006, 2014, 2018) of the HBSC study. Their analyses reveal that the family context significantly influences the prevalence of adolescents' risk behaviours. In particular, adolescents living in one-parent families and those from high socio-economic status families in Bulgaria are more likely to report risky behaviours compared to those from low socio-economic status families.

According to the UNICEF Innocenti Report (2020a), Bulgaria ranks near the bottom regarding children's physical health and skills, child wellbeing policies, and context. It ranks 39th place in terms of education policies, 37th in children's health care, and 19th in social policies (UNICEF, 2020a). This report compares ratings of 41 countries. In terms of mental health, in most countries less than four-fifths of children say they are satisfied with their lives. Life satisfaction is lowest in Turkey (53%), followed by Japan, and the United Kingdom. Bulgaria's ranks in the middle, 18th place, regarding mental wellbeing. UNICEF is also concerned about children's insufficient level of social skills. It turns out that rich countries do not always afford a good childhood. Experts explain this phenomenon with poor-quality relationships, lack of resources (poverty), gaps in services, gaps in family policy, etc. Above, we already mentioned the importance of children's relationships with significant others in their lives (parents, teachers, peers, etc.). The authors of the report also conclude, "Children view good relationships as crucial. Those with more supportive families have better mental wellbeing" (UNICEF, 2020a, p. 3).

A nationally representative survey of students' wellbeing was carried out in 2018 in Bulgaria by the Centre for Inclusive Education (CIE) in cooperation with G Consulting research agency and experts from the Bulgarian Academy of Sciences. More than 3,200 seventh-graders from 100 Bulgarian schools across the country completed questionnaires regarding their mental and social wellbeing, satisfaction with school, and how comfortable they feel there. The results show that only 4% of Bulgarian schools succeed in attaining both high grades and high student wellbeing (Centre for Inclusive Education, 2018). Iva Boneva, the CIE Executive Director, states: "It is often the case that by 'good school' we only mean that students there have high grades. However, schools have other tasks too; they should have children prepared for a full life as adults" (Centre for Inclusive Education, 2018). Experts set criteria and define a "good school," as one that cares about both children's academic success and wellbeing. These are schools where teachers are well-meaning and supportive, many extracurricular activities take place, the level of acts of aggression is low, and a school community exists. Only 10% of the surveyed schools meet the criteria. Additionally, 38.4% of Bulgarian seventh-graders exhibit very low to moderate levels of school wellbeing. Most of the 7th-grade students are more satisfied with their life outside school than with that in school (59.4%). According to the survey, the most important factors driving satisfaction are: (1) satisfaction with teachers (40%), (2) satisfaction with the school environment (38%), and (3) satisfaction with classmates (22%). The experts found a pronounced correlation between wellbeing and learning. Wellbeing influences academic success and the latter impacts wellbeing. "Regretfully, this correlation is broken in many of the schools: either wellbeing is sacrificed to high academic performance, or much effort is put in making children feel well but at the expense of educational function," said research manager Zhivko Georgiev (Centre for Inclusive Education, 2018). Given equal other conditions, students with higher levels of wellbeing and satisfaction index have higher academic results, higher attitudes towards learning and continuing education to higher levels, and greater satisfaction with their own success.

The Centre for Inclusive Education study (2018) provides further proof regarding the teachers' role at school and students' wellbeing and satisfaction. Teacher-student relationships are an issue studied by researchers for decades (Rohner, 2021). Numerous studies within Rohner's Interpersonal Acceptance-Rejection Theory (IPARTheory) have proven the importance of these relationships (Koltcheva, 2023). According to IPARTheory postulates, when students perceive rejection by their teachers, they start to act accordingly—have bad behaviours, underachieve in class, and overall act poorly in school. Research regarding teacher-student relationships done in Bulgaria by N. Koltcheva reveals similar results. There is a correlation between the child's subjective perception of acceptance or rejection by the teacher and the occurrence of behavioural manifestations ($r = 0.279$; $p = 0.01$) (Koltcheva, 2023). It is not a surprise a result in another study regarding the negative correlation between students' academic success and behaviour at school ($r = -0.369$; $p = 0.01$) (Koltcheva, 2023). A warm and accepting attitude towards the child certainly supports both the child's learning and his/her personal development and growth.

Teachers' wellbeing also is an important aspect. Results from a survey ordered by the Ministry of Education and Science in 2016 show that most of the teachers do not feel sufficiently supported by society, including students and parents (52%) (Gallup International, 2016). Gallup International collected data twice in 2016 among 716 teachers from different grades, educational institutions, and settlements throughout Bulgaria. The results are similar in both waves. Gallup International is another organization with traditions in surveying the topic of wellbeing. They have undertaken numerous surveys all over the world collecting data on various aspects of wellbeing. One of their newest surveys revealed that poor wellbeing is linked to the formation of new chronic conditions (Witters & Agrawal, 2023). They tracked 3,654 working adults over a three-year period. They found not only that lower wellbeing is linked to numerous health conditions but also estimated huge amounts of new annual healthcare costs that are needed (Witters & Agrawal, 2023).

6.10 Conclusions. Implications for Educational Policies

There is no doubt that wellbeing matters—it matters for both children and adults. The dynamics of today's world, characterized by intense global and local transformations, present many challenges for children. We must equip them with the skills and tools necessary to navigate these rapid and complex changes. Failing to do so jeopardizes the future strength of our society and its strong future.

Over the past decades, substantial evidence has accumulated demonstrating the importance of wellbeing and its benefits—not only within educational institutions but also more broadly. As Fayaz King, Deputy Executive Director for Field Results and Innovation at UNICEF, stated: "Wellbeing for children must be the top priority. … Such reports provide all of us with evidence of what happens to our children and also what happens to our future" (UNICEF Innocenti, 2020b, 8:50).

The UNICEF Innocenti Report (2020a) outlines three key recommendations for improving children's wellbeing: consult, connect, and create. Consulting children emphasizes the value of relationships and empowerment. Connecting policies—through integrated, cross-sectoral approaches—is essential. As King notes, "There is no doubt policy matters for children. And good policies pay off" (UNICEF Innocenti, 2020b, 8:19). Creating strong foundations is the third pillar. However, as Senator Rosemary Moodie (Canada) highlights: "It is not just the policies for children, it is about the policies in the country in general" (UNICEF Innocenti, 2020b, 36:30). Denitsa Sacheva, Bulgaria's former Minister of Labour and Social Policy, emphasized the need to "connect and create," stating, "We need to connect all the different dots and all the different systems, all the different actors in the field of child welfare, and we need to be more creative with the political solutions we provide for the benefit of children" (UNICEF Innocenti, 2020b, 47:30). The Bulgarian Ministry of Education and Science continues to take steps to improve the quality of education and children's wellbeing. A new education quality standard is currently under development (Germanova, 2024). According to the Minister of Education, this new vision will focus not only on developing students' skills and competencies but also on enhancing their wellbeing, strengths, and personalities.

Despite these efforts, Bulgaria still faces several obstacles to delivering quality preschool and school education. These include teacher shortages and training, unequal access to education, curriculum limitations, disparities in educational outcomes, insufficient early childhood programs, the digital divide, and underfunding. Addressing these challenges requires a comprehensive and coordinated approach involving national policy reforms, increased investment, professional development for teachers, and targeted actions to reduce socio-economic inequalities.

Different types of measures could be applied at national, regional, and local levels. At the national level, efforts could focus on curriculum review and reform, teacher development programs, early childhood education initiatives, increased funding, equalization of educational opportunities, and more. Addressing the obstacles to quality education requires a coordinated effort at multiple levels, involving government, communities, and educators working together to create a supportive and enriching learning environment for all students.

A holistic approach, supported by extensive research (Center for Child and Family Wellbeing, 2023; UNICEF Innocenti, 2020a), is essential. The integration of services and policies across levels aligns with Bronfenbrenner's Bioecological Model. Governments must commit to significant, well-coordinated investments. As Fayaz King states: "Investments in children lead to smarter, stronger, and more resilient societies that are better for all of us" (UNICEF Innocenti, 2020b, 9:09).

Policies supporting families, improving children's physical and mental health services, and enhancing the quality of education are urgently needed. Yet, much remains to be done in Bulgaria. The National Children's Network, in its 2023 report, criticizes the lack of a unified framework. "Although the Law on Preschool and School Education provides for the existence of a state educational standard for quality management in institutions, the education system in Bulgaria still lacks a comprehensive vision… The existing normative texts leave ambiguities… mechanisms remain only articles and paragraphs without practical application" (National Children's Network, 2023, p. 87). Improvements at the national level are needed.

Measures that can be applied at the regional or local level could improve children's wellbeing as well. The experts from the Centre for Inclusive Education advocate for "a whole school approach." Such an approach includes the development of a caring and supportive school atmosphere, partnerships with parents and the community, and a curriculum that addresses social and emotional issues. They emphasize measures like targeted teaching of social and emotional learning as a key curriculum competency, building a caring and inclusive classroom community focused on healthy relationships, a whole school environment conducive to mental health and wellbeing for all the parties at school (children, teachers, administration, etc.).

The Centre for Inclusive Education study (2018) derives factors that could propel the improvement of children's wellbeing at school. They put emphasis on factors that influence the relationship with peers, teachers, and parents, and the collaboration with families and communities. Among the multitude of factors, they point out: "fair, well-meaning, demanding, but also giving teachers; the extent to which the class has become a community; low levels of harassment and aggression; satisfaction with the grades as a measure of the academic performance; an environment offering a wide range of opportunities for proving oneself and manifest one's talents; a sense of own contribution to the community and the school, hence significance for the others; the school offers various forms of development, self-fulfilment and togetherness" (extracurricular forms, out-of-school lessons, camps, sports events, excursions, etc.) (Centre for Inclusive Education, 2018).

At the school level, a lot could be done in the field of relationships. Students benefit greatly from good relationships with their teachers, and teachers benefit from these relationships as well (Koltcheva, 2023). Teachers, who feel good about their workplace, have higher job satisfaction, commitment, and a sense of wellbeing. School psychologists could take advantage of these findings and apply them to improving school climate, preventing aggressive or victim behaviour, dropping out of school … improving children and teachers' wellbeing. Cefai and colleagues (2023), authors of the Resilience in Schools Factsheet (2023) also emphasize caring school and classroom community. "Resilience supportive classrooms are characterised by caring teacher-student relationships, supportive and inclusive peers, equal access to necessary resources, active and meaningful engagement, learner voice and choice, personalised learning, culturally responsive pedagogy, and positive beliefs and high expectations, promoting a sense of belonging, competence and control" (Resilience in Schools Factsheet, 2023, p. 2).

Cefai and colleagues (Resilience in Schools Factsheet, 2023) point out protective factors for resilient outcomes. They list factors at different levels starting from individual factors (positive self-concept, emotional regulation, problem-solving skills, sense of purpose), school factors (caring teachers, positive classroom relationships, learning support, high expectations for all learners), family factors (secure attachment, stable family environment, authoritative parenting (warmth and control) and the broader social context (prosocial and caring adults in the community, prosocial peer group, safe neighbourhoods). However, children's wellbeing depends not only on the sum of protective factors but also on the interaction between the individual child's qualities and personality and the contexts in which the child is growing up.

As UNICEF (2007) reminds us: "The true measure of a nation's standing is how well it attends to its children – their health and safety, their material security, their education and socialization, and their sense of being loved, valued, and included in the families and societies into which they are born."

Children have only one childhood. Let them enjoy it. But also, let's allow them to get the most out of their childhood! We must do more—and we must do better—now. Change is needed—and it is needed now—for our children, for ourselves, for our society, for our future.

Competing Interests The author has no conflicts of interest to declare that are relevant to the content of this chapter.

References

Bradshaw, J., Rees, G., Keung, A., & Goswami, H. (2010). The subjective wellbeing of children. In C. McAuley & W. Rose (Eds.), *Child wellbeing: Understanding children's lives*. Jessica Kingston Publishers.

Bronfenbrenner, U. (1979). *The ecology of human development: Experiments by nature and design*. Harvard University Press.

Bronfenbrenner, U., & Morris, P. A. (2006). The ecology of developmental processes. In W. Damon & R. M. Lerner (Eds.), *Handbook of child psychology* (6th ed., Vol. 1, pp. 793–828). Wiley.

Center for Child and Family Wellbeing. (2023). *The bioecological model*. https://ccfwb.uw.edu/about-us/the-bioecological-model/

Centre for Inclusive Education. (2018, September 13). *Only 4% of the Bulgarian schools report both high grades and high student wellbeing*. https://www.ela-bg.eu/en/what-is-good-school

Collaborative for Academic, Social, and Emotional Learning (CASEL). (2005). *Safe and sound: An educational leader's guide to evidence-based social and emotional learning (SEL) programs* (Illinois ed.). Author.

Council of Ministers, Republic of Bulgaria. (2022). *National programs for the development of education (No. 1 to No. 21)* [Decision No. 302 of May 13, 2022]. https://web.mon.bg/bg/101106

Gallup International. (2016, July 8). *Second part of the teacher survey. Culture and education*. https://www.gallup-international.bg/34778/second-part-of-opinion-poll-among-teachers/ (in Bulgarian)

Germanova, T. (2024, January 11). *The Ministry of Education and Science is preparing a new standard for the quality of schools*. Economic.bg. https://www.economic.bg/bg/a/view/mon-podgotvja-nov-standart-za-kachestvo-na-uchilishtata

Georgieva, S. (2023, January 6). *The Ministry of Education and Science did not find the strength to seriously change the curricula*. Newspaper Sega. https://www.segabg.com/hot/category-education/mon-ne-nameri-sili-za-seriozna-promyana-na-uchebnite-programi

Hair, E. C., Moore, K. A., Garrett, S. B., Ling, T., & Cleveland, K. (2008). The continued importance of quality parent-adolescent relationships during late adolescence. *Journal of Research on Adolescence, 18*(1), 187–200. https://doi.org/10.1111/j.1532-7795.2008.00556.x

Helseth, S., & Haraldstad, K. (2014). Child wellbeing. In A. C. Michalos (Ed.), *Encyclopedia of quality of life and wellbeing research* (pp. 746–749). Springer. https://doi.org/10.1007/978-94-007-0753-5

Inchley, J., Currie, D., Budisavljevic, S., Torsheim, T., Jåstad, A., Cosma, A., et al. (Eds.). (2020). *Spotlight on adolescent health and wellbeing. Findings from the 2017/2018 Health Behaviour in School-aged Children (HBSC) survey in Europe and Canada*. International report. Volume 1. Key findings. Copenhagen: WHO Regional Office for Europe; 2020. Licence: CC BY-NC-SA 3.0 IGO, ISBN 9789289055000.

Ivanov, P. (2023, January 6). *How does the quantity of teachers in the country affect the quality of education? Together in Class*. https://zaednovchas.bg/pedagozite-v-stranata-komentar/

Kateliev, S., Tsankova, E., Georgiev, R., & Tsoneva, V. (2023). *Education in the Republic of Bulgaria 2023* [Report]. National Statistical Institute, Demographic and Social Statistics Directorate, Education and Culture Statistics Department. https://www.nsi.bg

Khan, S., Hassan, S., Husain, G., & Gul, I. (2011). Relationship of parental acceptance and rejection with psychological wellness in young adults. *Journal of Rawalpindi Medical College (JRMC), 15*(1), 24–26.

Koltcheva, N. (2021). Relationships with parents and peers and subjective wellbeing in adolescents. *Bulgarian Journal of Psychology, 2*(4), 182–192. ISSN 0861-7813 (in Bulgarian)

Koltcheva, N. (2022). Bulgaria, country overview. In N. Koltcheva & V. Coelho (Eds.), *Social and emotional development for children aged 0 to 7 years old: European countries overviews compendium* (pp. xx–xx). EU-SELF Project. ISBN 978-619-233-213-6

Koltcheva, N. (2023). *The significant others in a person's life*. New Bulgarian University Publishing House. ISBN 978-619-233-281-5 (in Bulgarian)

Koltcheva, N., & Coelho, V. (2022). *Social and emotional development for children aged 0 to 7 years old: European countries overviews compendium*. EU-SELF Project. ISBN 978-619-233-213-6

Koltcheva, N., Wastijn, B., Achten, M., Van Rossem, L., & Costa, I. S. (2022). *Programs for social and emotional skills development for early and preschool children applied in European countries* [Compendium]. EU-SELF Project. ISBN 978-619-233-211-2

Kotzeva, T., & Dimitrova, E. (2022). Risk behaviours: Tracking youth health and wellbeing in Bulgaria 2006–2018. In A. Heinen, R. Samuel, C. Vögele, & H. Willems (Eds.), *Wohlbefinden und Gesundheit im Jugendalter* (pp. 665–687). Springer VS. https://doi.org/10.1007/978-3-658-35744-3_30

Ministry of Agriculture, Republic of Bulgaria. (2023). *National strategy for the implementation of a scheme for offering fruits, vegetables, milk and dairy products in kindergartens, schools and centers for special educational support in the Republic of Bulgaria from 2023/2024 to the end of 2028/2029 academic year* (Approved 30 March 2023). https://www.mzh.government.bg/bg/politiki-i-programi/politiki-i-strategii/obshta-selskostopanska-politika/obsha-organizaciya-na-pazarite-na-selskostopanski-produkti/uchilishni-shemi/

Ministry of Education and Science, Republic of Bulgaria. (2015). *Ordinance No. 5 of 30.11.2015 on general education* [State Gazette, issue 95, 08.12.2015; amended issue 75, 01.09.2023]. https://web.mon.bg/bg/59#N5-2016

Ministry of Education and Science, Republic of Bulgaria. (2016a). *Ordinance No. 5 of 03.06.2016 on pre-school education* [State Gazette, issue 46, 17.06.2016; amended issue 12, 11.02.2022]. https://web.mon.bg/bg/59#N5-2016

Ministry of Education and Science, Republic of Bulgaria. (2016b). *Ordinance No. 10 of 01.09.2016 on organization of activities in school education* [State Gazette, issue 73, 16.09.2016; amended issue 19, 28.02.2023]. https://web.mon.bg/bg/59#N5-2016

Ministry of Education and Science, Republic of Bulgaria. (2016c). *Ordinance No. 13 of 21.09.2016 on the civic, health, environmental and intercultural education* [State Gazette, issue 80, 11.10.2016; amended issue 75, 01.09.2023]. https://web.mon.bg/bg/59#N5-2016

Ministry of Education and Science, Republic of Bulgaria. (2016d). *Ordinance on the state requirements for acquiring the professional qualification "Teacher"* [State Gazette, issue 89, 11.11.2016; amended issue 10, 05.02.2021]. https://web.mon.bg/bg/59#N5-2016

Ministry of Education and Science, Republic of Bulgaria. (2016e). *Ordinance No. 16 of 08.12.2016 on quality management in the institutions* [State Gazette, issue 100, 16.12.2016]. https://web.mon.bg/bg/59#N5-2016

Ministry of Education and Science, Republic of Bulgaria. (2017). *Ordinance on inclusive education* [State Gazette, issue 86, 27.10.2017; amended issue 91, 02.11.2021]. https://web.mon.bg/bg/59#N5-2016

Ministry of Education and Science, Republic of Bulgaria. (2019). *Ordinance No. 15 of 22.07.2019 on the status and professional development of teachers, school headmasters and other pedagogical specialists* [State Gazette, issue 61, 02.08.2019; amended issue 52, 05.07.2022]. https://web.mon.bg/bg/59#N5-2016

Ministry of Education and Science, Republic of Bulgaria. (2020). *Ordinance No. 24 of September 10, 2020 on the physical environment and information and library provision of kindergartens, schools and personal development support centers* [State Gazette, issue 84, 29.09.2020]. https://web.mon.bg/bg/59#N5-2016

National Children's Network. (2023). *Notebook 2023. What is the country's average success in child care?* (April 2023). ISSN 1314-9970. https://www.nmd.bg

National Statistical Institute. (2022). *Children in Bulgaria in 2022* [Report]. https://www.nsi.bg

National Statistical Institute, Republic of Bulgaria. (2023a). *Population by districts, age, place of residence and sex as of 31.12.2022.* https://www.nsi.bg/en/content/2979/population-districts-age-place-residence-and-sex

National Statistical Institute, Republic of Bulgaria. (2023b). *Ethno-cultural characteristics of the population as of September 7, 2021* [Final data]. Published 21 December 2022. https://www.nsi.bg/en/content/ethno-cultural-characteristics-population-september-7-2021

National Statistical Institute, Republic of Bulgaria. (2023c). *Children enrolled at kindergartens by sex and age.* Published 26 April 2023. https://www.nsi.bg/en/content/3419/children-enrolled-kindergartens-sex-and-age

National Statistical Institute, Republic of Bulgaria. (2023d). *Students enrolled at general schools by grade groups, sex and ownership of the school.* Published 26 April 2023. https://www.nsi.bg/en/content/3440/students-enrolled-general-schools-grade-groups-sex-and-ownership-school

National Statistical Institute, Republic of Bulgaria. (2023e). *Children in kindergartens by organization of the learning process and location.* Published 26 April 2023. https://www.nsi.bg/en/content/3417/children-enrolled-kindergartens-organization-learning-process-and-location

National Statistical Institute, Republic of Bulgaria. (2023f). *Pedagogical staff in pre-primary education by age*. Published 26 April 2023. https://www.nsi.bg/en/content/3426/pedagogical-staff-kindergartens-age

National Statistical Institute, Republic of Bulgaria. (2023g). *Teaching staff in general schools by age*. Published 26 April 2023. https://www.nsi.bg/en/content/3468/teaching-staff-general-schools-age

National Statistical Institute, Republic of Bulgaria. (2023h). *Teaching staff in general schools by teaching level and sex*. Published 26 April 2023. https://www.nsi.bg/en/content/3464/teaching-staff-general-schools-teaching-level-and-sex

Prepodavame.bg. (2023). *Develop social-emotional skills in your classroom*. https://prepodavame.bg/resursi-za-razvivane-na-sotsialno-emotsionalni-umenia/

Pre-school and School Education Act, promulgated State Gazette, issue 79, 13.10.2015, effective since 01.08.2016, last amended and supplemented, State Gazette, issue 11, 02.02.2023. Ministry of Education and Science, Republic of Bulgaria. https://web.mon.bg/bg/57

Putnick, D. L., Bornstein, M. H., Lansford, J. E., Malone, P. S., Pastorelli, C., Skinner, A. T., Sorbring, E., Tapanya, S., Uribe Tirado, L. M., Zelli, A., Alampay, L. P., Al-Hassan, S. M., Bacchini, D., Bombi, A. S., Chang, L., Deater-Deckard, K., Di Giunta, L., Dodge, K. A., & Oburu, P. (2014). Perceived mother and father acceptance-rejection predict four unique aspects of child adjustment across nine countries. *Journal of Child Psychology and Psychiatry, 56*(8), 923–932. https://doi.org/10.1111/jcpp.12366

Regulation for extracurricular activities in municipal schools on the territory of the Metropolitan Municipality. (2017, June 4). *Adopted by Decision No. 136 under Protocol No. 30 of 04/06/2017, amended and adopted Decision No. 118 under Protocol No. 49 of March 15, 2018*. https://sofia.obshtini.bg/doc/3073240

Regulation for the implementation of additional educational activities in municipal kindergartens on the territory of the Metropolitan Municipality. (2017, June 4). *Adopted by Decision No. 135 under Protocol No. 30 of 04/06/2017, amended and adopted Decision No. 166 under Protocol No. 13 of 14.05.2020*. https://sofia.obshtini.bg/doc/3073241

Regulation on the creation, structure and activity of public councils for kindergartens and schools. (2016, September 27; amended 2023, May 9; updated 2023, June 1). *State Gazette, issue 75, 41*. https://web.mon.bg/bg/60

Regulation on the terms and conditions for the implementation of fruit and vegetable and milk and dairy products schemes in educational institutions – "School Fruit" Scheme and "School Milk" Scheme. (2016, September 27). *Adopted by PMS No. 251, promulgated State Gazette, issue 77 of 4.10.2016; amended following Decision No. 8272 of the Supreme Court of the Republic of Bulgaria, No. 59 of 16.07.2021*.

Report of the National Education Development Programs for 2022. (2023, April 20). https://web.mon.bg/bg/101106

Resilience in Schools. (2023). *Factsheet prepared by NESET experts: C. Cefai, C. Nada, H. Cowie, & L. van der Graaf*. European Union, Luxembourg: Publications Office of the European Union. https://doi.org/10.2766/154803

Rohner, R. P. (2021). *Introduction to Interpersonal Acceptance-Rejection Theory (IPARTheory) and Evidence*. Online Reading. https://csiar.uconn.edu/introduction-to-partheory/

Rothenberg, W. A., Ali, S., Rohner, R. P., Lansford, J. E., Britner, P. A., Di Giunta, L., Dodge, K. A., Malone, P. S., Oburu, P., Pastorelli, C., Skinner, A. T., Sorbring, E., Steinberg, L., Tapanya, S., Uribe Tirado, L. M., Yotanyamaneewong, S., Alampay, L. P., Al-Hassan, S. M., Bacchini, D., … Deater-Deckard, K. (2021b). Effects of parental acceptance-rejection on children's internalizing and externalizing behaviors: A longitudinal, multicultural study. *Journal of Child and Family Studies*. https://doi.org/10.1007/s10826-021-02072-5

Rothenberg, W. A., Lansford, J. E., Alampay, L. P., Al-Hassan, S. M., Bacchini, D., Bornstein, M. H., Chang, L., Deater-Deckard, K., Di Giunta, L., Dodge, K. A., Malone, P. S., Oburu, P., Pastorelli, C., Skinner, A. T., Sorbring, E., Steinberg, L., Tapanya, S., Uribe Tirado, L. M., & Yotanyamaneewong, S. (2019). Examining effects of mother and father warmth and control on child externalizing and internalizing problems from age 8 to 13 in nine countries. *Development and Psychopathology*, 1–25. https://doi.org/10.1017/s0954579419001214

Rothenberg, W. A., Lansford, J. E., Bornstein, M. H., Chang, L., Deater-Deckard, K., Di Giunta, L., Dodge, K. A., Malone, P. S., Oburu, P., Pastorelli, C., Skinner, A. T., Sorbring, E., Steinberg, L., Tapanya, S., Uribe Tirado, L. M., Yotanyamaneewong, S., Alampay, L. P., Al-Hassan, S. M., & Bacchini, D. (2020). Effects of parental warmth and behavioral control on adolescent externalizing and internalizing trajectories across cultures. *Journal of Research on Adolescence*, 1–21. https://doi.org/10.1111/jora.12566

Rothenberg, W. A., Lansford, J. E., Bornstein, M. H., Uribe Tirado, L. M., Yotanyamaneewong, S., Alampay, L. P., Al-Hassan, S. M., Bacchini, D., Chang, L., Deater-Deckard, K., Di Giunta, L., Dodge, K. A., Gurdal, S., Liu, Q., Long, Q., Malone, P. S., Oburu, P., Pastorelli, C., Skinner, A. T., … Steinberg, L. (2021a). Cross-cultural associations of four parenting behaviors with child flourishing: Examining cultural specificity and commonality in cultural normativeness and intergenerational transmission processes. *Child Development, 92*(6), 1–16. https://doi.org/10.1111/cdev.13634

Savova, T., & Koltcheva, N. (2018). *Interrelationship between perceived parental acceptance/rejection and behavioral problems in primary school-age children* [Master's thesis, New Bulgarian University]. (In Bulgarian)

Shriver, T. P., & Weissberg, R. P. (1996, May 15). No new wars! *Education Week, 15*(34), 33–37.

Strategic Framework for the Development of Education, Training and Learning in the Republic of Bulgaria. (2021–2030). Ministry of Education and Science. https://web.mon.bg/bg/143

Together in Class. (2021). *Learning together 2021: Overcoming the educational challenges caused by the pandemic.* https://zaednovchas.bg/uchim-zaedno-2021/

Together in Class. (2023). *Learning together 2023: Enhancing self-regulated learning and social-emotional skills.* https://zaednovchas.bg/uchim-zaedno/

UNICEF. (2007). *Child poverty in perspective: An overview of child wellbeing in rich countries* (Innocenti Report Card 7). UNICEF Innocenti Research Centre. ISBN 978-88-89129-43-2

UNICEF, Bulgaria. (2018). *The situation of children in Bulgaria: Challenges.* https://www.unicef.org/bulgaria/en/situation-children-bulgaria

UNICEF Innocenti. (2020a). *Worlds of influence: Understanding what shapes child wellbeing in rich countries* (Innocenti Report Card 16). UNICEF Office of Research – Innocenti. ISBN 978-92-1-103307-6

UNICEF Innocenti. (2020b, September 3). *Worlds of influence: Shaping policies for child wellbeing in rich countries [Video].* YouTube. https://www.youtube.com/watch?v=Q4wPYii3zO8

Witters, D., & Agrawal, S. (2023, October 24). *Poor wellbeing linked to formation of new chronic conditions.* Gallup. https://news.gallup.com/poll/512750/poor-wellbeing-linked-formation-new-chronic-conditions.aspx

Chapter 7
Challenges and Opportunities for Enhancing Wellbeing in Croatian Kindergartens and Schools

Sanja Tatalović Vorkapić

7.1 Introduction

The fundamental role of early childhood and preschool education is to create the conditions for the complete and harmonious development of the child's personality and to contribute to the quality of the child's education, thus ensuring the highest level of child wellbeing (Ben-Arieh et al., 2014; National Curriculum for Early Childhood & Preschool Care & Education in Croatia, 2015; Tatalović Vorkapić, 2019a, 2019b). However, in today's world—characterized by numerous changes such as shifts in family structure, extended working hours, everyday stress, a hectic lifestyle, and the increasing dominance of digitalization—this role is becoming increasingly demanding, especially because the changes are faster, more intense and affect different aspects of life, such as economic, social, and cultural. Children are confronted with refugee crises, problems in the lives of ethnic minorities, a pandemic caused by a virus, special individual educational needs, war, but also with many other risks that children face today, such as divorce, abuse, poverty, peer violence and cyber-bullying, etc. The consequence of all these challenges is that children's wellbeing can be significantly affected, which is associated with impaired mental health (Cefai et al., 2018). This is supported by various negative reports on children's mental health today, which point to a steady increase in the number of children who present with various mental health difficulties and whose mental wellbeing and life satisfaction are significantly reduced (2022b; Cavioni et al., 2023; Cefai, 2022a). In the last twenty years, mental health difficulties in children have increased worldwide and have become the most common cause of disability (WHO, 2018). The prevalence of diagnosed mental, emotional, or behavioral disorders among school-aged children is estimated to be between 10 and 20% (Erskine et al., 2015). The proportion of young people presenting with mental health problems before the age of 14 and before the

S. T. Vorkapić (✉)
Faculty of Teacher Education, University of Rijeka, Rijeka, Croatia
e-mail: sanjatv@uniri.hr

A. A. Colomeischi (ed.), *Wellbeing in Schools of Southeastern Europe*, Human Well-Being Research and Policy Making, https://doi.org/10.1007/978-3-032-10525-7_7

age of 18 was 35% and 48%, respectively, with the highest incidence at the age of 14.5 years (Solmi et al., 2022). Depression and anxiety are among the top five causes of illness (Liu et al., 2024). In addition, the outbreak of the COVID-19 pandemic led to a significant global increase in reported symptoms of anxiety, depression, and post-traumatic stress disorder (Singh et al., 2020). These findings were also confirmed by domestic studies conducted among adults, children, and adolescents in Croatia (Jokić Begić et al., 2020).

Professionals involved in care and education of preschool and primary school-aged children are in a position where they must think daily about the ways and means to create the best possible conditions. This is especially challenging for children's transitions from home to kindergarten, and from kindergarten to primary school, and their adjustment in kindergarten and school, which has been determined in the national five-year scientific project on the Well-being of children during transitions (uniri-drustv-18-11; Tatalović Vorkapić, 2024) and has still been explored within the new national scientific project Adjust_Well (uniri-iz-25-115). Since ensuring the best interests of the child is one of the fundamental goals of the National Curriculum for Early Childhood and Preschool Education (2015), early childhood and preschool education settings should provide a considerate, reliable, and safe environment, reducing the stress caused by various challenges. Every child has a right to development in which adults reinforce their inner strength and use their power to create a shield between the child and the risks that threaten them. In this process, adult support is crucial. The role of educational professionals responsible for children's growth and development is to reflect on the possibilities of enriching educational work through the implementation of programs that can simultaneously contribute to the prevention of deviations from the normal developmental process and the development of competencies necessary for children to grow up healthy and successful future young generations, thus contributing to the emotional and social wellbeing of the entire community. A specific strategic goal articulated by WHO in the area of mental health support around the world clearly recognizes the key role of the education system in addressing the mental health needs of children and adolescents and improving their quality of life and mental wellbeing. WHO recommends that kindergartens and schools act as one of the foundational systems for supporting children's mental health, providing promotion, prevention, and intervention (Cefai et al., 2022a, 2022b). About half of mental health problems develop before the age of 14, when children and adolescents are still in school (WHO, Regional Office for Europe, 2018), which opens up opportunities for the active promotion of mental health and wellbeing in kindergartens and schools, as well as the timely prevention of mental health problems during critical stages of child and adolescent development. In this context, it is crucial to ensure, within the framework of pedagogical work in kindergartens and schools, high-quality competency development of early childhood educators and primary school teachers, as well as their positive mental health and wellbeing (*Well teachers, well students:* McCallum & Price, 2010), where the quality of their initial training and professional development programs is crucial.

7.1.1 The Concept of Children's Wellbeing

Before delving into the key determinants of children's wellbeing, it is essential to first provide a clear definition of the concept. However, there are certain challenges to this effort. The concept of child wellbeing is very complex and challenging when it comes to its clear definition and theoretical determination. Until recently, research directions, which within positive psychology mostly dealt with research into the well-being of adults, contributed to this (Ben-Arieh et al., 2014). On the other hand, it is completely clear that two areas of science are dominant when it comes to the conceptual determination of children's wellbeing, namely: developmental psychology and positive psychology. Therefore, with the aim of defining and conceptualizing the child wellbeing, two directions are determined: developmental theories which define child wellbeing based on existing child development, learning and contextual theories, and wellbeing theories which define child wellbeing based on existing adult wellbeing theoretical models. The relevant scientific literature is undoubtedly abundant in scientific and professional knowledge about studies on the wellbeing of adults (Ben-Arieh et al., 2014). Empirical research on the wellbeing of adults, in its theoretical determination and measurement, has a rather long history, which cannot be claimed when it comes to the concept of the wellbeing of children. This fact is actually surprising considering that quite a number of different policy documents as well as international and national documents such as the National Curriculum for Early and Preschool Education (2015), base their activities and work plans precisely on the achievement and higher quality of both general wellbeing and socio-emotional wellbeing of children. Contemporary discourses of child wellbeing today include a very wide range of challenges in relation to the needs of the contemporary child and childhood. They range from intense reflections on the discrepancy between natural upbringing and controlled upbringing; about overloading of children in the education system; on the (in)balance of local and global actions on children and childhood; through the determining effect of the complexity of children's wellbeing and the method of its measurement; to questions about quality and useful policies that determine the living conditions of families and thus children and their childhood. The diversity and multidimensionality of the aforementioned discourses indicate that when it comes to children's wellbeing, we are entering a very complex area that is significantly more difficult to conceptually determine and define, unlike the wellbeing of adults. Nevertheless, over the past decade, significant progress has been made—primarily in one dimension of children's wellbeing: their subjective wellbeing (Ajduković et al., 2020). This is the result of new studies in the field of childhood theories, children's rights legislation, and a reorientation toward positive social sciences (Savahl et al., 2021), such as positive psychology. Having in mid these discourses, it is extremely important to clearly define the wellbeing of children, especially the psychological wellbeing of children.

Wellbeing of adults, understood as optimal psychological functioning and experience, is defined within three theoretical frameworks (Raghavan & Alexandrova, 2015). Within the framework of the hedonistic direction or Mental states theories, the subjective wellbeing of an individual consists of pleasure or happiness. According to Desire-based theories, wellbeing consists of the realization of one's own desires, which are the product of subjective perception. Finally, the eudaemonist direction or Needs-based theories points out that wellbeing is realized by actualizing human potential, that is, those needs that arise as a product of people's objective perception (e.g., because something is valuable in itself and not just because we think so or we experience pleasure within it). Although briefly listed theoretical models validly define the concept of people's wellbeing, they all have in common that they lack a developmental component, and are only partially applicable when understanding children's wellbeing.

On the other hand, the foundations of the modern child wellbeing model can be traced to two well-known developmental theories: Bronfenbrenner's ecological systems model (1979) and Bennett's model of the child in society (2004). Both models emphasize two key components in defining child wellbeing: the developmental and the contextual (socio-cultural) component. The first model emphasizes the role of context in a child's life and the importance of relationships that shape their environment. In this theory, the environment is conceptualized as a set of complex "layers," each influencing a child's development—from the immediate microsystem to the more distant macrosystem. The second model focuses on social identity as a major factor influencing a child's development. A child's social identity is shaped by their membership in various groups—such as family, nation, and religion—which together help define the child's place in society. This theory explains social identity through children's perceptions of social group membership, variations in the specific content of those identities, and their subjective identification with collectives. Critically looking at existing developmental and wellbeing models, Ben-Arieh et al. (2014) pointed out several aspects to be discussed and resolved: insufficient integrity and complexity; although happiness is a fundamental indicator of wellbeing, it is very difficult to measure; the answers to the questions about whether I have a quality life and whether I am satisfied are very complex; in addition to personal, subjective factors, objective and environmental factors are equally important; focus on adults and not on children; strong cultural determination of defining wellbeing (being well in different countries does not mean the same thing); neglect of children's perspective (no one asks children what it means for them to be happy); indicators of children's wellbeing (perspective indicators, measurement techniques and instruments and indicators of children); and significant changes in the perspective of monitoring children's wellbeing. Regarding the last aspect of changes in perspective of monitoring children's wellbeing, it is important to briefly mention each of the four changes that are in the basis of contemporary model of children's wellbeing. The first is a change in perspective from survival to wellbeing, that is, from basic survival and ensuring the satisfaction of children's basic needs with avoiding negative effects to the perspective of determining how to increase the level of quality of life. The second is a change of perspective from negative to positive, that is, from measuring and monitoring risk factors and negative/non-functional behaviors to the perspective of measuring and monitoring protective factors and positive/functional behaviors. The third refers to the change of perspective from well-becoming to wellbeing. By changing this perspective, a development perspective is more emphasized because, in addition to the how to become well as an accomplishment current model is more focused on current wellbeing of children and how to achieve it. Finally, when looking at children's wellbeing, it is necessary to determine what is good for the child now (being) and what is good for the child now and has strong consequences for his later life (becoming). The fourth change in perspective involves a shift in focus from the traditional view of domains of wellbeing to a new, contemporary view of domains of child wellbeing related to the domains defined by UNICEF (Lajoie & Leveille, 2007), as they are the most widely agreed upon among experts in this area. Child wellbeing represents a holistic view of the child and encompasses several domains: material wellbeing, health and safety, educational wellbeing, family and peer relationships, behavioral risks, and subjective wellbeing. It is precisely in the last domain of wellbeing, which focuses on the voice and opinion of children, that the greatest progress has been made, which is confirmed by a large number of studies that directly ask children about their wellbeing and life satisfaction (Ajduković et al., 2020; Tatalović Vorkapić & Anđić, 2023; Velan & Tatalović Vorkapić, 2020).

In conclusion, and taking into account the previous considerations by Ben-Arieh and associates (2014), a multifaceted model of child wellbeing proposed was developed and it includes multiple perspectives on child wellbeing; multiple approaches to child wellbeing; theoretical approaches to child wellbeing; children's activities and wellbeing; arts, creativity and child wellbeing; spirituality and religion; an ecological perspective on child wellbeing; economy/material wellbeing; life course and child wellbeing; interpersonal relations; media and communication and child wellbeing; wellbeing and the family; health and child wellbeing; wellbeing and children's rights; risk and vulnerability; methods, measures and indicators; interventions and policies that promote child wellbeing; global issues in child wellbeing. Regarding the model's complexity, one could observe that child wellbeing has various multiple approaches: child wellbeing: a philosophical perspective; child wellbeing: children's rights perspective; neuroscience and child wellbeing; educational science and child wellbeing; geographies of children's wellbeing: in, of, and for place; child healthcare and child wellbeing: from the past to the future; public health aspects of child wellbeing; wellbeing of children: a criminological perspective; economics of child wellbeing; social work and child wellbeing; children's wellbeing and politics; mediated wellbeing from the perspective of media and communication studies; child wellbeing: anthropological perspectives; social psychology and child wellbeing; psychology of child wellbeing. The last one, Psychology of child wellbeing is mostly connected with the psychological wellbeing of children, their socio-emotional wellbeing and mental health (Holte et al., 2014) what is the main focus of this chapter. So, within this model, Psychology of child wellbeing has its roots in positive psychology and framework of subjective wellbeing, resilience and adaptation and prosocial behavior. Additionally, other contextual variables are important when considering the psychology of child wellbeing—such as research methodology and the development of more effective indicators, measures, and approaches to assessing children's wellbeing. The topics covered include parents' perceptions of children's wellbeing, health-related quality of life, and subjective wellbeing in children and adolescents from cross-cultural and evolutionary perspectives, as well as the influence of genetics and cognitive factors on wellbeing. In addition, it addresses themes such as the happy personality, the happy family, and positive parenting, along with children's play and peer relationships. Finally, it encompasses contemporary discourses on the psychological aspects of children's wellbeing within institutional contexts, such as early childhood education and care, as well as schools (Holte et al., 2014).

7.1.2 Social and Emotional Development, Learning, Competencies, and Wellbeing of Children

Socio-emotional wellbeing is most often associated with the concepts of socio-emotional development, learning, socio-emotional competencies, and mental health; it is therefore important to define them more clearly. Socio-emotional development is a developmental process through which children acquire a set of skills essential for success in kindergarten, school, and life in general. These skills include the ability to recognize and understand others' feelings and emotional states, manage intense emotions and their expression, develop empathy, and establish and maintain relationships (Berk, 2015). The process of acquiring socio-emotional knowledge and skills within the framework of socio-emotional development is called socio-emotional learning, and it results in socio-emotional competencies. According to the CASEL (2013) definition, it includes five domains of learning, and thus the resulting skills of children: (a) self-awareness (the ability to assess and recognize one's emotions and thoughts and their influence on behavior); (b) self-management (the ability to effectively express and control one's emotions, thoughts, and behavior in various situations); (c) social awareness (the ability to understand and accept others and empathize with others of different cultures, beliefs, and attitudes); (d) relationship skills (the ability to establish and maintain healthy interpersonal relationships of some duration, resolve conflicts constructively, seek and offer help when needed, and the individual's ability to resist peer pressure and resolve conflicts meaningfully); and e) responsible decision-making (the ability to make decisions about personal behavior and social interactions that are consistent with ethical standards while contributing to the wellbeing of the community in which they live, with a sense of responsibility and respect for others. Within the socio-emotional learning, children "*acquire and apply the knowledge, skills, and attitudes to develop healthy identities, manage emotions, and achieve personal and collective goals, feel and show empathy for others, establish and maintain supportive relationships, and make responsible and caring decisions*" (Skoog-Hoffman et al., 2023: 6).

Depending on the quality of all the mentioned processes and the competencies themselves in a certain environmental context, children will have a certain level of socio-emotional wellbeing. Socio-emotional wellbeing—alongside physical-motor and cognitive-linguistic wellbeing—is an integral component of children's overall wellbeing. It reflects their optimal functioning and experience at the socio-emotional level and is significantly influenced by both intrapersonal factors (such as individual child characteristics) and interpersonal factors (including the environment, the society in which the child lives, and the child's relationships with that environment). Socio-emotional wellbeing of children encompasses a developmental dimension that has only recently become the focus of scientific research, as described above. Concepts close to socio-emotional wellbeing are mental health, which is a syndrome of symptoms of wellbeing, and resilience, which refers to the capacity of a dynamic system for successful adaptation regardless of risk factors and disturbances in the environment that threaten the sustainability, function or development of that system (Masten, 2018). Psychologically resilient children manage to achieve their developmental tasks at an optimal level regardless of the influence of risk factors in their lives. The characteristics of a resilient child are: easy temperament and sociability; the ability to evoke positive emotions in others; positive self-concept and self-esteem; autonomy and independence; proactive approach to problem solving; persistence and high concentration; satisfaction in new experiences; high curiosity and need for research; empathy and prosocial orientation; positive social relations; the ability to delay gratification; positive processing and restructuring of negative experiences; affect control; adequate expression of feelings and desires; optimism, cheerfulness and energy, a large number of hobbies and interests; the ability to quickly recover from stressful events; calmness and relaxation; and a sense of the meaning of life and a focus on the future. In other words, the characteristics of resilient children can be summarized in four categories: social competence, problem-solving skills, autonomy, and a sense of purpose and future. Resilience is, therefore, considered a multidimensional construct, which includes important psychological skills and abilities, but also the individual's ability to use the support of family, society, and the system as a whole to better cope with stress (Miljević-Riđički et al., 2017).

A prerequisite for the effectiveness of achieving the socio-emotional wellbeing of children of early and preschool age is knowledge of developmental milestones within the framework of children's socio-emotional development (Sindik & Boban, 2016). Keeping in mind the characteristics of socio-emotional development and age norms, as well as the recommended optimal conditions for encouraging and ensuring the same domain of development, it is possible to nurture and empower children's mental health. One of the contemporary models of socio-emotional wellbeing and resilience (Mayr & Ulich, 2009), which is specifically oriented only to the domain of the development of social skills, understanding and regulation of emotions and resilience, is based on three theoretical concepts: mental health as a result of adequate adopted life skills (those that enable appropriate interaction with others and easy coping with stressful situations); resilience as a characteristic of children who manage to achieve their developmental tasks at an optimal level regardless of the influence of risk factors in their lives; and readiness for school as an ability of children that enables self-regulation at different levels and aspects: cognitive, speech, socio-emotional, and physical-motor, which is visible through assertiveness, prosocial behavior, and social inclusion. According to the model they developed, the authors describe six dimensions of socio-emotional wellbeing and resilience of children: making contact and social skills; self-control and thoughtfulness; assertiveness; emotional stability and coping with stress; task orientation; and enjoyment of research. In a validation study (Tatalović Vorkapić & Lončarić, 2014) on a preschool sample of children ($N = 1792$; 939 girls and 853 boys) with an average age of $M = 4.891$ years, in which educators ($N = 112$) assessed children's behavior, 5 subscales were confirmed almost identical structures to those from the original research with the exception of the Task Orientation subscale, which was not retained. Age and gender differences in the assessed dimensions showed the expected direction (increasing results on all scales with increasing age, and significant differences in favor of girls). A significant contribution of this research lies in the development of a valid measurement instrument with exceptional applicability in working with preschool-aged children—an effectiveness that has been confirmed by numerous studies in which it has been used (Tatalović Vorkapić, 2020, 2023, 2024).

Considering the theoretical concepts presented, an important question arises: how can the optimal level of children's socio-emotional wellbeing be achieved? The answer lies in encouraging and strengthening socio-emotional learning, which fosters the development of socio-emotional competencies and ultimately supports the highest level of mental health in children. The presented theoretical models indicated WHAT is important. By following three key steps, we can begin to answer the question of HOW to implement these concepts in educational practice: (a) understanding the developmental milestones of children's socio-emotional development; (b) being familiar with the principles that support the development of preschool-aged children; and (c) possessing the skills and knowledge related to early and preschool education methods.

7.1.3 Social and Emotional Learning as an Efficient Solution for Mentally Health Children in Kindergartens and Schools

Social-emotional learning is a type of learning in which children acquire attitudes, skills, and knowledge in the domains of recognizing and managing emotions, effective decision-making, self-regulation, effective establishment, and maintenance of relationships with other people (Munjas Samarin & Takšić, 2009). It assumes that the best learning occurs in the context of supportive relationships that make learning challenging, engaging, and meaningful. Skills that result in social-emotional learning are crucial for a child to be a good student and citizen. Many different risky behaviors can be prevented or reduced when social-emotional skills are developed through multi-year, integrated efforts based on social-emotional learning. Learning and developing these skills is best achieved through effective activities in educational groups, children's participation in activities inside and outside early childhood and preschool education institutions, and when parents and the community are involved in the planning, implementation, and evaluation of the program. An effective SEL program begins in preschool age and continues through elementary school education and high school (CASEL, 2013). OECD (2015) uses the term "social and emotional skills" to define the type of skills involved in achieving goals, working with others, and managing emotions. The terms "life skills" of "self-care skills" are also used, which are defined as abilities for adaptive and positive behavior that enable people to effectively cope with the demands and challenges of everyday life. These skills encompass psychological and social abilities that influence behavior, as well as reflective skills such as problem-solving and critical thinking. They are also referred to as personal skills, which include self-awareness and interpersonal abilities such as sociability and tolerance. UNICEF identifies all of these as essential components of high-quality education.

Effective implementation of social-emotional learning in practice requires attention to eight key components (Cefai et al., 2018). The first one refers to the curriculum. Children and young people can directly develop social and emotional competencies through competence-based experiential learning only if there are appropriately defined and distributed goals and if a sufficient amount of focused time is provided in the curriculum. Social-emotional learning competencies should also be embedded in other content areas of the curriculum. Educators should be adequately trained and supported in performing social-emotional learning at the curricular level. The second includes the climate, because social and emotional learning in the curriculum must be accompanied by a positive climate in the group and the entire institution. In other words, the active participation of the entire institution and community is essential. The third is early intervention, since social and emotional learning is most effective when it is started in early childhood because then it will have important outcomes in adolescence and adulthood. The fourth part is related to targeted interventions, because social and emotional learning should follow the needs of children at risk or with difficulties, especially those with chronic and complex difficulties. The whole policy of the institution will also include both universal and targeted interventions. Just as this includes a contemporary understanding of children's wellbeing, effective implementation should be sensitive and receptive to children's voices. Namely, children should actively participate in the planning and implementation of initiatives, including the design, development, and evaluation of curriculum and resources. At the same time, educators' competencies and their own wellbeing are essential, as the social and emotional competence, health, and wellbeing of educators and other staff play a crucial role in the effective implementation of social-emotional learning (SEL) in kindergartens and schools. The seventh component is related to parental cooperation. Active cooperation and education of parents, made possible through an empowering approach, is crucial for the success of social and emotional learning. Finally, quality implementation and adaptation are crucial, what implies adequate and continuous education of educators at the level before and during work, appropriate preparation and provision of financial and human resources, as necessary conditions for effective implementation of social and emotional learning. Social and educational programs should also be sensitive and respond to the particularities of the institution's culture and the needs and interests of the children. This includes linguistic, cultural, social, and other areas. However, quality adaptation needs to find a balance between preserving the integrity of the intervention and adapting it to the needs of a new context.

A pleasant and safe family environment is a prerequisite for the successful development of children and shaping the child's motor, cognitive, speech and socio-emotional development. Modern society and way of life require early and preschool education institutions to take over part of the educational function, including the development of the social and emotional competency of children of early and preschool age. It is concluded that a stable family environment and supportive relationships in kindergarten greatly influence the development of resilience in a child. Numerous studies have shown how important it is that educational institutions in their overall environment and requirements correspond to the child's developmental needs, as well as possibilities. A developmentally appropriate, structured, and stimulating environment in which children will develop their competencies and relationships with others can act as a "safe harbor" for vulnerable children. In accordance with the goals of the National Curriculum for Early and Preschool Education (2015) in Croatia, one of the basic tasks of the institution for early and preschool education is to create a context in which an optimal development of all children will be achieved. Therefore, it is necessary to pay special attention to children who for some reasons can be labelled as vulnerable groups (children from families affected by poverty, marginalized ethnic minorities, immigrant children, especially gifted children, children with developmental disabilities, diverse children overall…).

Educational environments that promote resilience are inclusive communities that offer a responsive and flexible learning environment adapted to the individual needs of children (Cefai et al., 2015). Educators play the most important role in creating and sustaining inclusive communities. By focusing on the child, they provide opportunities for choice, encourage growth and active learning, and support diverse learning styles with understanding and care. Educators in inclusive communities promote ideas and values of mutual help, create an environment of respect and integration, convey positive attitudes, and set high but reasonable expectations for children. In an educational environment where resilience is encouraged, the values of collaborative learning and teamwork stand out. Children are encouraged to cooperate in smaller and larger groups, without competition where everyone is a winner. To improve and preserve the value of cooperative learning, the teamwork and collegiality of educators with each other, with other employees, and cooperation with parents is equally important. In order for an educational institution to become a community that promotes resilience, the atmosphere of encouraging and developing resilience should be permeated through all segments and throughout the entire educational institution, that is, the curricular approach to fostering resilience should be based on the idea of a complete educational institution (Cefai et al., 2015).

Durlak et al. (2015) stated that planned, continuous, and systematic social-emotional learning has seven basic features: (a) developing a common vision for social-emotional learning that prioritizes the promotion of social, emotional and academic learning for all children, (b) identifying existing strengths and support for social-emotional learning and building these strengths; (c) establishment of the central office and infrastructure of the institution and resources that provide continuous professional development, which includes how to build awareness of the importance of social-emotional learning, improving the social-emotional competencies of adults; (d) establishment of standards for social-emotional learning; (e) adoption and harmonization of emotional skills that are developed by programs based on scientific evidence and provide support in the development of social-emotional skills within the institution and community; (f) integration of social-emotional learning into school curricula, (g) use of research to improve practice and children's social-emotional learning. Children who are skilled in social-emotional competency are able to integrate feelings, thoughts, and behavior to master important tasks in school and life (Domitrovich et al., 2017). Such children competently recognize and manage their emotions, create healthy relationships with peers and adults, set realistic and positive goals, satisfy personal and social needs, and make responsible and ethical decisions (Oberle et al., 2016). The implementation of a social-emotional learning program provides a foundation for better adjustment and academic education, which is reflected in more positive social behavior and relationships with peers, fewer behavioral problems, less emotional stress, and improved academic success (Durlak et al., 2011; Greenberg et al., 2003). Cefai et al. (2018) stated that social-emotional learning has positive effects on social, emotional, and cognitive outcomes. They determined that social-emotional learning is associated with an increase in social and emotional competencies, positive attitudes, prosocial behavior, and mental health. It improves peer relationships, increases the level of readiness for school, as well as the level of general wellbeing among children (Moore et al., 2015). Social-emotional learning is associated with a reduction in mental health difficulties in children and young people, such as anxiety, depression, substance abuse, and anti-social behavior (Cavioni et al., 2023; Cefai et al., 2022a, 2022b; Colomeischi et al., 2022; Conte et al., 2023; Martinsone et al., 2022; Poulou et al., 2022).

7.1.4 Positive Psychology Programs in the Educational Context

In the Introduction part of his book, Noddings (2003: 1) wrote: "*In the past few months, when I have told people that I'm writing a book on happiness and education, more than one has responded with some puzzlement, "But they don't go together!" Indeed, the fact that the two seem increasingly opposed these days is one motive for tackling the topic. Happiness and education are, properly, intimately related: Happiness should be an aim of education, and a good education should contribute significantly to personal and collective happiness.*" So, when we consider how we can positively influence the effectiveness of the educational process, we must first reflect on the shared understanding of its purpose. This purpose should primarily aim to promote both current and future personal and social wellbeing. It is essential to foster the development of capable, emotionally stable, and happy young individuals. In addition to ongoing efforts focused on addressing problems such as violence, substance abuse, and alcohol use, every kindergarten or school should implement programs that explicitly promote emotional, social, and physical wellbeing. These programs should be holistically integrated into the curriculum. This requires a comprehensive approach that considers teaching content, instructional methods, assessment systems, school culture, the physical and social environment, and school leadership (Miljković, 2006). Furthermore, Seligman and colleagues (2009) identified three key reasons why happiness should be taught in schools: the rising rates of depression among children; the relatively consistent levels of happiness reported by children worldwide; and the fact that most children attend school, making it an ideal setting for implementing programs aimed at increasing overall wellbeing. The results of research in the field of positive psychology have been tried by many to translate into programs to encourage a variety of positive states in children. Some programs focus on encouraging positive emotions in general, while others focus on specific areas such as gratitude, optimism, hope, or wisdom. Although many programs have been developed and implemented, there are few whose effects have been scientifically evaluated, such as: the Positive psychology teaching program; Gratitude development program; Optimism development program; Hope development program; Flow development program; and the Wisdom development program.

Regarding the Positive psychology teaching program, Seligman and his colleagues (2009) developed and began to apply this program which covered a wide range of *positive concepts* (gratitude, forgiveness, enthusiasm, altruism, optimism) encouraging students in the final grades of primary school to apply them in everyday life. A program was applied at the Strath Haven School near Philadelphia throughout one year and more than twenty 90-min sessions were held. The main aim of the program was to help students realize their strengths and virtues and learn to use them in everyday life. By conducting the study evaluation at three time points, an increased level of curiosity, interest in learning, and creativity was observed among students. What is more, students' social skills (empathy, cooperation, assertiveness, self-control) were significantly higher with reduced behavioral problems. Rijavec and Miljković (2006) developed a similar Positive psychology program in Croatia with the aim of encouraging positive emotions. The program included topics such as noticing and remembering positive events, gratitude, forgiveness, counteracting pessimism, and the like. The aim of the study was to examine the effects of this program on students' feelings of happiness and depression. The program lasted one year (15–25 meetings during the school year) and was attended by 115 students from 5 high schools. The results of the evaluation study showed that, by the end of the program, students who participated had significantly higher scores on measures of general satisfaction and positive emotions compared to those who did not participate.

The *Gratitude development program* was developed since research has shown that gratitude has many positive outcomes that are extremely important for both the school and the students, such as increasing psychological wellbeing, school satisfaction, prosocial behavior, and encouraging setting and achieving meaningful goals (Bono &

Froh, 2009). In the Gratitude Program (Froh et al., 2008), two groups of younger adolescents kept a diary for two weeks. One group was instructed to write down five things they were grateful for each day, while the other recorded five things that made them angry. The results showed that the "gratitude group" experienced an increase in positive emotions both during and after the intervention, along with greater satisfaction with school.

The first and certainly best-known program for the *development of optimism* is Penn's program of optimism, which is described and well documented in the book *Optimistic Child* (Seligman et al., 1995). The program lasts 24 h in total and is implemented over 12 weeks, with sessions held for 2 h each week. Each key term is taught through the use of comics, plays, games, discussions, and videos. Two central characters—Aspiring Holly and Aspiring Howard—were created as an optimistic couple nicknamed "The Sparks." Throughout the program, each key concept was brought to life during the program through additional characters such as Gloomy Greg and Pessimistic Penny (the "Desperate Duo"), Clear Samantha, Brawler Brandi, and Sisi Pet. These characters appear in various scenes and stories to illustrate antidepressant techniques in an engaging and relatable way. It has two basic components: cognitive (thinking interventions) and social skills acquisition (quarrelsome/lazy). The program was implemented with 1,990 children and underwent a full evaluation process. At the beginning of the program, 24% of children in both the experimental and control groups exhibited moderate to severe symptoms of depression. Immediately after the program, this percentage decreased by 11%, with long-term positive effects observed in both groups. To date, more than 3,000 children and adolescents aged 8 to 22 have participated in the program.

The most important findings indicate that the program helps prevent symptoms of depression and anxiety, reduces feelings of helplessness and behavioral problems, increases optimism and overall wellbeing, and improves academic performance. Additionally, young adults who completed the program reported fewer health-related symptoms and adopted healthier lifestyle habits (e.g., engaging in regular physical activity). Some later studies have confirmed both the short-term and long-term positive effects of teaching optimism. However, the results of other studies have been less encouraging. Specific, targeted programs have proven to be more effective than general ones, with the most positive outcomes observed in preadolescent children.

Based on Snyder's Theory of hope (Snyder, 2000), some programs have been developed to *encourage hope* in children and young people. These programs include setting clear goals and finding different ways in which those goals could be achieved. This is followed by a phase of learning self-motivation to use these. The results of these programs have shown that although all students benefit from them, those who enter the program with the least developed hope benefit the most (Bouwkamp & Lopez, 2001). These programs are particularly significant because hope is associated with a variety of positive outcomes such as school success and less fear of school and testing (Rijavec & Marković, 2008; Snyder et al., 1997).

Realistically, in schools, passivity, individualism, teacher-controlled activities, and direct teaching are most common, so the kind of learning that students enjoy and that evokes intense positive emotions and enthusiasm is very rare. So, with the aim of experiencing enjoyment in school, a *Flow Activities Room* (FAR) was created in one school in Indianapolis. Students visit this room three times a week and participate in structured, self-selected activities. The main goal is to enable students to develop and use different competencies in a situation of intrinsic motivation, and to develop skills that would not be encouraged by the traditional curriculum. Whalen and Csikszentmihalyi (1991) showed that the choices students had in the FAR (Focused Attention Room) helped them discover and clarify their interests. Additionally, the experience of intense play led to meaningful learning of essential skills and improved attention.

Based on the balance theory of *wisdom*, Reznitskaya and Sternberg (2004) developed a program to teach students to make wise judgments. In doing so, they were put in situations to actively experience the various cognitive and affective processes that underlie wise decision-making. Sternberg (2001) emphasizes 16 pedagogical principles and 6 procedures that derive from his theory of wisdom. The basic idea is that children should not be taught what to think, but how to think and how to develop their abilities of reflexive, dialogical and dialectical thinking. What the student needs to be trained for in this regard is, for example, according to Ennis (1987): developing the ability to select information and infer which of them are important and which should be discarded because they are irrelevant or inaccurate; understanding how different information fits together, or could fit together; giving context to new insights; giving meaning to new experiences; converting information into meaningful settings that can then be applied in behavior.

Finally, it is interesting to mention the application of positive psychology in one school within the *Geelong project*. An interesting program was implemented by Seligman and Karen Reivich, along with 15 associates, in 2008 at Geelong High School in Australia (Seligman, 2011). The entire teaching staff participated in a two-week training during which they learned how to apply positive psychology skills in their own lives. Afterward, they were introduced to a detailed curriculum designed for working with children. Several team members remained in Australia throughout the entire year, while numerous other specialists in the field visited for a week or longer. Together, they developed an algorithm called: *Teach—Apply—Live Accordingly.* Within Teach component elements of positive psychology are taught in individual subjects and teaching units in several classes: psychological resilience, gratitude, human strength, meaning, enthusiasm, positive relationships, and positive emotions. In the *Apply* phase, teachers incorporate elements of positive psychology into the subjects they teach, sports activities, pastoral counseling, music, and religious activities. Finally, with regard to the "Live Accordingly" component, both teachers and students dedicate time during class to focus on positive behaviors, emotional shifts, and constructive thinking. For example, they might start by asking a simple question such as, "What went well yesterday?" After the children share their positive experiences, the teacher asks why it is important to talk about the good things that have happened to them. The children respond that it makes them feel good. This project is still ongoing, and the results of the evaluation studies will be available soon.

7.1.5 Programs of Social-Emotional Learning

"*Programs for social and emotional learning in children build the skills of recognizing and managing one's own emotions, establishing positive goals, making responsible decisions, dealing effectively with interpersonal relationships, and at the same time influence academic development, creating a positive and stimulating school environment*" (Munjas Samarin & Takšić, 2009: 357). According to Jones et al. (2017), six key features must be present for social-emotional learning (SEL) programs to be considered effective: a supportive environment, capacity-building for institutional staff, involvement of families and communities, a focus on key behaviors and skills, setting achievable goals, and adherence to the SAFE approach—sequenced, active, focused, and explicit (Durlak et al., 2011). Some of these programs are further described below.

Al's Pals is a social-emotional learning program for preschool children, aged three to eight. It enables the development of skills to prepare for life's challenges through interactive lessons, interesting puppets, original music, and impressive teaching approaches (Al's Pals, Kids Making Healthy Choices, https://teachingstrategies.com/product/als-pals-social-emotional-learning-curriculum/). This program consists of 46 core lessons delivered twice a week over a period of 23 weeks. Each lesson lasts 10 to 15 min and typically uses guided creative play, brainstorming, puppetry, songs, role-playing, and movement to model and practice lesson concepts and skills (Jones et al., 2021). This program enables the development of conflict resolution and problem-solving skills; supports children in managing their emotions and behaviors; fosters positive relationships and prevents peer violence; promotes a caring and cooperative classroom environment; encourages healthy decision-making; and strengthens authentic partnerships with families. Another example of a program is *Conscious Discipline*, which integrates social and emotional learning with the management of an educational group. It was designed to change the behavior of educators and children with the goal of creating an institution culture based on a sense of security, connection and problem solving instead of applying external rewards and punishments. This program builds School Family culture by consistently modelling routines, rituals, and structures designed to set expected behavior, build institution-group connectedness, and develop social and emotional skills during everyday moments (Jones et al., 2021).

An additional example of a program is *The Incredible Years*, which is a collection of interconnected, comprehensive, and developmentally based programs for parents, teachers, and children. They are based in the developmental theory about the role of multiple interrelated factors of risk and protection in the development of risky behaviors. The programs are designed to work together to promote emotional, social, and academic competency and to prevent, reduce, and treat behavioral and emotional problems in young children. In training programs for parents, teachers, and children, educated facilitators use video vignettes to structure content and encourage group discussions, problem solving, and initiating practices related to participants' goals (https://incredibleyears.com/programs/).

Finally, the program *Tools of the Mind* program provides educators with tools that ensure successful learning in every child, developing the fundamental cognitive, social, and emotional skills necessary to reach their highest potential (https://toolsofthemind.org/#). The program consists of activities and games carried out in different groups, including small group learning centers, pair activities, and large group activities throughout each day and throughout the pedagogical year. Activities vary in complexity and length, and educators can choose when during the year to conduct each activity based on their children's developmental needs and the guidance provided by Tools of the Mind.

7.2 Education System in Croatia

Early and preschool care and education in the Republic of Croatia encompasses non-compulsory programs for the education and care of young children. These programs integrate educational, health, nutritional, and social services for children from six months of age until they reach school age (typically six or seven years old). Preschool education marks the beginning of compulsory and free education in Croatia. It is intended for children in the year prior to their enrollment in eight-year elementary school, typically at the age of six. The program is organized to provide between 250 and 550 h per year and generally runs from October of the current year to June of the following year. Eight-year primary education in the Republic of Croatia is also compulsory and free for all children between the ages of six/seven and fifteen. Through primary education, the student acquires knowledge and skills for continuing education at the secondary school level. In the first four grades of elementary school, instruction is delivered through classroom teaching, while from the fifth to the eighth grade, subject-based teaching is introduced. Children can also receive parallel education in the form of basic art programs, such as music and dance. The schematic structure of education system in Croatia could be observed in Fig. 7.1.

Following primary education, secondary education in Croatia provides all individuals—on equal terms and according to their abilities—with the opportunity to acquire the knowledge and skills necessary for employment or further education. High school education is not compulsory. Depending on the type of program, secondary schools are categorized into gymnasiums, vocational schools, and art schools. Quality higher education is a precondition for a successful society. In accordance with the Bologna system, higher education in the Republic of Croatia has a three-cycle study model, including undergraduate, graduate, and postgraduate level of study. Like several other European higher education systems, the Croatian system has a binary structure comprising the professional and university profile of study programs and institutions.

National curricula for individual levels and types of education determine the purpose, values, goals, and principles of certain parts of the education system. They state the principles of the organization of the educational process, learning and teaching, as well as the evaluation and reporting, which are characteristic for a particular level or type of education. The Croatian national curricula

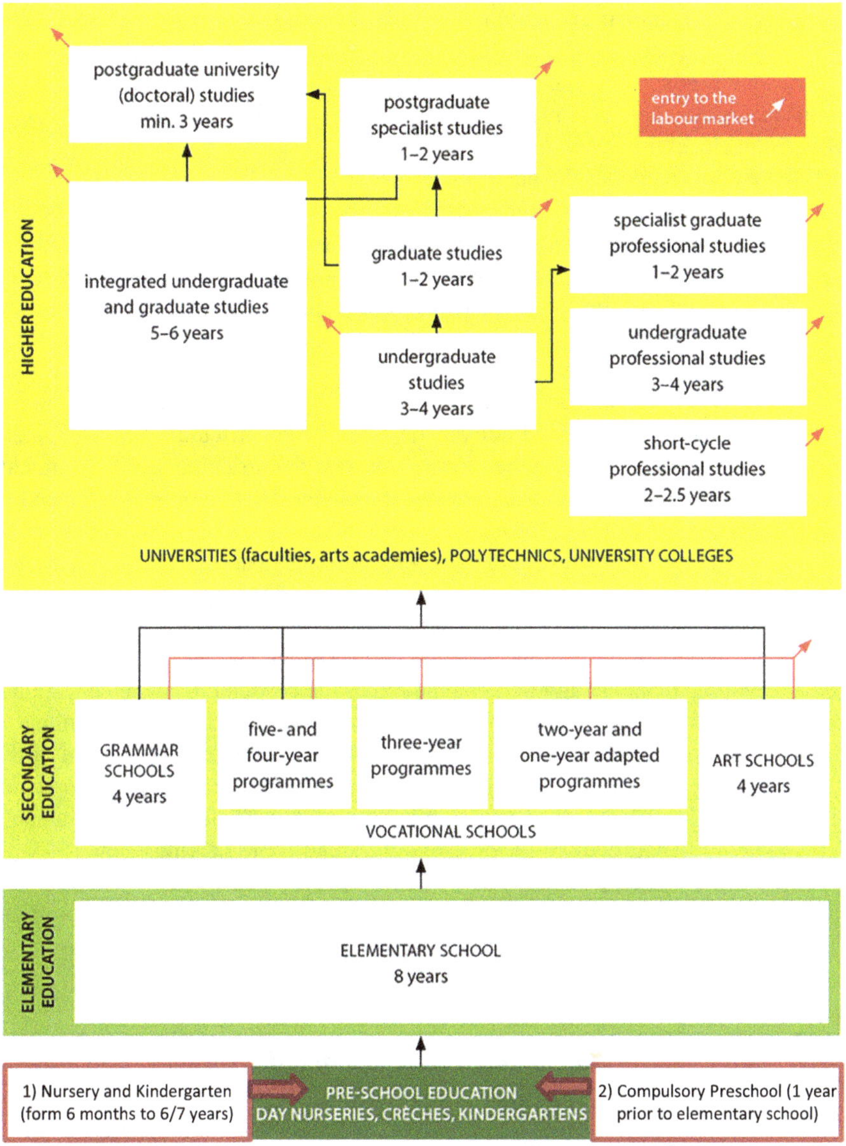

Fig. 7.1 Schematic overview of the entire education system in Croatia. *Source* https://croatia.eu/index.php?view=article&id=35&lang=2

consist of: the National curriculum for early and preschool care and education; the National curriculum for primary school education; the National curriculum for vocational education; the National curriculum for high school education; the National curriculum for art education (https://mzo.gov.hr/istaknute-teme/odgoj-i-obrazovanje/nacionalni-kurikulum/125).

National documents of the curriculum area determine the purpose, goals, structure, and educational expectations related to learning and teaching in wider educational areas. Curriculum area documents directly influence the creation of subject and modular curricula. In accordance with the National Framework Curriculum, the national documents of the curriculum area at the primary and secondary levels are: the Document of the language and communication area of the curriculum; the Document of the mathematical area of the curriculum; the Document of the natural science area of the curriculum; the Document of the technical and IT area of the curriculum; the Document of the social and humanistic area of the curriculum; the Document of the artistic curriculum areas; the Physical and health curriculum areas document. Educational expectations in curriculum area documents are determined at the end of individual educational cycles. National curricula of cross-curricular topics determine the purpose, goals, structure, educational expectations, learning and teaching, and evaluation of a specific cross-curricular topic at the primary and secondary levels through different ways and forms of educational work, whereby some of them are directly incorporated into the national subject curricula, while some are realized through the planning and implementation of the curriculum of the educational institution. National curricula of cross-curricular topics include: the Curriculum of the cross-curricular topic Personal and Social Development; the Curriculum of the cross-curricular topic Health (its domains are: physical health, mental and social health, help and self-help); the Curriculum of the cross-curricular topic Sustainable Development; the Curriculum of the cross-curricular topic Learning how to learn; the Curriculum of the cross-curricular topic Entrepreneurship; the Curriculum of the cross-curricular topic Use of Information and Communication Technology; the Curriculum of the cross-curricular topic topics Civic upbringing and education.

7.2.1 Socio-Emotional Learning as a Part of Croatian National Curriculum

Socio-emotional learning is recognized as part of the cross-curricular subject area within Croatia's educational reform initiative, School for Life (https://skolazazivot.hr/medupredmetne-teme/). Cross-curricular topics are topics of universal human values and competencies for life in the twenty-first century and, as such, are present in a special way on a daily basis in the educational work of the entire educational vertical. Interdisciplinary topics are realized by interconnecting educational areas and teaching topics of all subjects. The European Framework of Reference emphasizes that the competencies acquired during compulsory education are not limited to specific subjects but are connected to broader cross-curricular objectives, serving as a bridge between formal education and lifelong learning. Each of the mentioned cross-curricular topics is determined by the legally adopted curricula of cross-curricular topics. Curricula of cross-curricular topics are developed according to common guidelines. Each of the seven curricula of cross-curricular topics is organized by five educational cycles and domains: three cycles in primary school and two cycles in secondary school. Within each educational cycle and domain, educational expectations are listed and they are elaborated by stating the necessary knowledge, skills, and attitudes. All set expectations can be realized by different methods and forms of educational work within each individual subject or within joint class or school projects. It is important to emphasize that all subject teachers and professional associates participate in planning the realization of educational expectations of all interdisciplinary topics. Collaborative planning is recommended in order to achieve all the topics as comprehensively as possible in individual educational cycles. This means that it is necessary to achieve the educational expectations of all interdisciplinary topics through all subjects. Within each subject, the interdisciplinary topics that align closely with its content and learning outcomes will be addressed. Collaborative planning among all teachers and professional associates ensures the integration of all interdisciplinary topics throughout each educational cycle. The richness of educational expectations of interdisciplinary topics gives the opportunity to connect with the educational outcomes of each subject, considering the specifics of each student, as well as individual class communities. The implementation of all educational expectations related to interdisciplinary topics has been mandatory since the 2019/2020 school year in all grades of both primary and secondary schools. Cross-curricular theme *Personal and social development* encourages the holistic development of children and young people into healthy, creative, self-confident, productive, satisfied, and responsible persons who contribute to the community through mutual cooperation and action. The prominent values of this cross-curricular theme are knowledge, identity, integrity, entrepreneurship, respect, responsibility, and solidarity. This cross-curricular theme includes the development of responsible behavior and care for personal health and quality of life as well as the quality of relationships with others within the community. Educational expectations within the interdisciplinary topic of *Personal and Social Development* are divided into three domains: *Me and Society*, *Me and Others*, and *Me*. This division is visually represented in the graphical illustration of the domains (Fig. 7.2). Within this topic, students will develop a wide range of personal and social competencies. These include self-image, self-esteem, and self-confidence; the ability to recognize, accept, and manage their emotions and behavior; empathy, appreciation of diversity, and respect for others; as well as social and communication skills. Students will also strengthen their capacity for collaboration and teamwork, demonstrate responsible behavior toward themselves and others in the community, and enhance their decision-making and educational planning skills. Furthermore, the topic supports the development of lifelong learning habits, preparation for professional growth in modern society and the world of work, and the acquisition of problem-solving strategies and effective stress management techniques.

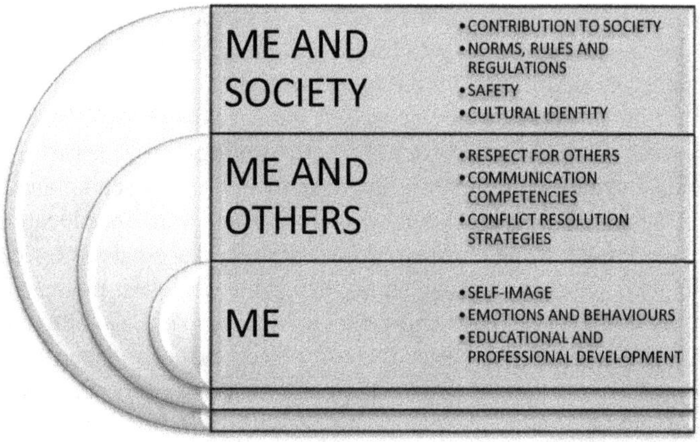

Fig. 7.2 Graphical representation of domains in the interdisciplinary topic Personal and social development

The National curriculum for preschool education, primary and secondary education in Croatia (2011: 17, http://mzos.hr/datoteke/Nacionalni_okvirni_kurikulum.pdf) identifies eight key competencies for lifelong learning. These are: competency in the mother tongue; competency in foreign languages; mathematical competency and basic competencies in science and technology; digital competence; learning to learn; social and civic competence; initiative and entrepreneurship; and cultural awareness and expression. Social and emotional competencies, which are essential for the socio-emotional wellbeing of children and youth, are explicitly emphasized in the National Curriculum for Early and Preschool Education (2015).

In general, it includes: personal, emotional and physical, educational, and social wellbeing of the child, which refers to the subjective feeling of health, satisfaction, and wellbeing. Personal, emotional, and physical wellbeing includes: development of motor skills; adoption of hygienic, dietary and movement habits as prerequisites for health; enjoying different interactions and activities; the child's openness to the world around him and to new experiences; calmness (absence of feelings of threat, restlessness, concern); self-acceptance of the child (not suppressing emotions, self-acceptance); self-esteem and self-awareness of the child; the ability to temporarily postpone meeting one's needs; development of the child's identity (personal and social); the readiness of the child to make decisions related to his activities; development of independent thinking and action; assessing the possible consequences of one's actions, that is, considering the way of their realization; initiative and innovation of the child; self-initiation and self-organization of own activities; and reflection and self-assessment of one's own activities and achievements. In addition, social wellbeing refers to successful interpersonal (social) functioning and development of social competencies, and includes: understanding and acceptance of others and their differences (arising from religious, racial, national, cultural and other differences or special needs); compliance with patterns, rules, norms and requirements of the social group/community; establishment, development and maintenance of quality relationships of the child with other children and adults; active participation, negotiation and constructive resolution of conflict situations; joint (coordinated) action of the child with others (children and adults); ethics, solidarity and tolerance of the child in communication with others; the ability of the child to adapt to new, changing situations and circumstances (flexibility and adaptability); the perception of oneself as an important part of the community/environment; feeling of acceptance and belonging; the perception of oneself as a member of the community who has the opportunity and opportunities to contribute to the community; responsible behavior of the child toward themselves and others.

The Croatian Ministry of Science and Education (https://mzo.gov.hr/en) is responsible for implementing school curricula. While local and regional governments serve as the founders of primary and secondary schools, they do not have the authority to intervene in the official curricula. However, they can support and implement extracurricular activities. Children with special needs have their teaching assistants and they are provided with food and transport. Children with a lower social and economic status are entitled to scholarships; free kindergartens; free extended stay at school; and free meals. Children from national minorities have access to educational programs in their minority languages, which support the preservation and cultivation of their language and cultural identity. In addition, cooperation with minority associations is constantly developing. Within the legal framework and policy of mental health protection, the Healthcare Act defines the principles and measures of healthcare, the rights and obligations of individuals when accessing healthcare services, the responsibilities of social welfare institutions in relation to public health, and the content and organization of healthcare activities, including their oversight. In 2008, mental health protection was, for the first time, formally recognized as a separate activity within the scope of primary healthcare services. Activities related to mental health care are entrusted to the Croatian Institute for Public Health and it emphasizes the role of psychologists. The National Strategy for the Protection of Mental Health provides guidelines for improving existing approaches and developing new methods for safeguarding mental health. Given that mental health issues in Croatia have been relatively marginalized, there has been a growing need to place greater emphasis on mental health within the national healthcare system. The envisioned mental health care system aimed to be significantly more effective than the traditional psychiatric model, with which it should function complementarily. It was intended to contribute more meaningfully to improving community mental health, preventing mental disorders, detecting at-risk populations early, and promoting the role of psychological and other non-pharmacological treatments. Achieving the goals and expectations expressed in the national curricula of cross-curricular topics is mandatory at all levels and in all types of education. Goals and expectations are realized and National Health Care Strategy 2012–2020 revealed data on mental disorders that contribute to the total hospital morbidity in Croatia with the share of about 7%. In addition, stress disorder (PTSD), as individual diagnostic categories, represent almost two thirds of all causes of hospital morbidity due to mental disorders. In hospital morbidity, there is a trend of increasing hospitalization rate per 100,000 inhabitants, especially concerning depressive disorders. Mortality rates due to suicide in Croatia have been continuously decreasing since 1998; however, they are still higher than in the "old" EU member states. The Croatian Institute for Public Health has several major role, including: Mental health protection (promotion, prevention, early recognition and treatment and rehabilitation of behavioral and mental disorders); Mental health promotion (activities on understanding mental health and raising awareness of the importance of mental health as part of general health, promoting good mental health and wellbeing, understanding mental health problems and mental disorders, combating stigma and discrimination; Activities that improve mental health through the strengthening of protective factors and by reducing the harming factors; effective promotion measures that result in better quality of life, better social functioning, better social inclusion, reduced human suffering, lower incidence and prevalence of mental disorders); Counseling aimed at protecting the mental health of children and adolescents (family counseling, counseling for school children and adolescents for healthy growth and better fit into the society; counseling and educational work with preschool and school staff teachers on healthy growth; participation in the implementation of health education); Preservation of mental health in children and adolescents with risky behaviors (counseling and care for those exhibiting high-risk behavior or experiencing stress. The goal is to enhance their ability to overcome the crisis situation, adapt to new circumstances, and prevent the occurrence of mental disorder; educational work with teaching staff of preschool and school institutions related to recognition and work with children and adolescents at increased risk); Early detection, diagnosis, and therapy of children and adolescents with behavioral disorders and mental health problems (sensitizing and educating primary health care for early detection of behavioral disorders and mental health problems; educating teachers in order to identify early behavioral disorders and mental health problems for children and adolescents; counseling, individual and group therapy for children and adolescents with behavior disorders and mental health problems; treatment and rehabilitation; involving the family in the therapeutic process).

7.2.2 Evidence-Based Preventive Programs Regarding Children's Psychological Wellbeing in Croatia

RESCUR is a response to numerous challenges faced by many children in Europe, such as cultural, social, and economic challenges. This program is actually "*a resilience curriculum for early and primary school schools in Europe to foster the academic, emotional and social learning of children who may be at risk of early school leaving, absenteeism, school failure, social exclusion and mental health problems amongst others, by providing them with the key tools to overcome the disadvantages and obstacles in their development whilst making use of their strengths*" (Cefai et al., 2015: 3). Through this curriculum, children are provided with key tools to help them overcome developmental obstacles and challenges by drawing on their personal strengths. It equips them with the skills needed to address various forms of adversity, including poverty, family stress, discrimination, general or peer violence, unemployment, and social exclusion. By providing opportunities and support to overcome such challenges, one invests in building future generations of resilient European citizens. The goals of the curriculum are: Developing and improving children's social and emotional learning and their resilience; Encouraging healthy relationships and positive and prosocial behavior of children; Encouraging mental health and children's wellbeing, especially children exposed to the risk of social exclusion; Improving children's academic engagement, motivation, and learning. The most important feature of this curriculum is the development of resilience through storytelling, which provides children with the opportunity to express their thoughts and feelings on specific topics. The implementation of the curriculum involves the active participation of children, parents, and preschool or primary school teachers. Through the storytelling approach, teachers can gain insight into their own behavior and reflect on it, allowing them to apply what they have learned to their personal and professional lives. The main characters in the stories for children of early and preschool age and for younger elementary school students are the squirrel Sherlock and the hedgehog Zelda. At the beginning of the activity, educators should present Sherlock and Zelda as rag dolls or finger corners. Throughout the story, it is recommended to introduce dialogues that facilitate the use of puppets, and the story itself can be transformed into a play in which children play the main roles. Building on the activity, children can create their own stories and act them out.

RULER stands for:**R**ecognizing, **U**nderstanding, **L**abelling, **E**xpressing, **R**egulating emotions (Brackett et al., 2013) and presents an acronym for the five skills of emotional intelligence. When recognizing emotions, the most important question is "*How do you feel?*" in order to become aware and recognize what we feel. Understanding emotions involves recognizing how we feel and gaining insight into why we feel that way. Naming emotions refers to understanding the complexity of the feelings we feel. We need to ask ourselves why we feel happy, sad, or angry and dig further and deeper to identify the complexity of the feeling we are feeling. Expressing emotions refers to the fact that we must first express our emotions and feelings to ourselves, and only then properly express them to other people. Emotion regulation refers to the way we deal with our emotions. We must not ignore or suppress them, but we should know how to use them wisely in order to achieve the desired goals (Brackett, 2019). The RULER program teaches emotional intelligence skills. Decades of research have shown that these skills are essential for effective teaching and learning, sound decision-making, physical and mental health, and success both in and beyond the classroom. RULER principles and tools are incorporated into day-care and community policies and practices, including mission statements, curricula and programs, staff professional development, facility improvement plans, discipline policies, and behavior support plans. Additionally, educators learn strategies for recognizing children's emotions and adapting their educational plans accordingly (Program Guide, RULER Approach, https://pg.casel.org/ruler-approach/). By involving all staff—educators, administrators, children, and families—RULER becomes an integrated part of daily life within an educational institution, rather than an add-on that may fade over time. The development of these five RULER skills relies on four core tools: the Mood Meter (children can draw on a mood meter to express how they're feeling), Meta-Moment (children learn to "press the pause bump" before responding to a trigger), and Blueprint (a problem-solving tool that helps children cope with conflicts). In early childhood and elementary school, RULER is embedded into existing academic curricula. Middle and high school content focuses on the intersection of social, emotional, and cognitive aspects of early and late adolescence. Validation studies indicate that the RULER program results in the development of emotional and interpersonal skills, a more positive classroom climate, and better student grades (Brackett et al., 2013).

PATHS—Promoting Alternative Thinking Strategies—is a social and emotional learning curriculum designed to support children in kindergarten through sixth grade to manage their behavior, understand their emotions, and work well with others. The program consists of a series of lessons covering topics such as recognizing and labelling feelings, controlling impulses, reducing stress, and understanding other people's perspectives. This curriculum is implemented through thirty-five to forty lessons per year and is supplemented with activities that support the application of newly acquired skills throughout the day within the educational institution, as well as take-home activities for parents. It is based on the ABCD (Affective—Behavioral—Cognitive—Dynamic) model of development, which gives primary importance to the developmental connection of behavior, affect, and cognitive understanding as they relate to social and emotional competence. The basic premise of PATHS is the belief that children's adjustment is a function of their skill level and the environmental context they live in. Emphasis is placed not only on teaching skills but also on creating meaningful, real-life opportunities for students to generalize those skills, promoting optimal internalization of concepts through practical application (Domitrovich et al., 2007). Furthermore, the PATHS curriculum also uses Feeling Face cards, which contain the four basic emotions: happiness, sadness, fear, and anger. Through the use of these cards, children are encouraged to talk about emotions and learn to understand them. At the core of the PATHS curriculum is psychoanalytic theory, which emphasizes respect for each child's integrity while encouraging active participation and interaction in the learning process. In other words, this curriculum does not aim to teach or condition children to conform to the external expectations of adults, but instead provides the conditions that will result in optimal internal integration, personality maturation, and cognitive growth. Children are encouraged to be aware of and express their emotions rather than suppress them to promote developmental integration. Jones et al. (2021) state that the PATHS program is primarily based on the emotional domain, and the secondary emphasis is on the social and cognitive domains. This program primarily uses the discussion method in instruction, followed by didactic teaching, visual displays, and social-emotional learning tools, while role-playing is used the least. Discussions usually start with a short introduction, followed by a discussion of the entire educational group led by the educator. Also, many lessons use group posters, for example, the Controlled Forces poster, which serves as a visual reminder and reinforcement of lesson strategies. The main features of this program are: Group activities outside the basic lessons; Supportive climate and culture; Applications for time outside of school; Flexibility and adaptability of the program; and Professional development and training. Within the framework of its implementation, it is crucial to ensure: support for implementation; tools for evaluating program outcomes: tools for evaluating implementation; family involvement; community engagement; and fair and inclusive education. In Croatia, Josipa Bašić and colleagues from the Education and Rehabilitation Faculty in Croatia have been developing and implementing PATHS within the project "Communities that care—development, implementation, and evaluation of the model of prevention within the community" since 2002. The program was conducted by preschool and primary school teachers on a weekly basis in educational groups or in the classroom. The project started in 2010 in collaboration with scientists from Penn State University. The primary goal of the PATHS-RASTEM project is to implement PATHS in 6 preschools and 15 primary schools in Zagreb, Rijeka, and Istria (Novak et al., 2017). Based on a rigorous evaluation of a social-emotional learning curriculum conducted in 29 schools ($N = 568$ children), results showed significant changes in eight out of nine targeted behaviors among lower-risk children. This study highlights the need to supplement universal preventive interventions with selective preventive interventions that can provide more intensive and targeted skill practice for higher risk children.

Fostering social and emotional learning in kindergartens (KA220-BE-23-36-157220) is an Erasmus + project co-financed by the Erasmus + program under Key Action 220: Cooperation between organizations and institutions. Since previous research and educational practice confirm that social and emotional skills can be taught, and given that not all kindergartens have access to high-quality programs and materials in this area, it is essential to enhance opportunities for the continuous and systematic development of children's social and emotional competencies within institutional settings. Based on this need, eight organizations from different countries are collaborating on this international project. All participating organizations believe that kindergartens are capable of fully integrating social-emotional learning (SEL) into their educational practice. They should have access to high-quality, freely available materials and a variety of approaches to the topic, allowing them to choose the method best suited to their institution and specific groups of children. This project aims to develop an effective program and materials for the improvement of social-emotional competencies in kindergartens and thus contribute to a higher quality preschool education that focuses on a holistic approach to children by encouraging all their developmental domains (Tatalović Vorkapić et al., 2024). Also, the aim of the project is to scientifically evaluate the impact of the newly applied SEL-program in kindergartens, based on the LifeComp model (Caena & Punie, 2019), which emphasizes its core elements: personal, social, and learning to learn competencies. The project runs from October 1, 2023 to September 30, 2026. The project leader is Studio Gaus GmbH, an organization based in Berlin, Germany, dedicated to the improvement of education and culture. In addition to Germany, which is also represented by the partner organization Deutsche Liga für das Kind e.V., three other countries are participating in the project. From Slovenia, the partners are Inter-kulturo d.o.o. and Kindergarten Tezno Maribor. Italy is represented by Università degli Studi di Perugia and IC Montecastrilli. From Croatia, the participating institutions are the

Faculty of Teacher Education at the University of Rijeka and Kindergarten Pčelica in Zagreb.

A Box Full of Feelings (Kog & Moons, 2008) presents the application of simple drawings that show a certain situation, accompanied by a simple text of a short story. They can serve as an excellent foundation for questions in the field of encouraging emotional literacy in preschool and school children. The questions serve as a framework for creating a discussion within a group or class. Preschool and primary school teachers can make drawings and a story together with children/students. The main aim of this material is to support children's socio-emotional development. It is intended for children aged 2 to 7 to recognize their inner emotions and talk about them openly. There are twenty different interactive procedures for use in working with a group of children or individually. Using the box children can explore four basic emotions—happy, sad, angry, and scared—and the way they recognize, name, accept, and develop awareness of them. Being able to express and control emotions in an acceptable way is the foundation of developing emotional intelligence, building resilience, and helping children stay composed when faced with painful experiences. The results of applying the *Box full of feelings* in practice are: children are more careful in expressing their feelings, they have a richer vocabulary in expressing emotions, their intuition is more refined and the ability to experience other people's emotions is increased. The material contains 48 picture cards—12 for each emotion, with a short story and questions; 16 pictures illustrating 4 emotions; 4 posters; 17 finger puppets; 4 masks; 4 portable houses with emotions; emotion wheel (for games); CD with meditative music; activity manual; and a cardboard box for storage.

PROMEHS (Promoting Mental Health at Schools) could be perceived as a high-quality response to existing programs diversity in Croatia. It was created within the international Erasmus + KA3 project PROMEHS: Promoting Mental Health in Schools. It was led by University of Milano-Bicocca, Italy, and lasted three years (2019–2022). Project partners were members of the academic community, practitioners, and policy makers from six additional countries: Croatia, Greece, Latvia, Malta, Portugal, and Romania. The theoretical framework of the curriculum project includes three important areas that relate to all age groups of children, namely the promotion of resilience, the promotion of social-emotional learning, and the prevention of social, emotional, and behavioral difficulties. The goals of this project were: to provide a systematic theoretical framework for the development and implementation of a universal mental health curriculum based on research results in kindergartens and schools and to provide high-quality education for kindergarten and school teachers; improve the mental health of children and young people as well as preschool teachers and primary and secondary school teachers; provide the best practical advice and instructions to school and kindergarten employees, parents, legislators and others on how to promote mental health in schools and kindergartens; integrate the PROMEHS curriculum into national education and health policies; to promote innovation within educational policy in cooperation with national and international bodies of public authorities; develop an evidence-based curriculum with the aim of promoting positive mental health in schools and kindergartens. In the mentioned three-year period, more than 10,000 students from six different countries were included in the PROMEHS implementation. The conducted quasi-experimental research design, in general, determined a significant positive effect of the influence of the PROMEHS curriculum on the socio-emotional learning and resilience of children and students, as well as teachers, and a significant reduction of behavioral difficulties in children and students (Cefai et al., 2022a, 2022b). This validates the PROMEHS curriculum as a systematic template for the development and implementation of an evidence-based general mental health curriculum in schools and institutions for early and preschool education, including high-quality teacher education, meetings, manuals, and guidelines for school staff, students, parents, and holders of educational policies. Also, PROMEHS, with the participation of the entire school, recognizes the importance of improving living conditions and environments that support mental health within the context of the institution, enabling children, institution staff, families and communities to adopt and maintain optimal emotional functioning (Cefai et al., 2022a, 2022b). The curriculum was implemented by trained teachers, and included activities aimed at strengthening self-awareness, self-regulation, social awareness, responsible decision-making, interpersonal skills, and social understanding. In the context of Croatian culture and the implementation of PROMEHS in 32 educational institutions, the results have demonstrated a significant positive impact of the PROMEHS curriculum on the mental health of children, youth, and teachers. This success was achieved through the effective synergy of the academic community, educational practitioners, and policy representatives. Given the significant positive impact of the PROMEHS curriculum on the mental health of children, youth, and educators, it was concluded that the Croatian Ministry of Science and Education will support the introduction of the PROMEHS curriculum as a universal prevention program in all kindergartens and schools across Croatia. With this in mind, PROMEHS is prepared to be launched as a lifelong learning program at the Faculty of Teacher Education in Rijeka, and after completing the necessary training, all interested teachers will be able to implement the PROMEHS curriculum in their institutions. This final step was initiated through a new, one-year university project, which is currently ongoing, with the launch of a lifelong learning program planned for March 2024 under the title Educational Work for the Enhancement of Mental Health and Wellbeing. In this way, the sustainability of the PROMEHS curriculum is ensured by enabling the continued implementation of its principles in educational practice. Although PROMEHS has proven to be a promising universal mental health program—both in Croatia and in other partner countries—for early childhood, primary, and secondary education in Europe, particularly in enhancing children's social and emotional competencies, promoting prosocial behavior, reducing internalized and externalized behaviors, and strengthening the sense of self-efficacy and resilience of preschool, primary school and secondary school teachers, questions remain about its overlap with existing cross-curricular topics in the Croatian education system. In other words, how can PROMEHS be systematically implemented in schools, and how should existing overlaps be addressed within Croatia's already burdened education system? The research question, methodology, and findings related to this issue are presented in the following text.

7.3 Study Aim

Building on the theoretical background related to wellbeing, socio-emotional learning, and children's mental health—as well as the contextualization of the Croatian education system and related programs—the main aim of this chapter is twofold: (a) to present the results of a qualitative analysis of educational and preventive programs and methodologies addressing mental health currently implemented within the Croatian education system; and (b) to present the results of a quantitative analysis of teachers' perspectives on the sustainability of the PROMEHS curriculum, particularly its potential for integration into the education system, with a focus on alignment with cross-curricular themes in schools.

By presenting a more holistic and systematic program—namely, PROMEHS—as a potential solution to the fragmentation of preventive programs likely to be identified in the analysis, the second part of the results will focus on a quantitative analysis of teachers' responses concerning the feasibility of implementing PROMEHS and its overlap with intra-curricular subjects in Croatian schools.

7.4 Results

7.4.1 Educational and Preventive Programs and Methodologies on Mental Health in Croatia

According to the National Office for Drug Abuse Prevention of Croatia (http://www.programi.uredzadroge.hr/), there are currently 262 educational programs in Croatia aimed at promoting and preventing mental health issues among children. However, only 79 of these programs are actually implemented in educational institutions such as kindergartens, primary schools, and secondary schools. In kindergartens (for children aged 6 months to 6/7 years), 3 programs are designed for preschool children, 2 for their parents, and 1 for preschool teachers. In primary schools (for children aged 6/7 to 13/14 years), 30 programs target primary school children, 11 are intended for their parents, and 1 is aimed at primary school teachers. In secondary schools (for students aged 14/15 to 17/18 years), 24 programs are developed for students, 6 for their parents, and 1 for secondary school teachers.

7.4.1.1 Kindergartens

None of the educational programs have been implemented in kindergartens in Primorje-Gorski Kotar County, which is noteworthy given that this county will serve as the target sample for the upcoming project research. In other counties, the program "Where Are You From, Child?" ("Oklen si dite?") has been implemented. This program focuses on promoting the importance of early childhood development and family values through the active involvement of adults—particularly parents, educators, and expert associates. Its activities include lectures for parents aimed at fostering cultural heritage and traditional customs, as well as raising public awareness about access to public health services. The program is intended for early childhood educators, children in early and preschool age groups, and their parents. *The Youth for youth in the prevention and elimination of addiction* project is also being applied. This project educates young people (students), who in turn have to educate their peers about healthy lifestyles in the context of drug addiction prevention; it also targets children of early and preschool age and their parents. The National Office for Drug Abuse Prevention also applies the Program on drugs and addiction issues across the country, which aims to inform and sensitize the public, with activities targeted at all levels of the education system.

7.4.1.2 Primary Schools

The School Preventive Program (SPP) is designed for children from first to eighth grade and is implemented through the education of teachers and parents. Its primary goals are the prevention of addiction and violence, as well as the promotion of health and civic education. The program focuses on enhancing problem-solving abilities, improving self-image, supporting decision-making and social integration, and increasing motivation for healthy lifestyles. It targets school teachers, parents of school children, and children from 6 to 11 years old. Other programs applied in primary schools are Open Umbrella (focuses on educating children in 6th grade and their parents; drug abuse prevention), Healthy Living (targets first through eighth grade students and their parents; strengthening of self-confidence, social skills and the positive self-image), Cyberbullying (dangers of the Internet, targets sixth grade students and their parents), Emica (development of emotional intelligence through games, emotional adaptation, and preservation of the students' mental health; targets school children and their parents), SPARK (Strengthening Parents' Competencies for Harmonization of Private and Professional Life), SPARK PLUS (strengthening of parents' competencies, prevention of emotional abuse and neglect during divorce), LA(R)A-CHAIN (RE)ACTION (workshops with the aim of developing social skills: getting to know, listening to, recognizing, and expressing feelings, empathy and compassion, and controlling anger; targets students and their parents), Youth for youth in the prevention and elimination of addiction (same as for kindergartens, described previously), Positive Mom, Positive Dad! (the overall objective is to empower parents in carrying out their parental responsibilities and capacities with an emphasis on the prevention of addiction, that is, the improvement of parental skills; improvement of parental competence; educating parents about the importance of and the way to achieve quality communication in the family; establishing and encouraging better relationships within the family; neutralizing risk factors in families; sensitization of parents to recognize the needs of the child and its positive potential), Positive parenting program Sunflower—Universal prevention of Addiction (involves working with children and parents, co-operating with the school and the local community for the prevention and suppression of alcohol and smoking addiction and addiction to psychoactive substances in children and young people; targets fifth-grade students and their parents).

Programs that focus exclusively on educating the children include:

- Totally Healthy (prosocial behavior, socio-emotional skills, drug abuse prevention; targets eighth-grade students),
- Early recognition of risk behavior in youth (aimed at emotional and communication difficulties; seventh-grade students),
- Life Skills Training (prevention of behavioral disorders and addiction; includes workshops on: self-esteem, decision-making, smoking, media influence, anxiety, coping with stress, confronting anger, assertiveness, communication skills, social skills, conflict resolution, peer pressure, smoking addiction, alcohol addiction, marijuana addiction; aimed at third to eighth-grade students),
- For a better world without violence (prevention of violence),
- Knowledge against addiction (development of social skills and creative socialization groups),
- Be brave and say no to tobacco (smoking prevention, targets fifth to eighth-grade students),
- Quality free time utilization (introduction of a series of extracurricular activities),
- Affirmation of positive values against violence and addiction (individual approach gives the possibility of self-realization, which increases self-esteem and reduces auto destruction),
- Fairytale Games (through children's psychodrama, which children themselves create, socio-emotional development of children is enhanced),
- Benjamin (prevention of computer addiction, targets fifth-grade students),
- Be independent, be yourself (communication and social skills development, free time, and prevention of addiction),
- Magic recipes for health and happiness (prevention of addiction, organization of free time, healthy lifestyle),
- Internet Security Day (prevention of cyberbullying via the Internet and mobile phones, targets fifth to eighth-grade students),
- Children and Media (development of critical thinking toward the media),
- Health through education (an integral part of education, development of life skills, positive thinking, critical thinking, prevention of addiction; first to eighth-grade students),
- Electronic violence and addiction (prevention of peer-to-peer violence over the Internet, prevention of Internet addiction),
- Apple (promotion of healthy and prevention of unhealthy behaviors with a focus on smoking),
- You are not alone (prevention of violence among children and youth via the Internet and social networks; fifth-grade students),
- Encouraging positive development of children via emotional literacy (the adoption of fundamental emotional knowledge and understanding (Maurer et al.,

2004); children learn to name, compare, evaluate their own opinions, feelings in comparison to the behavior of others),
- Preventive programs-miscellaneous activities (Prevention of addiction through lectures and workshops by professors, expert associates, and police officers),
- Program of prevention of risk behavior (developing feelings of own value, strengthening self-confidence, recognizing, understanding, and expressing feelings in an acceptable way, learning conflict resolution in non-violent ways, developing behavioral responsiveness, cooperation, tolerance, accepting diversity, improving communication skills, helping parents in their children's education through individual conversations and interactive lectures),
- Programs of health and social protection of pupils-informative-educational characteristics - Health Education (implementation of the Health education curriculum in primary and secondary schools through contents integrated in existing curricula: Nature, Nature and Society, Biology, Physical and Health Culture, Psychology-and separate classes),
- Development of social skills (the program aims to further develop and strengthen the social skills that pupils have learned in the previous class, thereby increasing the likelihood of adoption and application in everyday life).

7.4.1.3 Secondary Schools

Education program for professors on the prevention of addiction (EPPPA) is a seminar for secondary school teachers focused on acquiring knowledge and adopting practical skills needed for prevention of addiction and addictive behaviors in young people. Other programs that are applied in secondary schools are:

- SPARK (Strengthening Parents' Competencies for Harmonization of Private and Professional Life; targets parents),
- SPARK Plus (targets parents; aims to strengthen parents' competencies and prevent emotional abuse and neglect during divorce),
- Youth for Youth in the prevention and elimination of addiction (same as for kindergartens and primary schools, as described before; targets students and parents as well),
- New Addictions: Watch out for gambling!—Betting isn't a game (targets parents and students; includes workshops with students on "new addictions"; aims to sensitize, inform and educate about gambling/betting risks and ways of preventing addiction development), Positive mom, positive dad (same as for primary schools),
- Skretničar III-Switchman (targets parents and students; provides support regarding the mental and psychophysical health of adolescents and promotes healthy lifestyles; consists of workshops, lectures, advisory support, marking of important dates).

Programs that target students exclusively are:

- Gornjogradska Higschool Activities (it's goal is gambling/betting and drug abuse prevention, tolerance and accepting differences),

- Be Cool, Be Strong (positive self-image and self-respect),
- The Strongest Stance (drug abuse prevention),
- No, because no (targets 1st graders; drug abuse prevention), Early discovery of risk behavior in youth (targets first-graders; emotional and communicational difficulties),
- Testing for psychoactive substances in schools (throughout high school), Healthy (developments of healthy habits, targets first-graders),
- Be informed, be active (developing responsibility for oneself, social skills, decision-making, resisting social influences, preventing addiction; targets students),
- 3PO-Trust-Connection-Support (promotion of healthy lifestyles, prevention of addiction and violence, development of communication skills),
- Affirmation of positive values against violence and addiction (individual approach gives the possibility of self-realization which increases self-esteem and reduces auto destruction),
- Gain in favor of loss (prevention of gambling; targets second-grade students),
- EVO (development and promotion of volunteering and inclusion in volunteering),
- Games of chance in photo finish (prevention of gambling and betting; targets first-graders),
- I have a stance, I choose health (smoking prevention; targets first-graders),
- Young men initiative—H-Hommen program (developing responsibility), Internet addiction and the youth (prevention of Internet addiction),
- Construction of the community by rhythm and sound-Drumming therapy workshops (development of fine and crude motor skills, development of visual-motor coordination, exercise of concentration, attention and memory, alleviation of emotional and psychological difficulties, development of discipline, and respect for behavioral rules),
- Strengthening life skills (consists of a set of workshops that are conducted in home-room classes; affirmation of positive values and strengthening of self-esteem/self-confidence of students, self-assessment and assessment of others; strengthening of communication skills),
- How to resist bad influences? Totally Healthy (carried out through psychological workshops through which students learn about the ways to resist negative pressures and stresses; aims to make students aware of the positive goals in life and develop their skills needed to resist peer pressure),
- Prevention of addiction (improves the level of students' knowledge about the dangers of various forms of addiction with an emphasis on alcohol, drugs, smoking, gambling, the Internet, and their impact on the growth and development of young people),
- Programs of health and social protection of pupils-informative-educational characteristics/Health Education (implementation of the Health education curriculum in secondary schools planned through contents integrated in existing curricula and separate classes; aims to better inform the youth on youth related issues regarding health and social protection),

- Project "Healthy Living" (workshops during the school year on the subject prevention of addiction and violent behavior; aims to direct students toward the socially acceptable forms of behavior and raise healthy persons capable of dealing with life problems; promotes healthy lifestyles).

7.4.1.4 Prevention Programs in the Primorje and Gorski Kotar County—Conclusion on the Qualitative Results

A total of 36 prevention programs are currently implemented in primary schools. These include: Healthy for five; Affirmation of positive values; Healthy living youth; All different, all equally worthy; In a healthy body, healthy mind; Addiction Prevention Program "How to cope with bad social pressures"; Violence Prevention Program: Conflict and Communication; Internet Violence Prevention Program; Program for Prevention of Violence in Youth Relations; An addiction prevention program "What do parents need to know about marijuana?"; A lively library; Extracurricular activities of the volunteer core; Mountaineering Group—Extracurricular Activity; Preventive lectures by a school doctor; School sports club GEK; Health Education Program; The Gifted Program; Who's in the mirror: Look at yourself; We live with a smile; Why and how to say NO to alcohol; The second that changes life; Open Door Counseling; 3-PO (trust-connectivity-support); Prevention of Addiction and Promotion of Healthy Living; Promotion of security and public health awareness SAM; School Preventive Programs; Prevention of Violence in Youth Relations; Week of Psychology; Mind the mind; You think you can think; Together against addiction; Youth Initiative; Internet, addiction, youth; The Program of Prevention of Persons' Trafficking; and the Traffic Preventive Program.

In secondary schools, there are 35 preventive programs, including the following: Life skills training; School angels; Small creative socializations' groups; TEEN CAP; Basic CAP; Love on the move; Development of social competencies and non-violent conflict resolution; I can if I want 1 - MAH1; I can if I want 2 - MAH2; Identifying and expressing emotions; Prevention of Violence - Violence through the Internet; Work program with intellectual gifted children; School Preventive Programs; Together we can do more; By affirming positive values against addiction; Development of the model of social pedagogical intervention.

To conclude, the basic aims of programs are: drug abuse prevention, alcohol and smoking prevention, violence prevention, coping strategies, managing peer influence, healthy life styles, organization of free time, creativity, social skills, cyberbullying, positive self-image, self-esteem, parenting skills. Regarding the programs' methodologies, most programs are created based on the examples of good practice from other countries. Some of the programs have been developed as outcomes of projects (such as Erasmus or other international initiatives), while others are based on prior research analyses of risk behaviors among children and families—for example, the Life Skills Training Program. However, only a few of these programs have undergone formal evaluation, with Life Skills Training being one of the exceptions. A key limitation of many of the presented programs is that they are not grounded in fundamental quality principles, such as the whole-school approach, holistic approach, S.A.F.E. (Sequenced, Active, Focused, and Explicit) approach, and an inclusive, systematic framework. In addition, many of these programs focus only on specific aspects of wellbeing and mental health rather than addressing the full spectrum. They often target either students or teachers, but not both. In contrast, PROMEHS simultaneously engages students (from the age of 3 to 18), teachers, and parents. It takes a comprehensive approach by covering all key components of wellbeing and mental health, including socio-emotional learning, resilience, and the prevention of risk behaviors. Even though mental health is one of the main domains within the National Health Strategy in Croatia, there is no universal, evidence-based prevention program that would serve to strengthening all basic aspects of mental health in children and youth. There are many programs that vary in content and methodology, and the majority of them have not been formally evaluated. Some, such as those developed through Erasmus projects, are still in the phases of implementation and evaluation. Within the current theoretical framework, only one program to date—the PROMEHS curriculum—systematically addresses mental health for children aged 3 to 18. It targets key areas such as self-awareness, self-esteem, resilience, motivation, responsible decision-making, relationship skills, social awareness, and self-management. None of the existing programs comprehensively and systematically cover all of these aspects of mental health.

7.4.2 Results on Sustainability of the PROMEHS Curriculum: Possibilities of Implementation in the Croatian Education System

During December 2021 and January 2022, an online survey was conducted with kindergartens and schools that were involved in the implementation of the PROMEHS project, whose goal was to examine attitudes toward the possibilities of integrating the PROMEHS curriculum into existing (pre)school curricula. 74 subjects participated, all female, average age 44.5 years and 19 years of work experience. Respondents from the following cities in Croatia were included (all cities are in Primorje & Gorski Kotar County): Bakar, Crikvenica, Čabar, Čavle, Kastav, Kostrena, Kraljevica, Mali Lošinj, Matulji, Novi Vinodolski, Opatija, Rijeka, Ravna gora, Selce, Tribalj, Vrbovsko. Regarding their profession, subjects were: Pedagogues or psychologists ($N = 7$), school or kindergarten principals ($N = 5$), early childhood educators ($N = 25$), primary school teachers for 1–4 grade ($N = 17$), primary school teachers for 5–8 grade ($N = 10$) and high school teachers ($N = 5$), what can be observed at Fig. 7.3.

The online survey was completely anonymous. Before completing it, participants were provided with the following instruction: *Dear educators, please take five minutes to assess your level of agreement or disagreement with the statements below. They refer to the current state of cross-curricular topics in the educational*

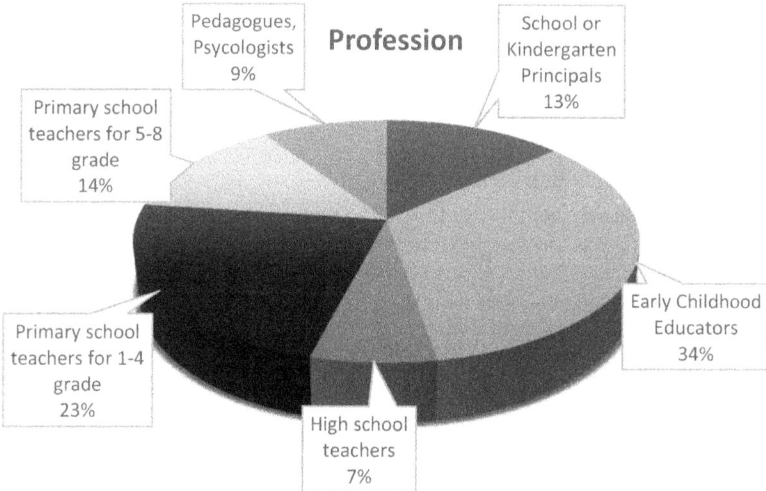

Fig. 7.3 Distribution of participants by profession (in percentages)

curriculum, as well as the opportunities and challenges involved in integrating promotional and preventive programs—particularly the PROMEHS curriculum you may have implemented. The collected data will be used to develop proposals on how to position the role of the PROMEHS curriculum within the existing education system. Your opinion and participation are extremely valuable, and I kindly ask for your engagement. The survey is anonymous, and responses will be analyzed only at the group level. Please be honest and critical, as that is the only way we can work toward meaningful change. I am available for any questions, and I thank you in advance. Feedback on the survey results was shared during the PROMEHS project's Closing National Conference, held in January 2022. (https://www.ufri.uniri.hr/hr/naslovnica/202-hr/promehs/4267-zavrsna.html). The results of the conducted online survey are presented in Table 7.1 and Fig. 7.4. The table shows the response frequencies that indicate the level of agreement with the statements in the survey. Although respondents answered using a 5-point Likert-type scale, for clarity and practicality, the results were grouped into three categories by combining complete and partial (dis)agreement. Figure 7.4 presents the arithmetic means of responses to each statement, which are also displayed in the final column of the accompanying table. The first question in the survey was open-ended and read: *In my opinion and/or experience, the most effective preventive program so far is (insert name).* Considering this, the subjects' answers are: Life skills training (16); PROMEHS (37); CAP program (6); I don't know (10); Solidarity with people with disabilities (1); MAH (1); Violence and addiction prevention programs (1); PATHS program (1); Traffic safety, safety protection programs (2); The existing curriculum is sufficient (1); early intervention (1); and a program only for a specific institution (1). It can be seen that the largest number of respondents mentioned the PROMEHS program, followed by Life Skills Training and the CAP program. Interestingly, 10 respondents reported that they were not aware of which preventive programs related to wellbeing and mental health were being implemented in their school or kindergarten. This is a significant finding, highlighting the need to improve communication and ensure that all educators are informed and actively involved in the implementation of such programs.

Furthermore, as shown in Table 7.1 and Fig. 7.4, participants expressed total and/or partial agreement on the majority of items—specifically, 18 of them. Respondents largely agreed that greater collaboration is needed between practitioners, researchers, and policymakers to support the systematic contribution of kindergartens and schools in promoting the mental health of children, youth, and teachers. They also recognized the importance of implementing preventive programs and emphasized that cross-curricular subjects and preventive initiatives should be better aligned. They also expressed a high level of positive attitudes toward the PROMEHS curriculum for mental health of children from 3 to 18 years of age; in other words that PROMEHS is a quality program characterized by a whole-school and holistic approach. Also, they perceive many advantages of PROMEHS implementation, such as: its flexibility regarding the choice of topics and the methods of implementing them with students; its possibility to work with children from 3 to 18 years of age; its possibility to enhance not only socio-emotional, resilience, and mental health competencies in children but also in teachers; its very high level of methodological-didactical structure and the possibility of including parents in education what implies the continuation of PROMEHS work from kindergarten/school to home. Since pedagogues and psychologists were not directly involved in PROMEHS—serving only as kindergarten and school coordinators—it was noteworthy to observe that participants perceived a need for their more intensive involvement. The suggestion that these professionals should have a defined role in the program will be taken into consideration when planning the further implementation of PROMEHS in Croatia. They agreed with the statement that, in general, preventive programs should be an integral part of the school curriculum. Regarding PROMEHS, they also agreed that it should be integrated in the school curriculum, regardless to cross-curricular subjects and that it should be systematically integrated in schools along with providing training support for teachers involved in the program. Additionally, participants recognized the strength of the PROMEHS program not only in fulfilling its primary purpose, but also in addressing the socio-emotional needs of both children and teachers during the COVID-19 pandemic. They are aware of their competencies, and the lack of competencies in the field of socio-emotional learning, resilience, and prevention of risk behaviors, so they agreed with the fact that they should be educated to apply PROMEHS in their classrooms. Importantly, and in line with the principles of the whole-school approach, participants emphasized the importance of building strong connections and collaboration among all stakeholders involved in the life of a school or kindergarten. They expressed agreement that scientists, practitioners, and policymakers should work together to align different curricula. Additionally, participants recognized the vital role of scientific research in improving educational programs and the education system as a whole. They strongly agreed that program selection should

Table 7.1 Frequencies of responses to survey items by three categories and corresponding means

Items	Complete and partial disagreement	Maybe	Complete and partial agreement	Mean
More collaboration is needed between practitioners, scientists, and policy makers	0	2	72	4.73
It is very important to run preventive programs	0	4	70	4.77
PROMEHS is a quality program	2	3	69	4.55
PROMEHS is holistic	2	3	69	4.54
Cross-curricular subjects and preventive programs should be aligned	0	6	68	4.58
The advantage of PROMEHS is in its flexibility	1	5	68	4.55
The advantage of PROMEHS is work with children from 3 to 18 years of age	0	7	67	4.58
In PROMEHS implementation, pedagogues and psychologists should be included besides teachers	1	6	67	4.55
Teachers should be educated to apply PROMEHS	1	7	66	4.4
The advantage of PROMEHS is in its focus on mental health of students and teachers also	3	5	66	4.5
Scientists, practitioners, and policy makers should align different curriculums	1	8	65	4.59
Preventive programs should be integral part of school curriculum	1	9	64	4.47
PROMEHS should be systematically integrated in schools with training support for teachers	4	6	64	4.39
Choosing programs should be based on their evaluation	2	9	63	4.45
The advantage of PROMEHS is in its methodical-didactic structure	3	8	63	4.17
PROMEHS should be integrated in school curriculum, regardless to cross-curricular subjects	3	9	62	4.36
PROMEHS is a quality program, especially reconsidering the COVID pandemic	5	13	56	4.03
The advantage of PROMEHS is that it includes the work with parents	5	14	55	4.08
There are too many preventive programs	10	14	50	3.78
Various preventive programs are applied in my school	11	22	41	3.72

(continued)

Table 7.1 (continued)

Items	Complete and partial disagreement	Maybe	Complete and partial agreement	Mean
PROMEHS is overlapping with cross-curricular subject Personal and social development	3	42	29	3.4
Cross-curricular subjects are applied consistently in schools	7	39	28	3.32
There are a small number of evidence-based programs	3	46	25	3.43
Preventive programs are not needed due to cross-curricular subjects	32	28	14	2.72
Cross-curricular subjects are enough support for mental health	29	37	8	2.64

be based on evaluations, and that only evidence-based programs should be implemented in schools. Although to a lesser extent, participants expressed agreement with the statement that there are too many preventive programs and that various such programs are implemented in their kindergartens or schools. They showed agreement and disagreement that PROMEHS is overlapping with the cross-curricular subject Personal and social development and that cross-curricular subjects are applied consistently in schools. In addition, participants held rather divergent opinions about the statement that there is a small number of evidence-based programs, as well as the idea that preventive programs are unnecessary due to the existence of cross-curricular subjects. The lowest level of agreement was observed in response to the statement that cross-curricular subjects alone provide sufficient support for mental health. This suggests that, although cross-curricular subjects—particularly Personal and Social Development—theoretically include socio-emotional learning, their practical implementation is not at a satisfactory level. In this context, PROMEHS makes a significant contribution. Ultimately, this provides strong evidence that the development and implementation of the PROMEHS curriculum in Croatian kindergartens and schools represents a major advancement in enhancing educational curricula with high-quality programs focused on wellbeing and mental health for both children and teachers.

7.5 Conclusions

In order for a child to be able to function successfully in their later life and participate in society, they must undergo social-emotional development and learning and thus possess various social-emotional skills and competencies. Through social-emotional learning, children acquire and use knowledge, attitudes, and skills through which they understand and manage emotions, effectively recognize other people's emotions,

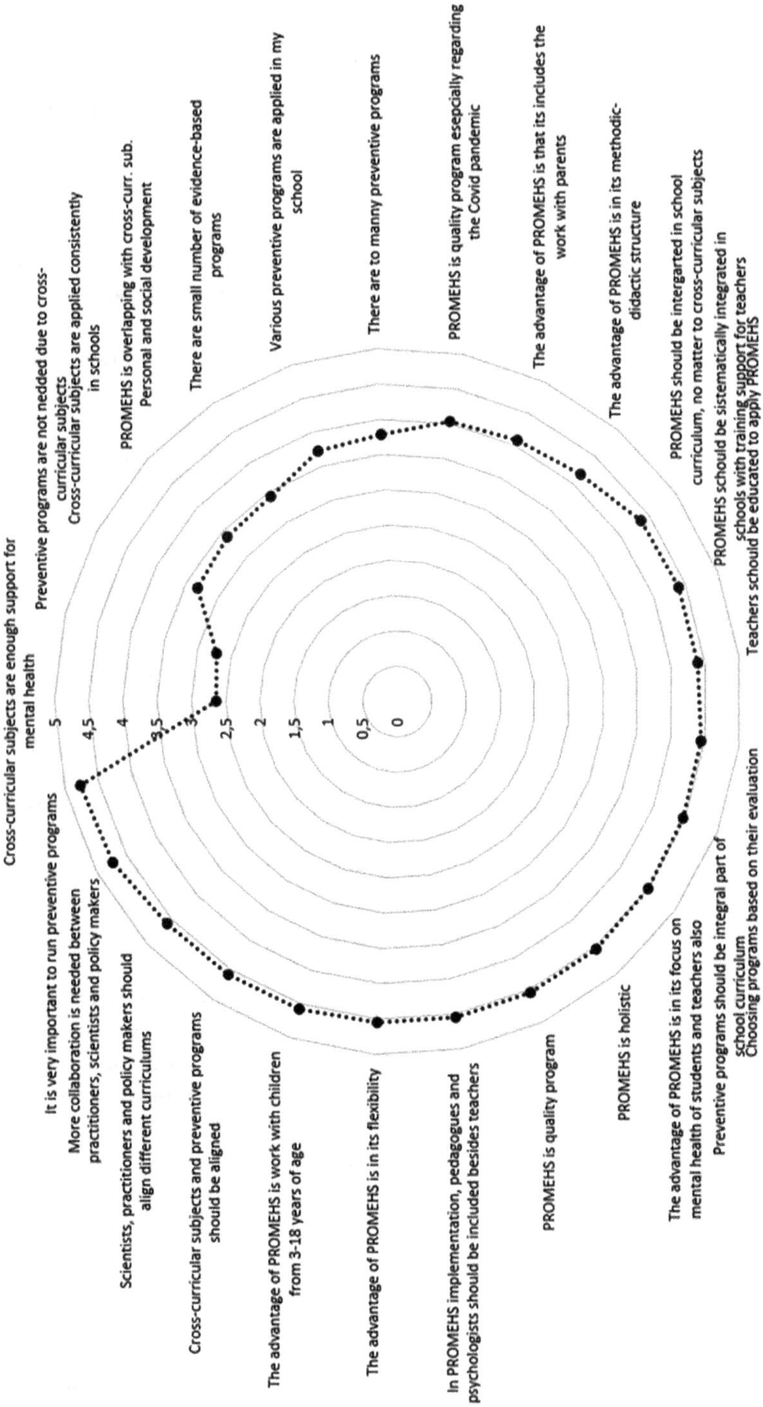

Fig. 7.4 Mean values of participants' responses to each survey item on the sustainability of PROMEHS in Croatia

create, and nurture positive relationships and empathy, successfully manage their own behavior, and make responsible decisions. Likewise, through social-emotional development, the child develops their resilience in different life situations, and the greater the challenges in the environment, the greater the risks for the appearance of certain difficulties in children. Therefore, in addition to learning strategies to avoid the development of risky behaviors, students also learn how to promote their own wellbeing and that of others, as well as ways to sustain it and maintain a high quality of life. In order to make all of the above as effective and accessible as possible, it is the responsibility of adults—primarily families, followed by educators, researchers, and policymakers—to ensure that children receive an education that serves not as a risk factor in their development, but rather as a protective factor. In doing so, it helps us understand the wellbeing of children, their socio-emotional needs, and the timely detection of risk and protective factors of development with the aim of preventing behavioral difficulties that may develop. In addition, good knowledge of the education system in each country and the cultural context in which children live is important, as well as the variety of programs for social-emotional learning, resilience, and prevention of behavioral difficulties. This chapter presents a wide range of programs used internationally, and the analysis conducted in Croatia revealed a similarly large number of programs with diverse content and methods, most of which are primarily aimed at children and students. However, the fact is that there is no systematic coordination in the application of these programs. In addition, there is no systematic implementation of evidence-based evaluations to assess the effects of programs implemented in schools. As a result, it is not guaranteed that only effective programs are being adopted in kindergartens and schools. Each school and kindergarten typically select programs based on pragmatic criteria—such as prior implementation, staff training, positive feedback from children, teacher preference, or ease of implementation. However, this practice should shift toward a single, evidence-based criterion: the scientific evaluation of a program's effectiveness. Some of these programs are evidence-based, such as Life Skills Training, Paths and PROMEHS. Given that PROMEHS includes a number of unfulfilled criteria until now, such as holism, inclusiveness, whole-school approach, use of the S.A.F.E. approach to learning, comprehensiveness of the entire development period from 3 to 18 years, cooperation between development systems, cultural sensitivity, circularity, easy implementation, universality, potential for prevention and promotion, engagement of all important subjects: children, parents, teachers and principals based on scientific evidence and sustainability, a survey was conducted on the perception of the educational staff about the possibility of its implementation and sustainability in relation to similar content within the cross-curricular subject *Personal and Social Development* in Croatian schools. Although, theoretically, there is a noticeable overlap between cross-curricular subjects and PROMEHS, due to different experiences in the implementation of cross-curricular subjects (on the scale from high systematic implementation to low systematic implementation), PROMEHS showed a very high level of efficiency, both in the original evaluation study (Cefai et al., 2022a, 2022b) and in the framework of the survey whose results are presented in this chapter. In view of the established findings about the high positive impact of the PROMEHS curriculum on the wellbeing and mental health of children and teachers, and the positive attitudes of respondents about its further implementation, a project is being implemented at the Faculty of Teacher Education in Rijeka named Development of the Program for the acquisition of micro-qualifications in educational work for the improvement of mental health and wellbeing. This project is developing a module titled Mental Health and Wellbeing in Education, which will be integrated into two existing study programs: the graduate-level Early and Preschool Care and Education program, and the Integrated Primary School Education program. At the same time, this module will be delivered through a new lifelong learning program for educational practitioners. In this way, both pre-service and in-service kindergarten and primary school teachers will learn together, exchanging experiences and knowledge. This collaboration will not only support the effective implementation of PROMEHS but also foster a better understanding of the roles and practices across different educational levels—kindergarten and primary school. The course is being developed during this academic year and is scheduled to begin in March 2024. It will enable all teachers who complete the module to implement PROMEHS in their schools and kindergartens. In this way, the sustainability of PROMEHS implementation in Croatian educational institutions is ensured.

Acknowledgements This work has been supported in part by the University of Rijeka under the project number (uniri-iz-25-115): "ADJUST_WELL: Adjustment in kindergarten: Enhancement of educational practice as a facilitator of early transitions and children's well-being" Many thanks to Asist. Prof. PhD Matea Butković for her support in proofreading.

Competing Interests The author has no conflicts of interest to declare that are relevant to the content of this chapter.

References

Ajduković, M., Rajhvajn Bulat, L., Sušac, N., & Vejmelka, L. (2020). *Subjektivna dobrobit djece u Hrvatskoj* (Subjective wellbeing of children in Croatia. In Croatian). Office for UNICEF-a for Croatia.

Ben-Arieh, A., Casas, F., Frønes, I., & Korbin, J. E. (2014). Multifaceted concept of child wellbeing. *Handbook of Child Wellbeing, 1*, 1–27. https://doi.org/10.1007/978-90-481-9063-8_13

Bennett, M. J. (2004). Becoming interculturally competent. *Toward Multiculturalism: A Reader in Multicultural Education, 2*, 62–77.

Berk, L. E. (2015). *Dječja razvojna psihologija* (Child developmental psychology. In Croatian). Naklada slap.

Bono, G., & Froh, J. J. (2009). Gratitude in school: Benefits to students and schools. In R. Gilman, E. S. Huebner, & M. Furlong (Eds.), *Handbook of positive psychology in the schools: Promoting wellness in children and youth* (pp. 77–88). Lawrence Erlbaum.

Bouwkamp, J., & Lopez, S. J. (2001). *Making hope happen: A program for inner-city adolescents* (Unpublished master's thesis). University of Kansas, Lawrence.

Brackett, M. A. (2019). *Permission to feel: Unlocking the Power of emotions to help our kids, ourselves, and our society thrive.* Celadon Books.

Brackett, M. A., Floman, J. L., Ashton-James, C., Cherkasskiy, L., & Salovey, P. (2013). The influence of teacher emotion on grading practices: A preliminary look at the evaluation of student writing. *Teachers and Teaching, 19*(6), 634–646.

Brofenbrenner, U. (1979). *The ecology of human development*. Harvard University Press.

Caena, F., & Punie, Y. (2019). *Developing a European framework for the personal, social & learning to learn key competence(LifEComp)—Literature review and analysis of frameworks*, Publications Office. Retrieved from 1st Dec 2023, https://data.europa.eu/doi/10.2760/172528

CASEL: The Collaborative for Academic, Social, and Emotional Learning Guide (CASEL Guide) (2013).*Effective social and emotional learning programs: Preschool and elementary school edition.* Retrieved from 1st Dec 2023, https://ed.buffalo.edu/content/dam/ed/alberti/docs/CASEL-Guide-SOCIAL-EMOTIONAL-LEARNING.pdf

Cavioni, V., Grazzani, I., Orhaghi, V., Agliati, A., Gandellini, S., Cefai, C., Camilleri, L., Bartolo, P., Tatalović Vorkapić, S., Golob, L., Poulou, M., Martinsone, B., Supe, I., Simones, C., Lebre, P., Colomeischi, A., Rusu, P., Acostoaie, L., Vintur, T., & Conte, E. (2023). A multi-component curriculum to promote teachers' mental health: Findings from the PROMEHS program. *International Journal of Emotional Education, 15*(1), 1–19.

Cefai, C., Miljević-Riđički, R., Bouillet, D., Pavin Ivanec, T., Milanovic, M., Matsopoulos, A., Gavogiannaki, M., Zanetti, M. A., Cavioni, V., Bartolo, P., Galea, K., Simões, C., Lebre, Paula, L., Santos, A.C., Kimber, B., & Eriksson, C. (2015). *RESCUR surfing the waves—A resilience curriculum for early years and primary schools: A teachers guide.* Centre for Resilience and Socio-Emotional Health, University of Malta.

Cefai, C., Bartolo, P. A., Cavioni, V., & Downes, P. (2018). *Strengthening social and emotional education as a core curricular area across the EU*. Publications Office of the European Union.

Cefai, C., Camilleri, L., Bartolo, P., Grazzani, I., Cavioni, V., Conte, E., Ornaghi, V., Agliati, A., Gandellini, S., Tatalović Vorkapić, S., Poulou, M., Martinsone, B., Stokenberga, I., Simões, C., Santos, M., & Colomeischi, A. A. (2022a). The effectiveness of a school-based, universal mental health programme in six European countries. *Frontiers in Psychology, 13*, Article 925614. https://doi.org/10.3389/fpsyg.2022.925614

Cefai, C., Camilleri, L., Bartolo, P., Grazzani, I., Cavioni, V., Conte, E., Ornaghi, V., Agliati, A., Gandellini, S., Tatalović Vorkapić, S., Poulou, M., Martinsone, B., Stokenberga, I, Simões, C., Santos, M., & Colomeischi, A. A. (2022b). *Promoting mental health in schools: Evaluating the effectiveness of the PROMEHS Programme in improving students' and teachers' social and emotional competence, resilience and mental health.* Seventh Monograph in Resilience and Health by the Centre for Resilience and Socio-Emotional Health, University of Malta, Malta. ISBN: 978-9918-9510-5-5, ISBN: 978-9918-9510-4-8

Colomeischi, A. A., Duca, D. S., Bujor, L., Rusu, P. P., Grazzani, I., Cavioni, V. (2022). Impact of a school mental health program on children's and adolescents' socio-emotional skills and psychosocial difficulties. *Children, 9*, 1661. https://doi.org/10.3390/children9111661

Conte, E., Cavioni, V., Ornaghi, V., Agliati, A., Gandellini, S., Santos, M. F., Santos, A. C., Simões, C., & Grazzani, I. (2023). Supporting preschoolers' mental health and academic learning through the PROMEHS program: A training study. *Children, 10*(6), 1070. https://doi.org/10.3390/children10061070

Domitrovich, C. E., Cortes, R. C., & Greenberg, M. T. (2007). Improving young children's social and emotional competence: A randomized trial of the preschool "PATHS" curriculum. *Journal Od Primary Prevention, 28*, 67–91.

Domitrovich, C. E., Durlak, J. A., Staley, K. C., & Weissberg, R. P. (2017). Social-emotional competence: An essential factor for promoting positive adjustment and reducing risk in school children. *Child Development, 88*(2), 408–416. https://doi.org/10.1111/cdev.12739

Durlak, J. A., Weissberg, R. P., Dymnicki, A. B., Taylor, R. D., & Schellinger, K. B. (2011). The impact of enhancing students' social and emotional learning: A meta-analysis of school-based universal interventions. *Child Development, 82*(1), 405–432.

Durlak, J. A., Domitrovich, C. E., Weissberg, R. P., & Gullotta, T. P. (Eds.). (2015). *Handbook of social and emotional learning: Research and practice* (pp. 3–19). The Guilford Press.

Ennis, R. H. (1987). A taxonomy of critical thinking dispositions and abilities. In J. B. Baron & R. J. Sternberg (Eds.), *Teaching thinking skills: Theory and practice* (pp. 9–26). W H Freeman/ Times Books/Henry Holt & Co.

Erskine, H. E., Moffitt, T. E., Copeland, W. E., Costello, E. J., Ferrari, A. J., Patton, G., Degenhardt, L., Vos, T., Whiteford, H. A., & Scott, J. G. (2015). A heavy burden on young minds: The global burden of mental and substance use disorders in children and youth. *Psychological Medicine, 45*(7), 1551–1563. https://doi.org/10.1017/S0033291714002888

Froh, J., Sefick, W. J., & Emmons, R. A. (2008). Counting blessings in early adolescents: An experimental study of gratitude and subjective wellbeing. *Journal of School Psychology, 46*, 213–233.

Greenberg, M. T., Weissberg, R. P., O'Brien, M. U., Zins, J. E., Fredericks, L., Resnik, H., & Elias, M. J. (2003). Enhancing school-based prevention and youth development through coordinated social, emotional, and academic learning. *American Psychologist, 58*, 466–474.

Holte, A., Barry, M., Bekkhus, M., & Trommsdorff, G., Helmen Borge, A. I., Bowes, L., Casas, F., Friborg, O., Grinde, B., Headey, B., Jozefiak, T., Lekhal, R., Marks, N., Muffels, R., Bang Nes, R., Røysamb, E., Thimm, J. C., Torgersen, S., Trommsdorff, G., …, Veenhoven, R. (2014). Psychology of child wellbeing. In A. Ben-Arieh et al. (Eds.), *Handbook of child wellbeing* (pp. 555–631). Springer Science+Business Media Dordrecht. https://doi.org/10.1007/978-90-481-9063-8_13

Retrieved from 1st Dec 2023, https://teachingstrategies.com/product/als-pals-social-emotional-learning-curriculum/

Retrieved from 1st Dec 2023, https://incredibleyears.com/programs/

Retrieved from 1st Dec 2023, https://toolsofthemind.org/#

Retrieved from 1st Dec 2023, https://croatia.eu/index.php?view=article&id=35&lang=2

Retrieved from 1st Dec 2023, https://mzo.gov.hr/istaknute-teme/odgoj-i-obrazovanje/nacionalni-kurikulum/125

Retrieved from 1st Dec 2023, https://skolazazivot.hr/medupredmetne-teme/

Retrieved from 1st Dec 2023, https://mzo.gov.hr/en

Retrieved from 1st Dec 2023, https://pg.casel.org/ruler-approach/

Retrieved from 1st Dec 2023, http://www.programi.uredzadroge.hr/

Retrieved from 1st Dec 2023, https://www.ufri.uniri.hr/hr/naslovnica/202-hr/promehs/4267-zavrsna.html

Jones, S., Brush, K., Bailey, R., Brion-Meisels, G., McIntyre, J., Kahn, J., Nelson, B., & Stickle, L. (2017). *Navigating SEL from the inside out: Looking inside & across 25 leading SEL programs–A practical resource for schools and OST providers*. Harvard Graduate School of Education.

Jones, S. M., Brush, K. E., Ramirez, T., Mao, Z. X., Marenus, M., Wettje, S., Finney, K., Raisch, N., Podoloff, N., Kahn, J., Barnes, S., Stickle, L., Brion – Meisles, G., McIntyre, J., Cuartas, J. & Bailey R. (2021). *Navigating SEL from the inside out, Looking inside & across 33 leading SEL programs: A practical resource for schools and OST providers, Preschool & Elementary focus. Revised & expanded second edition.* Harvard Graduate School of Education.

Jokić Begić, N., Hromatko, I., Jurin, T., Kamenov, Ž., Keresteš, G., Kuterovac Jagodić, G., Lauri Korajlija, A., Maslić Seršić, D., Mehulić, J., Mikac, U., Tadinac, M., Tomas, J., & Sangster Jokić, C. (2020). Kako smo svi mi? Rezultati istraživanja psihičkog zdravlja za vrijeme pandemije COVID-19 u Hrvatskoj (How are we all? Results of mental health research during the COVID-19 pandemic in Croatia. In Croatian). In: A. Bogdan, (Ed.), *Coronavirus and mental health: Psychological aspects, advice and recommendations* (pp. 415–460). Croatian Psychological Chamber.

Kog, M., & Moons, J. (2008). *A box full of feelings*. Routledge.

Lajoie, J., & Léveillé S. (2007). T*he wellbeing of children in wealthy countries: UNICEF Report Card 7*. CECW Information Sheet #52E. McGill University, School of Social Work.

Liu, J., Ning, W., Zhang, N., Zhu, B., & Mao, Y. (2024). Estimation of the global disease burden of depression and anxiety between 1990 and 2044: An analysis of the global burden of disease study 2019. *Healthcare (Basel), 29;12*(17), 1721. https://doi.org/10.3390/healthcare12171721.

Martinsone, B., Supe, I., Stokenberga, I., Damberga, I., Cefai, C., Camilleri, L., Bartolo, P., O'Riordan, M. R., & Grazzani, I. (2022). Social Emotional competence, learning outcomes, emotional and behavioral difficulties of preschool children: Parent and teacher evaluations. *Frontiers in Psychology, 3*(12), Article 760782. https://doi.org/10.3389/fpsyg.2021.760782.PMID: 35185671;PMCID:PMC8852736

Masten, A. S. (2018). Resilience theory and research on children and families: Past, present, and promise. *Journal of Family Theory & Review, 10*, 12–31. https://doi.org/10.1111/jftr.12255

Maurer, M., Brackett, M. A., & Plain, F. (2004). *Emotional literacy in the middle school: A 6-step program to promote social, emotional and academic learning.* Dude Pub.

Mayr, T., & Ulich, M. (2009). Social-emotional wellbeing and resilience of children in early childhood settings - PERIK: An empirically based observation scale for practitioners. *Early Years: An International Journal of Research and Development, 29*(1), 45–57.

McCallum, F., & Price, D. (2010). Well teachers, well students. *Journal of Student Wellbeing, 4*(1), 19–34.

Miljković, D. (2006). Motivacijom i odgovornošću do uspješnijeg odgoja i obrazovanja (Motivation and responsibility for more successful upbringing and education. In Croatian). In H. Vrgoč (Ed.), *A child/student in the process of upbringing and education* (pp. 13–21). HPKZ.

Miljević-Riđički, R., Plantak, K., & Bouillet, D. (2017). Resilience in preschool children—The perspectives of teachers, parents and children. *International Journal of Emotional Education, 9*(2), 31.

Moore, J. E., Cooper, B. R., Domitrovichc, C. E., Morganc, N. R., Clevelandc, M. J., Shahc, H., Jacobsonc, L., & Greenberg, M. T. (2015). The effects of exposure to an enhanced preschool program on the social-emotional functioning of at-risk children. *Early Childhood Research Quarterly, 32*(3), 127–138. https://doi.org/10.1016/j.ecresq.2015.03.004

Munjas Samarin, R., & Takšić, V. (2009). Programi za poticanje emocionalne i socijalne kompetentnosti kod djece i adolescenata (Programs for encouraging emotional and social competencein children and adolescents. In Croatian). *Suvremena psihologija, 12*(2), 355–370.

National Framework Curriculum for Preschool Education and General Compulsory and Secondary Education (*Nacionalni okvirni kurikulum za predškolski odgoj i obrazovanje te opće obvezno i srednjoškolsko obrazovanje*). (2011). Ministarstvo znanosti, obrazovanja i športa RH (Ministry of science, education and sports, Zagreb, Republic of Croatia). Retrieved from 1st Dec 2023, http://mzos.hr/datoteke/Nacionalni_okvirni_kurikulum.pdf

National Curriculum for an Early and Preschool Care and Education (*Nacionalni kurikulum za rani i predškolski odgoj i obrazovanje*) (2015). Ministry of Science, education, and Sport, Zagreb, Croatia. Retrieved from 1st Dec 2023, https://mzo.gov.hr/UserDocsImages/dokumenti/Obrazovanje/Predskolski/Nacionalni%20kurikulum%20za%20rani%20i%20predskolski%20odgoj%20i%20obrazovanje%20NN%2005-2015.pdf

Noddings, N. (2003). *Happiness and education.* Cambridge University Press. https://doi.org/10.1017/CBO9780511499920

Novak, M., Mihić, J., Bašić, J., & Nix, R. L. (2017). PATHS in Croatia: A school-based randomised-controlled trial of a social and emotional learning curriculum. *International Journal of Psychology, 52*(2), 87–95. https://doi.org/10.1002/ijop.12262

Oberle, E., Domitrovich, C., Meyers, D., & Weissberg, R. P. (2016). Establishing systemic social and emotional learning approaches in schools: A framework for schoolwide implementation. *Cambridge Journal of Education, 46*, 1–21.

OECD. (2015). *Skills for social progress: The power of social and emotional skills.* OECD Publishing.

Poulou, M. S., Grazzani, I., Cavioni, V., Ornaghi, V. M., Conte, E., Cefai, C., Camilerri, L., & Bartolo, P. (2022). Teachers' and students' changes in social and emotional competencies following the implementation of PROMEHS: A European program for promoting mental health at schools. *Educational Research Applications, 7*, 205. https://doi.org/10.29011/2575-7032.100205

Rijavec, M., & Marković, D. (2008.), Nada, strah od ispitivanja i školski uspjeh (Hope, fear of examination and school success. In Croatian). *Metodika, 9*, 16, 8—17.

Rijavec, M., & Miljković, D. (2006). Pozitivna psihologija: psihologija čije je vrijeme (ponovno) došlo (Positive psychology: Psychology whose time has (again) come. In Croatian). *Društvena istraživanja, 15*(4–5)(84–85), 621–641.

Raghavan, R., & Alexandrova, A. (2015). Toward a theory of child wellbeing. *Social Indicators Research, 121*, 887–902. https://doi.org/10.1007/s11205-014-0665-z

Reznitskaya, A., & Sternberg, R. J. (2004). Teaching students to make wise judgments: The "teaching for wisdom" program. In P. A. Linley & S. Joseph (Eds.), *Positive psychology in practice* (pp. 181–196). Wiley.

Savahl, S., Casas, F., & Adams, S. (2021). The structure of children's subjective wellbeing. *Frontiers in Psychology, 12*, Article 650691. https://doi.org/10.3389/fpsyg.2021.650691

Seligman, M. E. P. (2011.). *Flourish.* Free Press.

Seligman, M. E. P., Reivich, K., Jaycox, L., & Gillham, J. (1995). *The optimistic child: Proven program to safeguard children from depression & build lifelong resilience.* Houghton Mifflin Company.

Seligman, M. E. P., Ernst, R. M., Gillham, J., Reivich, K., & Linkins, M. (2009). Positive education: Positive psychology and classroom interventions. *Oxford Review of Education, 35*(3), 293–311.

Sindik, J., & Boban, M. (2016). *Miljokazi razvoja predškolske djece: Studija na uzorku djece u Hrvatskom predškolskom institucionalnom kontekstu* (Milestones of preschool children's development: A study on a sample of children in the Croatian preschool institutional context. In Croatian). Institut za antropologiju & HAD, Zagreb.

Singh, S., Royb, D., Sinhac, K., Parveenc, S., Sharmac, G., & Joshi, G. (2020). Impact of COVID-19 and lockdown on mental health of children and adolescents: A narrative review with recommendations. *Psychiatry Research, 293*, Article 113429. https://doi.org/10.1016/j.psychres.2020.113429

Skoog-Hoffman, A., Coleman, B., Nwafor, E., Lozada, F., Olivo-Castro, S., & Jagers, R. (2023). Building Authentic School-Family Partnerships Through the Lens of Social and Emotional Learning. CASEL. Retrieved from 1st Dec 2023, https://casel.org/sel-innovations-1/

Snyder, C. R. (2000). The past and possible futures of hope. *Journal of Social and Clinical Psychology, 19*, 11–28.

Snyder, C. R., Hoza, B., Pelham, W. E., Rapoff, M., Ware, L., Danovsky, M., Highberger, L., Ribinstein, H., & Stahl, K. J. (1997). The development and validation of the Children's hope scale. *Journal of Pediatric Psychology, 22*(3), 399–421. https://doi.org/10.1093/jpepsy/22.3.399

Solmi, M., Radua, J., Olivola, M., Croce, E., Soardo, L., de Pablo, G. S., Shin, J. I., Kirkbride, J. B., Jones, P., Kim, J. H., Kim, J. Y., Carvalho, A. F., Seeman, M. V., Correll, C. U., & Fusar-Poli, P. (2022). Age at onset of mental disorders worldwide: Large scale meta-analysis of 192 epidemiological studies. *Molecular Psychiatry, 27*, 281–295.

Sternberg, R. J. (2001). Why schools should teach for wisdom: The balance theory of wisdom in educational settings. *Educational Psychologist, 36(*4), 227–245.

Tatalović Vorkapić, S., & Lončarić, D. (2014). Validacija hrvatske verzije ljestvice socio-emocionalne dobrobiti i otpornosti predškolske djece. *Hrvatska Revija Za Rehabilitacijska Istraživanja, 50*(2), 102–117.

Tatalović Vorkapić, S. (2019a). Socio-emocionalna dobrobit i otpornost djece rane i predškolske dobi: Kako omogućiti da djeca (p)ostanu dobro? (Socio-emotional wellbeing and resilience of of children at early and preschool age: How to ensure for children to be(come) well?). *Dijete, Vrtić, Obitelj, 89*, 2–6.

Tatalović Vorkapić, S. (2019b). Podrška socijalno-emocionalnoj dobrobiti djece u Hrvatskoj: Prikaz tri znanstveno-stručna projekta (Support for socio-emotional wellbeing and resilience of children at early and preschool age: Presentation of three scientific and professional projects). In: M. Orel (Ed.) *EDUVision 2019 – Sodobni pristopi poučevanja prihajajočih generacij* (pp. 69–83). EDUvision, Stanislav Jurjevčič s.p.

Tatalović Vorkapić, S. (2020). *Psihologija privrženosti i prilagodba u dječjemu vrtiću – Psihologija dobrobiti djece vol. 1.* (Psychology of attachment and adjustment in kindergarten—The

Psychology of children's wellbeing, Vol. 1, In Croatian). University of Rijeka, Faculty of Teacher Education, Rijeka, Croatia.

Tatalović Vorkapić, S. (2023). Children's socio-emotional wellbeing and resilience during transition from family home to kindergarten. In V. Chiou, L. Geunis, O. Holz, N. O. Ertürk, J. Ratkowska-Pasikowska, & F. Shelton (Eds.), *Contemporary challenges in education: Paradoxes & illuminations; voices from the classroom* (Vol. 3, pp. 68–79). Waxmann Verlag GmbH.

Tatalović Vorkapić, S. (2024). *Dobrobit djece tijekom prijelaznih perioda: Empirijska provjera Ekološko-dinamičkog modela; Psihologija dobrobiti djece vol. 3* (Children's wellbeing during transitions' periods: Empirical validation of ecological and dynamic model—The psychology of children's wellbeing, Vol. 3, In Croatian). University of Rijeka, Faculty of Teacher Education, Rijeka, Croatia.

Tatalović Vorkapić, S. (2025). Are we efficient in timely adjusting teachers' competencies to contemporary childhood? An overview of research studies from Croatia. In H. Harju-Luukkainen, S. Garvis, J. Kangas, J. Marôco, M. Maunula, & M. Maunumäki (Eds.), Generating sustainable futures through teacher education. Rethinking higher education (pp. 47–68). Springer. https://doi.org/10.1007/978-981-96-3329-6_4

Tatalović Vorkapić, S., & Anđić, D. (2023). Understanding transition through the children's voices: The application of puppet interview as the research method. In V. Chiou, L. Geunis, O. Holz, N. O. Ertürk, J. Ratkowska-Pasikowska, & F. Shelton (Eds.), *Contemporary challenges in education: Paradoxes & illuminations; Voices from the classroom* (Vol. 3, pp. 80–93). Waxmann Verlag GmbH.

Tatalović Vorkapić, S., Klarić, A., Smojver-Ažić, S., & Čepić, R. (2024). Kako poticati socijalno-emocionalno učenje u dječjim vrtićima: prikaz projekta EDUSKILLS+SEL (How to foster socio-emotional leraing in kindergartens: The presentaton of project EduSkills+SEL. In Croatian). In M. Tkalčić & I. Miletić (Eds.), Book of abstracts: 31. Annual conference on Croatian psychologists, Opatija, 6. - 9. 11. 2024. Contemporary challenges of mental health in various working contexts (p. 203). Crotian Psychological Association, Psychological Association of Primorje and Gorski Kotar county, Rijeka.

Velan, D., & Tatalović Vorkapić, S. (2020, July 6–7). The voices of the children: what do children have to say about the kindergarten? In L. Gómez Chova, A. López Martínez, I. Candel Torres (Eds.), *EDULEARN2020 Proceedings, 12th annual international conference on education and new learning technologies* (pp. 2367–2376). IATED, Palma de Mallorca.

Whalen, S. P., & Csikszentmihalyi, M. (1991). *Putting flow theory into education practice: The key school's flow activity room. A report to the Benton center for curriculum and instruction.* University of Chicago.

WHO. (2018). *Mental health: Strengthening our response.* Retrieved from 1st Dec 2023, https://www.who.int/news-room/fact-sheets/detail/mental-health-strengthening-ourresponse

WHO. (2020). *Guidelines on mental health promotive and preventive interventions for adolescents: Helping adolescents thrive.* Retrieved from 1st Dec 2023, https://apps.who.int/iris/handle/10665/33686

Chapter 8
Wellbeing and Mental Health in Schools: The Case of Greece

Maria Poulou

8.1 Wellbeing and Mental Health

The concept of wellbeing was first described by the ancient Greek philosopher Aristotle who described emotional wellbeing using the Greek word eudaimonia, meaning a state of having good indwelling spirit or happiness. Since then, emotional wellbeing has been described throughout history by ancient philosophers and modern-day psychologists with varying terminologies (Bradburn, 1969), and although the core essence of the concept has remained consistent, an adequate definition of wellbeing in youth has not yet been defined (Courtwright et al., 2019). Subjective wellbeing has been considered as a broad multidimensional construct encompassing the subcomponents of emotional, psychological, and social wellbeing (Keyes, 2006). Subjective wellbeing is categorized into hedonic/affective wellbeing, referring to the pursuit of pleasure and enjoyment, and into eudemonic wellbeing, referring to the living well or actualizing one's human potentials (Deci & Ryan, 2008; Diener, 1994, 2000; Diener & Emmons, 1985; Ryan & Deci, 2001). Emotional wellbeing in youth has been described as an overall positive state of emotions, self-esteem, and resilience that leads to self-actualization, self-efficacy, and health-promoting behaviors (Courtwright et al., 2019). The defining attributes of emotional wellbeing in youth are positive emotions, positive self-esteem, and resilience.

Mental health on the other hand has been defined as a state of wellbeing in which every individual realizes his or her own potential, copes with the normal stresses of life, works productively and fruitfully, and is able to make a contribution to her or his community (WHO, 2005). The relationship between mental health and wellbeing concepts is not adequately defined, with Norwich et al. (2021) arguing for a dual-factor mental health model which treats mental illness/disorder and wellbeing as two separate concepts and reflects two distinctive aims of school education

M. Poulou (✉)
Patras University, Patras, Greece
e-mail: mpoulou@upatras.gr

A. A. Colomeischi (ed.), *Wellbeing in Schools of Southeastern Europe*, Human Well-Being Research and Policy Making, https://doi.org/10.1007/978-3-032-10525-7_8

(wellbeing promotion and mental health services). Therefore, school education aims are about promoting personal and social wellbeing (cognitive, emotional, physical, spiritual, moral etc.) and mental health aims about preventing, coping, and helping mental health difficulties. Wellbeing and mental health of children and youth are of increasing concern worldwide, and they consist of constructs that should not be taken for granted (Cooper & Hornby, 2018). A growing body of evidence suggests that adolescents' subjective wellbeing is related to their school functioning (Shoshani & Slone, 2013). Adolescents who have more frequent experiences of positive emotions are more engaged in learning, adaptive coping, school achievements (Lewis et al., 2009) and school-related behaviors (Suldo et al., 2006; Poulou & Norwich, 2019). On the other hand, adolescents who rate themselves as feeling more depressed, unhappy, frustrated, worried/anxious, and angry/hostile experience more emotional, conduct, hyperactivity, and peer difficulties (Poulou & Norwich, 2020).

The incidence of mental, emotional or behavioral disorders is estimated between 10 and 20% among school children (Erskine et al., 2015; WHO, 2015), whereas half of mental health disorders begin before the age of 14 (Darling et al., 2021). Mental health difficulties can manifest as externalizing problems (disruptive behavior, attention deficit hyperactivity disorder, conduct disorders etc.) or internalizing problems (depression, anxiety, panic disorder, social phobia etc.), and can have an opposing effect on children's and youth different aspects of life, if they go unnoticed.

8.2 Wellbeing and Mental Health in Greece

WHO (2005) highlighted the importance of mental health promotion and urged governments worldwide to include mental health in their primary healthcare. Research evidence in Greece aligns with international data, suggesting that the levels of mental health and wellbeing of young people are linked to and predict immediate and long-lasting academic, emotional and social outcomes, and therefore suggesting that special attention should be paid to promoting the mental health of young people in schools (Madianos et al., 2011). The educational system in Greece is characterized by centralization and bureaucratic administration which is reflected in the curricula (Alahiotis & Karatzia-Stavlioti, 2006). New schemas of social construction towards globalization accompanied with diverse cultural, linguistic, national and socio-economic characteristics which took place in the Greek society were reflected in the goals formulation of the Greek official curriculum, which declares students' social and emotional development as one of its main goals (Ministry of Education and Religious Affairs, 2003a, 2003b). The role of school became the development of the individual: nurturing moral values, feelings of self-awareness, skills for personal and life-long growth and positive interpersonal and group relationships (Pedagogical Institute, 2003).

A plethora of prevention programs consistent with CASEL's (2013) framework were developed by individual researchers or research centers to support teachers promote students' mental health (Amal Aliance, 2022; Cefai et al., 2015;

Chiementi & Triliva, 1994; Doni & Giotsa, 2017; Kourmousi et al., 2017, 2018; Triliva et al., 2014). One of the largest school-based program implemented in Greece was the School and Social Life program, created by the Greek Educational Policy Institute, with guidelines for teachers. It was implemented nationally in 2011–2012, in ninety-six schools in primary and secondary education (Babalis et al., 2013). The ultimate goal of the curriculum was to prevent violence and social exclusion, and to promote the physical, mental health and wellbeing of students. Steps for Life was another universal teacher-taught program designed to improve learners' personal and social skills. It was implemented to 998 kindergarten students (5–6 years old) and 2,439 elementary school students to help them in learning how to think for themselves and find their own solutions to their everyday problems (Kourmousi et al., 2017, 2018).

The devastating economic crisis and the long-lasting recession which some southern European countries including Greece have gone through in 2009, had profound consequences for young people's social and emotional development and mental health (Madianos et al., 2011). This situation has created additional stressors to the psychosocial prosperity and mental health of young people. The risk to mental health was further exacerbated by the general limited availability and access to counselling, support, and mental health services (Giannakopoulos et al., 2009). However, in this economic crisis and political turmoil, over half of the Greek adolescent students were flourishing and only a small proportion of them were languishing, suggesting a minor crisis on students from an even though limited urban area of Greece (Didaskalou et al., 2018).

8.3 Wellbeing and Mental Health During Pandemic

At the end of 2019, a new type of previously unidentified coronavirus appeared in the Chinese city of Wuhan, officially named Coronavirus Disease-2019 (COVID-19). Due to the growing rate of reporting cases in Chinese and international locations, on January 30, 2020, the WHO Emergency Committee declared a global health emergency (Velavan & Meyer, 2020). To eliminate the spread of COVID-19 many countries around the world have implemented restrictions on population movement or partial lockdowns, police-enforced curfew, strict travel bans and closed borders (Vujčić et al., 2021) establishing a new way of living.

The severity of the COVID-19 pandemic posed a new challenge to mental health. The effects of the novel coronavirus disease in many parts of the world, have been depicted in different aspects of society and people's lives: physical and mental health, economic activity, technological use, political action, and social interaction (Baker et al., 2020). As a result of COVID-19, a significant worsening of the mental health of children and young people was evidenced (Gillard et al., 2021). During the pandemic an estimated of 2.6 billion people was living under lockdown or quarantine which could be deemed as the largest psychological experiment ever conducted. Home isolation and social distancing emerged as the most effective measures for societies to restrict the COVID-19 pandemic (Mourelatos, 2023). Health and wellbeing have declined due to the coronavirus disease pandemic in many countries worldwide. Stressful negative life events such as the COVID-19 are known to contribute to the development of anxiety, depression, and loneliness levels, especially in vulnerable social groups such as students and the elderly (Xiong et al., 2020). People who were quarantined were in risk of developing a wide range of symptoms of psychological stress, including low mood, insomnia, stress, anxiety, anger, irritability, emotional exhaustion, depression, and post-traumatic stress symptoms (Cruwys et al., 2020). Depression, anxiety, and stress have been identified as basic negative indicators of mental health and some of the major health problems, and research interest has focused on understanding their nature, causes, and treatments (Lovibond & Lovibond, 1995). Studies assessing stress, anxiety and depression during quarantine caused by COVID-19 revealed the presence of severe psychological distress and psychopathological factors and shown that the COVID-19 pandemic is associated with very significant levels of stress, which in many cases could reach the threshold of clinical importance (Xiong et al., 2020).

Literature shows that isolation associated with quarantine measure has negative psychological effects in adults, including confusion anger and post-traumatic distress (Magklara et al., 2021). Meta-analytic data denoted an overall increase in mental health symptoms in the general population which was most pronounced during the early stages of the pandemic (Magklara et al., 2021). The outbreak of the COVID-19 pandemic caused an increase in the prevalence of mental disorders by a massive 25%. The most common and important of these disorders were depression, anxiety, and various types of psychological distress. One of the main explanations for the increase in mental health problems is the unprecedented multiple stress caused by the social isolation resulting from the pandemic and the related stressors such as loneliness, fear of infection, suffering and death of loved ones, financial worries to name a few. A review of research literature from China, India, Nepal, Iran, Iraq, Japan, Nigeria, the United Kingdom, Italy and Spain showed that the average prevalence of depression in 14 studies with a sample size of 44,531 people was 33.7%, the prevalence of anxiety in 17 studies with a sample size of 63,439 was 31.9%, while stress rates in 5 studies with a total sample size of 9074 individuals were 29.6% (Salari et al., 2020). Similarity of results are also met in Europe. In Serbia it was found that of the 1057 adult participants, 28.9% reported moderate to severe depression, 36.9% moderate to severe anxiety, and 38.1% moderate to severe symptoms of stress. In Croatia, in a nationally representative sample of 1201 adult participants, 9.8% were at risk of adjustment disorders, 7.7% were at risk of developing depressive disorder, 7.8% were at risk for anxiety disorder, and 7.2% experienced high levels of stress (Ajduković et al., 2021).

Children and adolescents around the world experienced an unusual disruption of their everyday lives and daily routines due to the COVID-19 pandemic and the subsequent lockdown measures, whereas concerns about the effects of the pandemic on mental health and wellbeing of the youth population have been raised (Mazza et al., 2020). In many countries around the world, children and adolescents have experienced an unexpected and prolonged period of physical isolation from their friends, peers, teachers, extended family, and various community networks. COVID-19 has caused increases in levels of depression, confusion, anger child-related domestic violence, sleep-related issues, suicidal ideation, health-related anxiety, and psychotic symptoms in children (Mouratidis & Yiannakou, 2022). Rising depression, anxiety and loneliness rates were reported in China, Canada, Turkey, U.S, India, Italy, Spain, Germany, U.K (Magklaras et al. 2021). A review of 13 studies from different European countries showed that the overall combined prevalence rate for students was 55% for anxiety, 63% for depression, and 62% for stress Oliveira Carvalho et al., 2021).

A significant increase in anxiety, depression and stress has been identified among university students across Europe. A study conducted in 338 University students in Serbia during COVID-19 pandemic showed significantly higher ratings of depression, anxiety and stress comparing to their ratings before the pandemic (Safiye & Vukčević, 2020). Research in University students in Spain revealed similar finding (Odriozola-González et al., 2020). During the outbreak of COVID-19, a percentage of 15.2% among 3936 French students experienced anxiety-related symptoms (Bourion-Bédès et al., 2021).

8.4 Wellbeing and Mental Health During Pandemic in Greece

In Greece, regulatory lockdown measures have been introduced in the spring of 2020. The long-lasting strict lockdown measures and the risks linked to isolation along with the collateral threat from the same invisible enemy of our physical health revealed the enemy of our mental health as well. The coronavirus disease pandemic has led to dramatic changes in quality of life (Mouratidis & Yiannakou, 2022). The campaign message "we stay home" undoubtedly has overturned everybody's daily routine. As in any crisis, reorganization and reconstruction of concepts were the new challenges that we all had to face (Giannopoulou et al., 2020). The increased rate of internet addiction and e-gambling among young people was another collateral threat of the pandemic (Giannopoulou & Tsobanoglou, 2020).

The pandemic has placed enormous pressure on health systems around the globe, but particularly for the Greek health system, the pandemic added a significant load to the health system, which had only recently started recovering from the very deep fiscal crisis with profound socio-economic implications. Greece as one of the countries hardest hit by the economic crisis, after 10 years of recession, it now dives into another crisis, the COVID-19 pandemic. The current situation is having a dramatic negative impact on the economy with an associated risk to people's mental health. The 63% of Greeks believe that the pandemic will have a negative impact on their mental health and 57.9% on their income (Dianeosis, 2020). Child and adolescent mental health services and supportive policies underwent major budget changes due to COVID-19.

The Greek National Public Health Organization (EODY in Greek), Public Authorities and various civil associations have set up COVID-19 crisis hotlines. The provision of services to people with mental health problems and their families has been substantially affected.

Another sensitive and challenging issue which received detrimental dimensions was the living conditions of approximately 40.000 asylum seekers in the refugee camps on the Aegean islands (Giannopoulou et al., 2020). The situation met in these camps during pre-COVID-19 period did not allow to receive necessary precautions, such as social distancing and vigilant hygiene. Specialized medical teams were located to the camps for the creation of self-isolation areas and compulsory temperature checking.

The psychological distress caused by prolonged lockdown, along with evolving sense of inactivity, boredom, frustration, and uncertainty lead to psychosomatic or psychological problems. Alcohol drinking, dysfunctional personal and family coping strategies drove to ineffective parent–child communication patterns. Staying at home has placed some children and adults at increased risk of domestic violence, as evidenced by increased numbers of reported incidents. A dramatic increase in stress-related disorders, associated with increased levels of depression and anxiety in parents resulted from the financial hardship (Giannopoulou et al., 2020). In the imposed COVID-19 lockdown period in Greece, adults showed decreased physical activity, increased depressive symptoms, disturbed eating behavioral patterns and the lowest wellbeing across the 27 European union member states (European Foundation for the Improvement of Living Working Conditions, 2020). In addition, 35% of the Greek families reported that the well being of their kids (<18 years) decreased in the first lockdown during spring 2020, similar to other countries (Magklara et al., 2021).

Data reporting on the mental health effects of COVID-19 on children and adolescents in Greece are limited, but they are in accordance with the international worrying reports on the deleterious effects of COVID-19 to youth's mental health. Adolescents' daily life had dramatically changed during the COVID-19 due to the social restrictions that have been imposed, including closures of schools, leisure centers, and sport facilities. An online survey of 442 Greek senior high school students -a special category of students- revealed a rise in depression and anxiety levels in the time of home confinement (Giannopoulou et al., 2020). Senior high school students are in the final year of secondary education and they have to take university entrance exams. The pressure to score high in these exams in combination with the Greek society's contention that every student should get a University degree (Giannopoulou et al., 2020) is a highly demanding and stressful situation on its own. Giannopoulou and colleagues (2020) investigated the impact of the nationwide lockdown on the levels of anxiety and depression to this specific category of students. The results indicated a substantial and worrying increase in anxiety and depression symptoms from before the COVID-19 outbreak to the period of nationwide lockdown. The study also revealed that the most significant difficulty experienced by the children and adolescents during the lockdown was social isolation. The social isolation of their children was also one of the major concerns of the parents during the lockdown. In addition, parents were concerned about the limited physical activity and the increased screen time during the lockdown. Although study results can be subject to bias, the unexpected high rates of anxiety and depression warrant an urgent call to action especially for this group of adolescents. The Ministry of education, the educators, the parents need to be aware of the added stress experienced by already stressed young people preparing for highly competitive university entrance exams, in order to address more effectively the mental health impact of potential future restrictions measures in response to future waves of pandemic (Giannopoulou et al., 2020).

Research in Greece during the COVID-19 pandemic, pointed to an increase in anxiety, depression and psychological distress in students compared to the time before the pandemic (Patsali et al., 2020). During lockdown period, 25.9% of Greek young adults (University students) have shown increased depressive symptoms corresponding to a threshold for clinical depression (Kaparounaki et al., 2020). This information combined with the evidence that many Greek adolescents in the pre-COVID-19 era showed the lowest levels across 31 countries (Bruckauf, 2017) is worrying and needs prioritized efforts by decision-makers on effective policies for adolescents during a lockdown period. In the study of Morres and colleagues (2021), adolescents showed insufficient physical activity levels and moderate scores of healthy eating behavior. The most striking result however was the worrying low levels of wellbeing. The average score on wellbeing was below the threshold identified by WHO as requiring inspection for depressive symptoms (Parlapani et al., 2020).

8.5 Mental Health at Schools

The COVID-19 pandemic presents an interesting historical moment, which is now understood as a consequential societal crisis, especially for education (Wodon, 2020). During the years, schools have responded to different forms of crises such as like the influenza, the 2020 COVID-19 viruses, economic crisis, and wars like those in South Sudan, Sierra Leone, Afghanistan, Syria and Ukraine and the consequences for refugees and children. Often the concern is for how schools can continue to serve its purpose of educating children, given the constraints forced upon by different crises (Trinidad, 2021). There is evidence of the COVID-19 crisis worsening mental health problems (Fox et al., 2020), and reinforcing the perspective that schools have a central role (Norwich et al., 2021). Never in recent history there has been such a clear need for schools to implement the most effective mental health provision for children (Gillard et al., 2021).

In these circumstances, the importance of prevention and early-intervention in childhood is self-evident, with particular attention now paid to the pre-school and school years as foci of preventive and remedial interventions (Hornby & Atkinson, 2003). WHO recommends that schools function as one of the primary mental health support systems for students (WHO, 2007). Schools have been consistently identified by policymakers and other stakeholders as an ideal universal platform to promote and support mental health for all students, to identify and manage students with emerging mental health issues early and to target interventions for students with significant mental health problems (Darling et al., 2021; UK Department of Health & Education, 2017). Schools should arrange provision to promote children's wellbeing and make provision to proactively promote the wellbeing of all of their students (Gillard et al., 2021).

During the Greek economic crisis, teachers were able to create a sense of stability for their schools through resilience and positive school climates (Botou et al., 2017), whereas teachers of students with mental health issues and special education needs used school routines and school social connections as important coping mechanisms (Lee, 2020). However, the solution for mental health difficulties come into conflict with the physical health need to socially distance and contain the spread of the COVID-19 pandemic (Lewnard & Lo, 2020). In this situation of limited social interaction and uncertainty for the implications of pandemic, educators addressed the need for social emotional learning strategies to help students cope with the implications of isolation, lack of structure and other adverse conditions (Trinidad, 2021). Many of the studies on schools during times of crises focused on the effects of these crises on student learning, teacher employment and other educational outcomes. Research has shown that there were substantial and sustained effects on students and their families during these periods of home learning, struggling with work and domestic life (Wang et al., 2021). However, less research exists on teachers' and school leaders' concerns in response to crises and the competing values inherent in these concerns (Trinidad, 2021). Trinidad (2021) pointed out the need to understand the school staff perspectives about their needs, priorities and the deeper values during a societal crisis and provide a shared vocabulary of equity, engagement and health between central administration and school staff.

8.6 Teachers' Mental Health

Teachers' wellbeing is defined as a positive emotional state, which is the result of balance and harmony between environmental factors and personal needs and expectations (Aelterman et al., 2007). Teaching had always been a difficult process for educators. Teaching under normal situations is a stressful job per se (Montgomery & Rupp, 2005), with teachers reporting an increased risk of developing mental health difficulties (Kidger et al., 2016). It was a general consensus long before COVID-19 that teachers experience high levels of stress and negative emotions (Hargreaves, 2000; Hodge et al., 1994; Kariou et al., 2021), especially those who teach in low-resource, high poverty schools (Hakanen et al., 2006). The problem of teacher stress is pervasive. It is evident across all sectors of education and across countries (Gray et al., 2017). In fact, there is an association between better teacher wellbeing and lower student psychological difficulties, and an association between lower teacher depression and better student wellbeing (Harding et al., 2019). Poor teacher wellbeing could therefore be problematic for students' wellbeing (Harding et al., 2019) and children's learning and progress (Glazzard & Rose, 2020). Teachers' levels of stress can diminish instructional effectiveness, interfere with the ability to implement appropriate classroom management practices, and lower motivation for teaching (Frenzel et al., 2009; Gilmour et al., 2022), factors that contribute to teachers' burnout. Teacher burnout is conceptualized as prolonged work-related stress response characterized by negative attitudes, beliefs, and emotions towards individuals with whom one works (i.e., depersonalization as it relates to students), the job itself (i.e., reduced personal achievement), and emotional exhaustion (i.e., feeling fatigued because of negative workplace emotions; Maslach et al., 2001). Research demonstrates that teachers with poor mental health give lower ratings to their ability to support the wellbeing and mental health of their students (Sisask et al., 2014), particularly if they are struggling with their own wellbeing and mental health. Emotionally exhausted early childhood teachers tend to have lower quality interactions and relationships with children in their classrooms, an association that may be influenced by years of education (Aboagye et al., 2020; Ansari et al., 2020). Teacher burnout is also negatively associated with observers' ratings of teachers' provision of emotional support and classroom organization (Braun et al., 2019). Studies have also shown that teachers who report high levels of burnout tend to have difficulty moderating their displays of negative emotion in the presence of their students (Fiorilli et al., 2017). Greek teachers on the other hand tend to be satisfied with their work and experience low-to-moderate levels of burnout, depression, and role conflict ambiguity, though country-level indicators suggest that they may be on the rise (Kourmousi & Alexopoulos, 2016; Papastylianou et al., 2009).

From the spring of 2020 and during the entire academic year 2020–2021, COVID-19 pandemic, caused a variety of changes, new demands, and challenges in the education system. Teachers across the world had to adapt, continue schooling, and protect students and their own wellbeing. The changes in teaching with the modification of traditional methods of knowledge sharing and the introduction of entirely new technologies with the peculiarities and problems associated with them certainly affected the mental health of teachers. Teaching staff had to accept the responsibility to adjust their practices and negotiate unfamiliar synchronous online platforms for teaching and learning, as well as deal with their own isolation and the needs of their families (Brooks et al., 2022; Zagkas et al., 2023). A survey of 1330 Canadian teachers in May 2020, revealed that teachers were concerned about the vulnerable students in their classrooms, the inequities among them and the provision of materials and instruction to meet their needs (Sokal & Eblie Trudel, 2020). The survey also showed that the increased demands placed on teachers in learning to teach virtually, working full-time from home adopting new technologies, while caring for their own families, and engaging students through remote learning were key stressors during pandemic education. The study of Baker et al. (2021) also showed that teachers were challenged by their lack of familiarity with online teaching and the rapidly changing methods for conducting their work and communicating with students and parents. Many teachers were challenged to engage students with online learning or to maintain student learning without technology resources. Teachers also felt concern about their students' basic needs which were unable to address. They also felt concern about educational inequity as it became clear that the most vulnerable students were likely to be impacted the most from the pandemic (Baker et al., 2021). It is not surprising therefore that teachers experienced emotional distress with negative impact to teachers' wellbeing (Ciprianno & Brackett, 2020).

Specifically during pandemic, teaching directly depended on teachers' wellbeing, was linked to teaching performance and was a key prerequisite for education. Teachers need to feel well with themselves in order to be able to effectively function in the teaching–learning process, create appropriate conditions for students in the new educational context, conducive to learning and further promote students' wellbeing. However, teachers' wellbeing has not been sufficiently examined as studies measuring subjective wellbeing largely focused on students (Lee, 2020) and were limited to the professional group of teachers (Zagkas et al., 2023). Understanding teachers' wellbeing is important by itself, because poor wellbeing can have serious consequences for teaching profession, driving teachers to stress, burnout and leaving the profession (Madigan & Kim, 2021). Under COVID-19 conditions though, the level of teachers' stress had increased (Zagkas et al., 2023). Anxiety about the pandemic and lack of administrative support were important predictors of teachers' stress, anxiety, depression (Alves et al., 2021) and burnout (Pressley, 2021).

The existing research on teachers' wellbeing during pandemic revealed worrying results for teachers' wellbeing and health in general. Early in the pandemic, a survey of over 5.000 US teachers revealed that the five most highly experienced feelings were anxiety, fear, worry, sadness and feeling overwhelmed (Cipriano & Brackett, 2020). A longitudinal qualitative study examining the trajectories of teachers' wellbeing during COVID-19 revealed decline of teachers' wellbeing throughout the pandemic, especially for primary school leaders. It identified uncertainty, workload, negative perceptions of the profession, concern of others' wellbeing, health struggles and multiple roles as the job demands which negatively influenced teachers' wellbeing, and social support, work autonomy and coping strategies as the job resources which positively influenced teachers' wellbeing (Kim et al., 2022). Studies of professional groups during the COVID-19 revealed that during the early months of the pandemic's emergence, poor sleep quality and reported stress were prevalent among healthcare personnel. Two years into the pandemic, teachers' reported stress decreased as sleep quality deteriorated. High stress was related with severe sleep length and quality disruptions (Jahrami et al., 2022). High rates of overweight/obesity, weekly alcohol consumption and smoking were observed among 786 Greek primary teachers. The majority of participants reported being in the moderate stress category, while more than half of them experiencing sleep problems (Zagkas et al., 2023). Based on these findings we understand the need to support teachers' mental health and wellbeing with the aim of reducing their stress and improve their quality of life.

8.7 Promotion of Teachers' Mental Health and Wellbeing During Pandemic

Nevertheless, during the early months of the pandemic teachers noted positive changes. They reported for example feeling more appreciative of things they took for granted, finding greater meaning in their work, the importance of feeling supported by family and friends and connected to students (Baker et al., 2021), factors all of which have been found to foster resilience in the face of crisis (Fredrickson et al., 2003). Teachers also highlighted the importance of support received by the administration and colleagues, and the role of technology which allowed them to stay connected to people (Baker et al., 2021).

At present, there is evidence that female, under 40 years old (Lei et al., 2020), student status, unemployment or poor economic status, lower level of education (Lei et al., 2020; Vujčić et al., 2021), presence of chronic illness and history of medical or psychiatric illness (Mazza et al., 2020), consist of the demographic characteristics with the highest risk of mental health problems related to COVID-19. Frequent exposure to social media and news related to COVID-19 (Lei et al., 2020), and inadequate information about the virus (Serafini et al., 2020) add risk to mental health status.

Besides these demographic characteristics, there were significant individual differences in adapting to stressful situations such as the COVID-19 pandemic, which depends on personality characteristics. There is evidence that psychological symptoms during the pandemic were related to personality traits, such as temperament, positive stress coping mechanisms (Moccia et al., 2020), secure and avoidant attachment styles (Wang et al., 2020), hope (Yildirim & Solmaz, 2022) and resilience (Serafini et al., 2020). Mourelatos (2023) showed that depression increased significantly in line with the escalation of the pandemic, with students with high levels of neuroticism, extraversion, and agreeableness to face a sense of loneliness, evolving into anxiety or depression over time. There is evidence that teachers who experience more stressors reported more serious mental health problems, whereas teachers who experience more protective factors were more likely to find teaching and coping with pandemic easier (Baker et al., 2021), emphasizing on the importance of resilience construct during crisis (Beltman et al., 2011).

Even before COVID-19, resilience in mental health promotion attracted research interest. Resilience implies successful adaptation, the ability to maintain or regenerate mental health despite obstacles as well as the ability to easily recover from a variety of difficulties (Wald et al., 2006). Resilience is negatively associated to depression and anxiety (Poole et al., 2017; Wells et al., 2001) and reduce the association between burnout syndrome and subjective wellbeing (Hu et al., 2020). Research during COVID-19 confirmed the significant protective role of resilience to mental health problems. A study of 220 adults, in the early stages of the COVID-19 pandemic, showed that hope and resilience had significant direct effects on mental health and subjective wellbeing (Yıldırım & Arslan, 2020).

Capacity for mentalizing is another construct considered to play a preventive role in maintaining mental health (Luyten et al., 2020; Manzano-García et al., 2020). Mentalizing consists of interpreting perceived human behavior based on intentional mental states such as needs, desires, feelings, beliefs, goals, purposes, and reasons. Mentalizing is a process that enables individuals to understand their own and other people's behavior in interpersonal relationships, as well as to regulate their own emotions and impulses (Luyten et al., 2020). Empathy, active listening, and authentic curiosity about mental states, both for oneself and the others, are expressed during direct communication. Mentalizing is positively associated with teachers' wellbeing and mitigates the negative impact of stress (Schwarzer et al., 2021), whereas lack of mentalizing reduces the ability of people to understand their own and others' behavior, which leads to interpersonal misunderstandings, conflicts, dissatisfaction and professional frustrations (Bateman et al., 2018; Manzano-García et al., 2020). The introduction of mindfulness, encourages teachers to focus on the present, manage attention with intention and observe situations in a nonjudgmental way (Roeser, 2016). Studies using mindfulness, transcendental meditation (Elder et al., 2014) or similar intervention programs that focus on physiological and psychological states showed reduction in teachers' stress and burnout, improving quality of teaching (Jennings et al., 2013) and improved sleep quality (Frank et al., 2013).

Beside the individual-focused interventions for teachers, interventions linking the school context and the individual through school-based programs promote wellbeing in the school context. Several prevention programs have been developed that mainly target the promotion of social and emotional learning skills, resilience and prevention of social and emotional difficulties (Ashdown & Bernard, 2012; Cefai et al., 2018; Durlak et al., 2011). It is well evidenced that students' social and emotional competences contribute to students' academic engagement and achievement (DiPerna et al., 2018), their psychosocial health (Van de Sande et al., 2019) and consist of an antidote for preventing negative outcomes (Green et al., 2021).

While there is acknowledgment that teachers' social and emotional competences influence the quality of teacher-student relationships, and the quality of learning environments (Morris et al., 2013), the role of teachers' own mental health promotion has been overlooked (Jones et al., 2013). This delay on teachers' own social and emotional competences may be attributed to the assumption that teachers are already competent and have the tacit knowledge to act as social and emotional competent models for their students (Elliot et al., 2011; Jennings & Greenberg, 2009). This assumption though was faltered during COVID-19 pandemic where teachers had to take care of their own mental health. Pandemic disclosed the need to promote teachers' mental health early on, starting from teacher preparation programs (Greenberg et al., 2016).

8.8 Promotion of Teachers' Mental Health and Wellbeing During Pandemic in Greece

Following the COVID-19 experience, SEL skills and resilience cultivation for teachers and students in schools became an outstanding need. The difficulties suffered by teachers and students highlighted the importance of social and emotional well-being for teaching and learning (Katz et al., 2020). The implementation of the Promoting Mental Health Program at Schools (PROMEHS), a school-based universal mental health curriculum was designed to address students' and teachers' mental health, during the 2020–2021 academic year, with the collaboration of parents, school directors and policy makers. The PROMEHS curricula activities met the quality criteria identified by CASEL (2020), and aimed to develop a set of social and emotional competences such as self-awareness, self-regulation, social awareness, relationship building, resilience and prevention of emotional and behavioral difficulties. These competences are particularly helpful in the face of challenging situations (Holtge et al., 2021) and serve as a protective factor for teachers' mental health (Hascher et al., 2021). Manuals for teachers, students and parents were provided along with guidelines. PROMEHS was implemented applying a pre- and post-training study in other 5 European countries at the same time (Italy, Portugal, Romania, Croatia and Latvia, see Cavioni et al., 2023; Colomeischi et al., 2022), and although it was not initially designed as such, it was administered online due to COVID-19 restrictions.

PROMEHS in Greece was delivered to 1558 kindergarten, primary and secondary students through teleconferencing due to Covid-19 policy restrictions (Poulou et al., 2022a). PROMEHS has been approved by the Ministry of Education and Religious Affairs (53971/17/05/2021). The implementation of PROMEHS to the experimental group of students revealed that students' social and emotional competences were significantly improved compared to their peers control group, a finding also confirmed by their teachers and parents (Poulou et al., 2022b). Similarly, positive impact on students' social and emotional competences, and prosocial behavior and decrease in externalizing and internalizing problems were found in all the European countries implemented PROMEHS mental health program (Cefai et al., 2022). In addition, 152 Greek teachers from kindergarten to secondary education who implemented PROMEHS curriculum to their students and studied the relevant material on teachers' mental health reported changes in their own social and emotional competences and resilience in accordance with their colleagues in the 5 European countries (Cavioni et al., 2023; Poulou et al., 2022a).

In September 2020, 218 schools and kindergartens across Greece piloted The 21st Century Skills Lab, with the aim of developing a new skills national curriculum (Ministry of Education and Religious Affairs, 2020). The 21st Century Skills Lab encompasses life skills, digital and science skills, and soft skills. The term soft skills is used to describe social skills, empathy, citizenship, adaptability, responsibility, resilience, social and self-awareness, self-control, decision making, mediation, and problem solving (OECD, 2019; Partnership for 21st Century Skills, 2009). In May 2021, The 21st Century Skills Lab received a Global Education Award from the

Global Education Network Europe. Following this pilot project, from September 2021, The 21st Century Skills Lab is being taught in kindergarten, primary and lower-secondary schools in Greece as part of the compulsory curriculum (Ministry of Education and Religious Affairs 2021). Teachers are responsible for the design of 20–28 programs to be implemented during the school year, stemming from four broad thematic areas (wellbeing, social awareness and responsibility, environment and creative thinking and innovation). An online platform is provided to schools by the Ministry of Education and Religious Affairs, along with a variety of approved SEL programs (PROMEHS included), teaching resources and suggested activities for teachers and students, assessment material and information for parents.

8.9 Final Suggestions

Teaching and learning build on the components of social, emotional, and academic wellbeing (Durlak et al., 2022). Schools have a fundamental role in providing students with the opportunity to gain social and emotional skills that promote positive mental health, academic progress and therefore encouraging a "whole-child" approach. School-based social and emotional programs and developing social, emotional and wellbeing school policies are among the key factors to address for the overall benefit of students. Gillard and colleagues (2021) for example argue for the need schools to select and implement universal wellbeing practices, and suggest the implementation of the Five Ways to wellbeing (connect, give, be active, take notice and keep learning) as a framework for organizing provisions.

Nevertheless, if we want to reach students, we need to support teachers (Schonert-Reichl et al., 2017). A strong start for helping teachers is to provide them opportunities for cultivating their own emotional competences (Oberle et al., 2020), whereas the social and emotional competences required for the classroom context can be developed through training (Jennings & Greenberg, 2009). In-service and pre-service teacher training need to enhance teachers' mental health and social and emotional skills as well as teachers' strategies and approaches to promote students' and families' wellbeing. Mental health training for teachers must be practical, simple, and interactive. Shelemy and colleagues (2019) based on teachers' perceptions have identified key factors that school training interventions should cover, such as practical strategies, resources tailored by teachers, communication with external services etc. Participants highlighted the need for teacher training on how to identify and provide early support for students who are struggling without taking on the perceived role of a therapist. They also emphasized the strong need for practical, interactive, and expert-led training that provides resources that can be adapted to individual settings.

To summarize, teachers experienced considerable stress as a result of the COVID-19 pandemic, which was related to poorer mental health, coping, and teaching. At the same time, they reported resilience, which was related to better coping and teaching (Baker et al., 2021). Research suggests that socially and emotionally competent teachers can understand and manage their own and others' emotions, they have strong relationship-building capabilities, report higher self-efficacy in teaching and less burnout (Jennings & Greenberg, 2009). By promoting teachers' social and emotional competences we avoid the devastating ripple effects of teacher burnout (Herman et al., 2017) and ameliorate teacher-student relationships (Poulou and Garner, submitted). Therefore, teachers should be empowered to develop better intrapersonal and interpersonal skills and experience a better quality of life (Zagkas et al., 2023). Supporting teachers' wellbeing is critical to prevent significant adverse consequences for teachers, their students, and the education system as a whole.

Competing Interests The author has no conflicts of interest to declare that are relevant to the content of this chapter.

References

Aboagye, M. O., Boateng, P., Asare, K., Sekyere, F. O., Antwi, C. O., & Qin, J. (2020). Managing conflictual teacher-child relationship in pre-schools: A preliminary test of the job resources buffering-effect hypothesis in an emerging economy. *Children and Youth Services Review, 118*, Article 105468. https://doi.org/10.1016/j.childyouth.2020.105468

Aelterman, A., Engels, N., Van Petegem, K., & Verhaeghe, J. P. (2007). The wellbeing of teacher in Flanders: The importance of a supportive school culture. *Educational Studies, 33*(3), 285–298. https://doi.org/10.1080/03055690701423085

Ajduković, D., Rezo Bagarić, I., Bakić, H., Stevanović, A., Frančišković, T., & Ajduković, M. (2021). Mental health status and risk factors during Covid-19 pandemic in the Croatia's adult population. *European Journal of Psychotraumatology, 12*, 1984050. https://doi.org/10.1080/20008198.2021.1984050

Alahiotis, S. N., & Karatzia-Stavlioti, E. (2006). Effective curriculum policy and cross-curricularity: Analysis of the new curriculum design of the Hellenic Pedagogical Institute. *Pedagogy, Culture and Society, 14*(1), 119–147. https://doi.org/10.1080/14681360600738277

Ashdown, D. M., & Bernard, M. E. (2012). Can explicit instruction in social and emotional learning skills benefit the social-emotional development, wellbeing, and academic achievement of young children? *Early Childhood Education Journal, 39*, 397–405. https://doi.org/10.1007/s10643-011-0481-x

Alves, R., Lopes, T., & Precioso, J. (2021). Teachers' wellbeing in times of Covid-19 pandemic: Factors that explain professional wellbeing. *International Journal of Educational Research and Innovation, 15*, 203–217.

Amal Alliance. (2022). *Colors of Kindness*. https://colorsofkindness.org/

Ansari, A., Pianta, R. C., Whittaker, J., Vitiello, V. E., & Ruzek, E. A. (2020). Preschool teachers' emotional exhaustion in relation to classroom instruction and teacher-child interactions. *Early Education and Development, 33*(2), 107–120. https://doi.org/10.1080/10409289.2020.1848301

Babalis, T., Tsoli, K., Artikis, C. T., Mylonakou-Keke, I., & Xanthakou, Y. (2013). The impact of social and emotional learning programs on the emotional competence and academic achievement of children in Greek primary school. *World Journal of Education, 3*(6), 54–63.

Baker, C. N., Peele, H., Daniels, M., Saybe, M., Whalen, K., Overstreet, S., & Trauma-Informed Schools Learning Collaborative The New Orleans. (2021). The experience of COVID-19 and its impact on teachers' mental health, coping and teaching. *School Psychology Review, 50*(4), 491–504. https://doi.org/10.1080/2372966X.2020.1855473

Baker, R., Bloom, N., Davis, S. J., Kost, K. J., Sammon, M. C., & Viratyosin, T. (2020). *The unprecedented stock market impact of COVID-19* (Working paper 26945). National Bureau of Economic Research. www.nber.org/papers/w26945

Bateman, A., Campbell, C., Luyten, P., & Fonagy, P. (2018). A mentalization-based approach to common factors in the treatment of borderline personality disorder. *Current Opinion in Psychology, 21*, 44–49. https://doi.org/10.1016/j.copsyc.2017.09.005

Beltman, S., Mansfield, C., & Price, A. (2011). Thriving not just surviving: A review of research on teacher resilience. *Educational Research Review, 6*(3), 185–207. https://doi.org/10.1016/j.edurev.2011.09.001

Botou, A., Mylonakou-Keke, I., Kalouri, O., & Tsegras, N. (2017). Primary school teachers' resilience during the economic crisis in Greece. *Psychology, 8*(1), 131–159. https://doi.org/10.4236/psych.2017.81009

Bourion-Bédès, S., Tarquinio, C., Batt, M., & Sorsana, C. (2021). Psychological impact of the COVID-19 outbreak on students in a French region severely affected by the disease: Results of the PIMS-CoV 19 study. *Psychiatry Research, 295*, Article 113559. https://doi.org/10.1016/j.psychres.2020.113559

Bradburn, N. M. (1969). *The structure of wellbeing*. Aldine Publishing Company.

Braun, S. S., Roeser, R. W., Mashburn, A. J., & Skinner, E. (2019). Middle school teachers' mindfulness, occupational health and wellbeing, and the quality of teacher-student interactions. *Mindfulness, 10*, 245–255.

Brooks, M., Creely, E., & Laletas, S. (2022). Coping through the unknown: School staff wellbeing during the COVID-10 pandemic. *International Journal of Educational Research*. https://doi.org/10.1016/j.ijedro.2022.100146

Bruckauf, Z. (2017). *Adolescents' mental health*. United Nations.

CASEL. (2020). *CASEL evidence-based social and emotional learning programs: CASEL criteria updates and rationale.*

Cavioni, V., Grazzani, I., Ornaghi, V., & Conte, E. (2023). A multi-component curriculum to promote teachers' mental health: Findings from the PROMEHS program. *International Journal of Emotional Education*. https://doi.org/10.56300/KFNZ2526

Cefai, C., Arlove, A., Duca, M., Galea, N., Muscat, M., & Cavioni, V. (2018). RESCUR Surfing the waves: An evaluation of a resilience programme in the early years. *Pastoral Car e in Education, 36*(3), 189–204. https://doi.org/10.1080/02643944.2018.1479224

Cefai, C., Cavioni, V., Bartolo, P., Simoes, C., Miljevic-Ridicki, R., Bouilet, D., Ivanec, T. P., Matsopoulos, A., Gavogiannaki, M., Zanetti, M. A., Galea, K., Lebre, P., Kimber, B., & Erickson, C. (2015). Social inclusion and social justice. A resilience curriculum for early years and elementary schools in Europe. *Journal of Multicultural Education, 9*(3), 122–139.

Cefai, C., Camilleri, L., Bartolo, P., & Colomeischi, A. (2022). The effectiveness of a school-based, universal mental health programme in six European countries. *Frontiers in Psychology*. https://doi.org/10.3389/fpsyg.2022.925614

Chiementi, G., & Triliva, S. (1994). Cognitive and behavioral effects of social skills training on Greek and Lebanese elementary-school children. *International Journal of Mental Health, 23*(4), 53–68.

Cipriano, C., & Brackett, M. (2020). *Teachers are anxious and overwhelmed. They need SEL now more than ever*. EdSurge News. https://www.edsurge.com/news/2020-04-07-teachers-are-anxious-and-overwhelmed-they-need-sel-now-more-than-ever

Collaborative for Academic, Social and Emotional Learning (CASEL). (2013). *Effective social and emotional learning programs. Preschool and elementary school edition*. CASEL.

Colomeischi, A. A., Duca, D. S., Bujor, L., Rusu, P. P., Grazzani, I., & Cavioni, V. (2022). Impact of a school mental health program on children's and adolescents' socio-emotional skills and psychosocial difficulties. *Children, 9*, 1661. https://doi.org/10.3390/children9111661

Cooper, P., & Hornby, G. (2018). Facing the challenges to mental health and wellbeing in schools. *Pastoral Care in Education, 36*(3), 173–175. https://doi.org/10.1080/02643933.2018.1488658

Courtwright, S. E., Makic, M., & Jones, J. (2019). Emotional wellbeing in youth: A concept analysis. *Nursing Forum, 55*, 106–117. https://doi.org/10.1111/nuf.12404

Cruwys, T., Stevens, M., & Greenaway, K. H. (2020). A social identity perspective on COVID-19: Health risk is affected by shared group membership. *British Journal of Social Psychology, 59*(3), 584–593. https://doi.org/10.1111/bjso.12391

Darling, S., Dawson, G., Quach, J., & Oberklaid, F. (2021). Mental health and wellbieng coordinators in primary schools to support student mental health: Protocol for a quali-experimental cluster study. *BMC Public Health, 21*, 1467. https://doi.org/10.1186/s12889-021-11467-4

Deci, E. L., & Ryan, R. M. (2008). Facilitating optimal motivation and psychological wellbeing across life's domains. *Canadian Psychology, 49*, 14–23.

Dianeosis. (2020). *Public opinion survey* (in Greek). https://www.dianeosis.org/wp-content/uploads/2020/03/tpe_2020_final.pdf

Didaskalou, E., Andreou, E., Roussi-Vergou, C., & Skrzypiec, G. (2018). Are Greek school students flourishing? *Pastoral Care in Education, 36*(3), 223–237. https://doi.org/10.1080/02643944.2018.1480185

Diener, E. (1994). Assessing subjective wellbeing: Progress and opportunities. *Social Indicators Research, 31*, 103–157.

Diener, E. (2000). Subjective wellbeing: The science of happiness, and a proposal for a national index. *American Psychologist, 55*(1), 34–43.

Diener, E., & Emmons, R. A. (1985). The independence of positive and negative affect. *Journal of Personality and Social Psychology, 47*(5), 1105–1117.

DiPerna, J. C., Lei, P., Cheng, W., Hart, S. C., & Bellinger, J. (2018). A cluster randomized trial of the social skills improvement system-classwide intervention program in first grade. *Journal of Educational Psychology, 110*(1), 1–16. https://doi.org/10.1037/edu0000191

Doni, E., & Giotsa, A. (2017). Prevention programs for the cultivation of social and emotional skills in preschool. *Scientific Journal the Department of Nursery Education of the University of Ioannina, 10*, 68–97 (In Greek).

Durlak, J. A., Mahoney, J. L., & Boyle, A. E. (2022). What we know, and what we need to find out about universal, school-based social and emotional learning programs for children and adolescents: A review of meta-analyses and directions for future research. *Psychological Bulletin, 148*(11–12), 765–782. https://doi.org/10.1037/bul0000383

Durlak, J. A., Weissberg, R., Dymnicki, A. B., & Schellinger, K. B. (2011). The impact of enhancing students' social and emotional learning: A meta-analysis of school-based universal intervention. *Child Development, 82*(1), 405–432. https://doi.org/10.1111/j.1467-8624.2010.01564x

Elder, C., Nidich, S., Morirty, F., & Nidich, R. E. (2014). Effects of transcendental mediation on employee stress, depression and burnout: A randomized control study. *Permanente Journal, 18*, 19–23.

Elliot, J. G., Stemler, S. E., Stenberg, R. J., Grigorenko, E. L., & Hoffman, N. (2011). The socially skilled teacher and the development of tacit knowledge. *British Educational Research Journal, 37*, 83–103.

Erskine, H., Moffitt, T., Copeland, W., & Scott, G. (2015). A heavy burden on young minds: The global burden of mental and substance use disorders in children and youth. *Psychological Medicine, 45*(7), 1551–1563. https://doi.org/10.1017/S0033291714002888

European Foundation for the Improvement of Living Working Conditions. (2020, April). *Living, working and COVID-19: First findings*. Publications Office of the European Union. https://www.eurofound.europa.eu/publications/report/2020/living-working-and-covid-19-first-findings-april-2020

Fiorilli, C., De Stasio, S., Di Chiacchio, C., Pepe, A., & Salmela-Aro, K. (2017). School burnout, depressive symptoms and engagement: Their combined effect on student achievement. *International Journal of Educational Research, 84*, 1–12. https://doi.org/10.1016/j.ijer.2017.04.001

Fox, E., Parsons, S., Todorovic, A., Songco, A., & Lim, M. (2020). *The Oxford ARC study: Achieving resilience during COVID-19-Psychosocial risk and protective factors amidst a pandemic in adolescents and their parents*. http://oxfordarcstudycom.files.wordpress.com/2020/05/oxfordarcstudy_report_1-1.pdf

Frank, J. L., Reibel, D., Broderick, P., Cantrell, T., & Metz, S. (2013). The effectiveness of mindfulness-based stress reduction on educator stress and wellbeing: Results from a pilot study. *Mindfulness, 6*, 208–216.

Fredrickson, B., Tugade, M., Waugh, C., & Larkin, G. (2003). What good are positive emotions in crises? A prospective study of resilience and emotions following the terrorist attacks on the United States on September 11, 2001. *Journal of Personality and Social Psychology, 84*(2), 365–376. https://doi.org/10.1037/0022-3514.84.2.365

Frenzel, A. C., Goetz, T., Ludtke, O., Pekrun, R., & Sutton, R. E. (2009). Emotional transmission in the classroom: Exploring the relationship between teacher and student enjoyment. *Journal of Educational Psychology, 101*(3), 705–716. https://doi.org/10.1037/a0014695

Giannakopoulos, G., Kazantzi, M., Dimitrakaki, C., Tsiantis, J., Kolaitis, G., & Tountas, Y. (2009). Screening for chidlren's depression symptoms in Greece: The use of the children's depression inventory in a nation-wide school-based sample. *European Child and Adolescent Psychiatry, 18*(8), 485–492.

Giannopoulou, I., Efstathiou, V., Triantafyllou, G., Korkoliakou, P., & Douzenis, A. (2020). Adding stress to the stressed: Senior high school students' mental health amidst the COVID-19 nation-wide lockdown in Greece. *Psychiatry Research*, 295. https://doi.org/10.1016/j.psychres.2020.113560

Giannopoulou, I., & Tsobanoglou, G. O. (2020). COVID-19 pandemic: Challenges and opportunities for the Greek health care system. *Irish Journal of Psychological Medicine, 37*, 226–230. https://doi.org/10.1017/ipm.2023.35

Gillard, D., Reid, A., Bull-Beddows, R., Mohamed-Goush, S., Stanley-Duke, M., & Cook, E. (2021). Universal wellbeing practices in schools: Framing evidence-informed practice within the five ways to wellbeing. *Educational Psychology Research and Practice, 7*(1).

Gilmour, A. F., Sandilos, L. E., Pilny, W. V., Schwartz, S., & Wehby, J. H. (2022). Teaching students with emotional/behavioral disorders: Teachers' burnout profiles and classroom management. *Journal of Emotional and Behavioral Disorders, 30*(1), 16–28. https://doi.org/10.1177/10634266211020258

Glazzard, J., & Rose, A. (2020). The impact of teacher wellbeing and mental health on pupil progress in primary schools. *Journal of Public Mental Health, 19*(4), 349–357. https://doi.org/10.1108/JPMH-02-2019-0023

Gray, C., Wilcox, G., & Nordstokke, D. (2017). Teacher mental health, school climate, inclusive education and student learning. *A Review. Canadian Psychology, 58*(3), 203–210.

Green, A. L., Ferrante, S., Boaz, T. L., Kutash, K., & Wheeldon-Reece, B. (2021). Social and emotional learning during early adolescence: Effectiveness of a classroom-based SEL program for middle school students. *Psychology in the Schools, 58*(6), 1056–1069. https://doi.org/10.1002/pits.22487

Greenberg, M. T., Brown, J. L., & Abenavoli, R. M. (2016). *Techer stress and health effects on teachers, students and schools.* Pennsylvania State University.

Hakanen, J. J., Bakker, A. B., & Schaufeli, W. B. (2006). Burnout and work engagement among teachers. *Journal of School Psychology, 43*(6), 495–513. https://doi.org/10.1016/j.jsp.2005.11.001

Harding, S., Morris, R., Gunnella, D., Ford, T., Kidger, J., et al. (2019). Is teachers' mental health and wellbeing associated with students' mental health and wellbeing? *Journal of Affective Disorders, 242*(2019), 180–187.

Hargreaves, A. (2000). Mixed emotions: Teachers' perceptions of their interactions with students. *Teaching and Teacher Education, 16*(8), 811–826. https://doi.org/10.1016/S072-051X(00)00028-7

Hascher, T., Beltman, S., & Mansfield, C. (2021). Teacher wellbeing and resilience: towards an integrative model. *Educational Research, 63*(4), 416–439. https://doi.org/10.1080/00131881.2021.1980416

Herman, K. C., Hickmon-Rosa, J. E., & Reinke, W. M. (2017). Empirically derived profiles of teacher stress, burnout, self-efficacy, and coping and associated student outcomes. *Journal of Positive Behavior Interventions, 2*, 90–100.

Hodge, G. M., Jupp, J. J., & Taylor, A. J. (1994). Work stress, distress and burnout in music and mathematics teachers. *British Journal of Educational Psychology, 64*, 65–76.

Holtge, J., Jefferies, P., Cowden, R. G., & Ungar, M. (2021). A cross-country network analysis of adolescent resilience. *Journal of Adolescent Health, 68*(3), 580–588. https://doi.org/10.1016/j.jadohealth.2020.07.010

Hornby, G., & Atkinson, M. (2003). A framework for promoting mental health in schools. *Pastoral Care in Education, 21*(1), 3–9.

Hu, D., Kong, Y., Li, W., Han, Q., Zhang, X., & Zhu, L. X. (2020). Frontline nurses' burnout, anxiety, depression, and fear statuses and their associated factors during the COVID-19 outbreak in Wuhan, China: A large-scale cross-sectional study. *EClinicalMedicine, 24*, Article 100424. https://doi.org/10.1016/j.eclinm.2020.100424

Jahrami, H., Haji, E. A., Saif, Z. Q., & Vitiello, M. V. (2022). Sleep quality worsens while perceived stress improves in healthcare workers over two years during the COVID-19 Pandemic: Results of a longitudinal study. *Healthcare, 10*, 1588.

Jennings, P. A., & Greenberg, M. T. (2009). The prosocial classroom: Teacher social and emotional competence in relation to student and classroom outcomes. *Review of Educational Research, 79*(1), 491–525. https://doi.org/10.3102/0034654308325693

Jennings, P. A., Frank, J. L., Snowberg, K. E., Coccia, M. A., & Greenberg, M. T. (2013). Improving classroom learning environments by cultivating awareness and resilienece in education (CARE): Results from two randomized, waitlist-control field trials. *Journal of Educational Psychology, 28*, 374–390.

Jones, S. M., Bouffard, S. M., & Weissbourd, R. (2013). Educators' social and emotional skills vital to learning. *Phi Delta Kappan, 94*, 62–65.

Kaparounaki, C. K., Patsali, M. E., Mousa, D., Papadopoulou, E., Papadopoulou, K., & Fountoulakis, K. N. (2020). University students' mental health amidst the COVID-19 quarantine in Greece. *Psychiatry Research, 290*, Article 113111.

Kariou, A., Koutsimani, P., Montgomery, A., & Lainidi, O. (2021). Emotional labor and burnout among teachers: A systematic review. *International Journal of Environmental Research and Public Health, 18*(23), 12760. https://doi.org/10.3390/ijerph182312760

Katz, D., Mahfouz, J., & Romas, S. (2020). Creating a foundation of wellbeing for teachers and students starts with SEL curriculum in teacher education programs. *Northwest Journal of Teacher Education, 15*(2). https://doi.org/10.15760/nwjte.2020.15.2.5

Keyes, C. M. (2006). Mental health in adolescence: Is America's youth flourishing? *American Journal of Orthopsychiatry, 76*(3), 395–402.

Kidger, J., Brockman, R., Tilling, K., & Gunnell, D. (2016). Teachers' wellbeing and depressive symptoms, and associated risk factors: A large cross sectional study in English secondary schools. *Journal of Affective Disorders, 192*, 76–82.

Kim, L. E., Oxley, L., & Asbury, K. (2022). "My brain feels like a browser with 100 tabs open": A longitudinal study of teachers' mental health and wellbeing during the COVID-19 pandemic. *British Journal of Educational Psychology, 92*, 299–318. https://doi.org/10.1111/bjep.12450

Kourmousi, N., & Alexopoulos, E. C. (2016). Stress sources and manifestations in a nationwide sample of pre-primary, primary, and secondary educators in Greece. *Frontiers in Public Health, 73*(4). https://doi.org/10.3389/fpubh.2016.00073

Kourmousi, N., Markogiannakis, G., Tzavara, C., Kounenou, K., Mandrikas, A., Christopoulou, E., & Koutras, V. (2018). Students' psychosocial empowerment with the "Steps for Life" personal and social skills Greek elementary program. *International Electronic Journal of Elementary Education, 10*(5), 535–549.

Kourmousi, N., Salagianni, M., Merakou, K., Tzavara, C., & Koutras, V. (2017). Evaluation of the "Steps for Life" personal and social skills Greek K-Curriculum. *Creative Education, 8*, 1912–1940. https://doi.org/10.4236/ce.2017.812131

Lee, J. (2020). Mental health effects of school closures during COVID-19. *The Lancet. Child and Adolescent Health, 4*, 421.

Lei, L., Huang, X., Zhang, S., Yang, J., Yang, L., & Xu, M. (2020). Comparison of prevalence and associated factors of anxiety and depression among people affected by versus people unaffected by quarantine during the COVID-19 epidemic in southwestern China. *Medical Science Monitor, 26*, e924609. https://doi.org/10.12659/MSM.924609

Lewis, A. D., Huebner, E. S., Reschly, A. L., & Valois, R. F. (2009). The incremental validity of positive emotions in predicting school functioning. *Journal of Psychoeducational Assessment, 27*, 397–408.

Lewnard, J., & Lo, N. C. (2020). Scientific and ethical basis for social-distancing interventions against COVID-19. *The Lancet. Infectious Diseases, 20*(6), 631–633. https://doi.org/10.1016/S1473-3099(20)30190-0

Lovibond, S. H., & Lovibond, P. F. (1995). *Manual for the depression anxiety stress scales* (2nd ed.). Psychology Foundation.

Luyten, P., Campbell, C., Allison, E., & Fonagy, P. (2020). The Mentalizing approach to psychopathology: State of the art and future directions. *Annual Review of Clinical Psychology, 16*, 297–325. https://doi.org/10.1146/annurev-clinpsy-071919-015355

Madianos, M., Economou, M., Alexiou, T., & Stefanis, C. (2011). Depression and economic hardship across Greece in 2008 and 2009: Two cross-sectional surveys nationwide. *Social Psychiatry and Psychiatric Epidemiology, 46*, 943–952.

Madigan, D. J., & Kim, L. E. (2021). Towards an understanding of teacher attrition: a meta-analysis of burnout, job satisfaction, and teachers' intentions to quit. *Teaching and Teacher Education, 105*, 10342. https://doi.org/10.1016/j.tate.2021.103425

Magklara, K., Lazaratou, H., Barbouni, A., Poulas, K., & Farsalinos, K. (2021). The impact of COVID-19 lockdown on children's and adolescents' mental health in Greece. *Children and Society, 37*, 469–484. https://doi.org/10.1111/chso.12605

Manzano-García, G., Ayala-Calvo, J. C., & Desrumaux, P. (2020). Entrepreneurs' capacity for Mentalizing: Its influence on burnout syndrome. *International Journal of Environmental Research and Public Health, 18*(3). https://doi.org/10.3390/ijerph18010003

Maslach, C., Schaufeli, W., & Leiter, M. P. (2001). Job burnout. *Annual Review of Psychology, 52*, 397–422.

Mazza, C., Ricci, E., Biondi, S., & Napoli, C. (2020). A Nationwide survey of psychological distress among Italian people during the COVID-19 pandemic: Immediate psychological responses and associated factors. *International Journal of Environmental Research and Public Health, 17*, 3165. https://doi.org/10.3390/ijerph17093165

Ministry of Education and Religious Affairs. (2003a). *A cross thematic curriculum framework for compulsory education and analytical curricula for primary and secondary education*. Official Gazzette, Issue B, no 303 and 304, 13-3-2003. Greek Pedagogical Institute.

Ministry of Education and Religious Affairs. (2003b). *A cross thematic curriculum framework for compulsory education and analytical curricula for primary and secondary education*. Official Gazzette, Issue B, (1366/18-10-2001), B (1373/18-10-2001), B (1376/18-10-2001). Greek Pedagogical Institute.

Ministry of Education and Religious Affairs. (2020). Reforms for primary, secondary education and Life-Long Learning. (FEK A111–12.06.2020)

Ministry of Education and Religious Affairs. (2021). *Curriculum framework for Skill labs in all types of the schools in preschool, primary and secondary education Official Gazzette* (FEK 3567, 4-08-2021).

Moccia, L., Janiri, D., Pepe, M., Dattoli, L., Molinaro, M., & De Martin, V. (2020). Affective temperament, attachment style, and the psychological impact of the COVID-19 outbreak: An early report on the Italian general population. *Brain, Behavior, and Immunity, 87*, 75–79. https://doi.org/10.1016/j.bbi.2020.04.048

Montgomery, C., & Rupp, A. (2005). A meta-analysis for exploring the diverse causes and effects of stress in teachers. *Canadian Journal of Education/revue Canadienne De L'education, 28*(3), 458–486. https://doi.org/10.2307/4126479

Morres, I. D., Galanis, E., Hatzigeorgiadis, A., Androutsos, O., & Theodorakis, Y. (2021). Physical activity, sedentariness, eating behaviour and wellbeing during a COVID-19 lockdown period in Greek adolescents. *Nutrients, 13*, 1449. https://doi.org/10.3390/nu13051449

Morris, C. A., Denham, S. A., Bassett, H. H., & Curby, T. W. (2013). Relations among teachers' emotion socialization beliefs and practices and preschoolers' emotional competence. *Early Education and Development., 24*, 979–999.

Mouratidis, K., & Yiannakou, A. (2022). COVID-19 and urban planning: Built environment, health, and wellbeing in Greek cities before and during the pandemic. *Cities*, 121. https://doi.org/10.1016/j.cities.2021.103491

Mourelatos, E. (2023). How personality affects reaction. A mental health behavioral insight review during the Pandemic. *Current Psychology, 42*, 8644–8665. https://doi.org/10.1007/s12144-021-02425-9

Norwich, B., Moore, D., Stentiford, L., & Hall, D. (2021). A critical consideration of "mental health and wellbeing" in education: Thinking about school aims in terms of wellbeing. *British Educational Research Journal, 48*, 803–820. https://doi.org/10.1002/berj.3795

Oberle, E., Gist, A., Cooray, M. S., & Pinto, J. B. (2020). Do students notice stress in teachers? Associations between classroom teacher burnout and students' perceptions of teacher social–emotional competence. *Psychology in the Schools, 57*(11), 1741–1756. https://doi.org/10.1002/pits.22432

Odriozola-González, P., Planchuelo-Gómez, Á., Irurtia, M. J., & de Luis-García, R. (2020). Psychological effects of the COVID-19 outbreak and lockdown among students and workers of a Spanish university. *Psychiatry Research, 290*, 13108. https://doi.org/10.1016/j.psychres.2020.113108

OECD. (2019). *Future of education and skills 2030 concept note*. https://www.oecd.org/education/2030-project/teaching-and-_learning/learning/skills/Skills_for_2030_concept_note.pdf

Oliveira Carvalho, P., Hülsdünker, T., & Carson F. (2021). The impact of the COVID-19 lockdown on European Students' negative emotional symptoms: A systematic review and meta-analysis. *Behavior Science, 12*(3). https://doi.org/10.3390/bs12010003

Papastylianou, A., Kaila, M., & Polychronopoulos, M. (2009). Teachers' burnout, depression, role ambiguity and conflict. *Social Psychology of Education, 12*, 295–314.

Parlapani, E., Holeva, V., Voitsidis, P., & Chatzigeorgiou, A. E. (2020). Psychological and behavioral responses to the COVID-19 pandemic in Greece. *Frontiers, Psychiatry, 11*, 821.

Partnership for 21st Century Skills. (2009). *Ohio department of education*. https://www.scribd.com/document/432204021/partnership-for-21st-century-skills-2009

Patsali, M. E., Mousa, D. V., Papadopoulou, E. V. K., Papadopoulou, K. K. K., & Diakogiannis, I. (2020). University students' changes in mental health status and determinants of behavior during the COVID-19 lockdown in Greece. *Psychiatry Research, 292*, Article 113298. https://doi.org/10.1016/j.psychres.2020.113298

Pedagogical Institute. (2003). *Introductory note by the president of the Pedagogical Institute*. Official Gazetta, issue B, nr 303/13-03-2003, issue B, nr 304/13-03-2003.

Poole, J. C., Dobson, K. S., & Pusch, D. (2017). Childhood adversity and adult depression: The protective role of psychological resilience. *Child Abuse and Neglect, 64*, 89–100. https://doi.org/10.1016/j.chiabu.2016.12.012

Poulou, M., & Norwich, B. (2020). Psychological needs, mixed self-perceptions, wellbeing and emotional and behavioral difficulties: Adolescent students' perceptions. *European Journal of Psychology of Education, 35*, 775–793. https://doi.org/10.1007/s10212-019-00457-1

Poulou, M. S., & Garner, P. W. (submitted). Students' other-oriented cognitions: The roles of teachers' emotional competence and classroom social support in a greek sample. *School Psychology International.*

Poulou, M. S., & Norwich, B. (2019). Adolescent students' psychological needs: Development of an existence, relatedness, and growth needs scale. *International Journal of School & Educational Psychology, 7*(supl), 75–83.

Poulou, M.S., Grazzani, I., Cavioni, V., Ornaghi, V., Conte, E., Cefai, C, Camilleri, L., Bartolo, P. (2022a). Teachers' and students' changes in social and emotional competences following the implementation of PROMEHS: A European program for Promoting Mental Health at Schools. *Educational Research Application, 7*(1). https://doi.org/10.29011/2575-7032.100205

Poulou, M.S., Grazzani, I., Cavioni, V., Ornaghi, V., Conte, E., Cefai, C, Camilleri, L., Bartolo, P. (2022b). Changes in students' social and emotional competences following the implementation of a school-based intervention program. *American Journal of Applied Psychology, 11*(5), 122–132. https://doi.org/10.11648/j.ajap.20221105.11

Pressley, T. (2021). Factors contributing to teacher burnout during COVID-19. *Educational Researcher, 50*, 325–327. https://doi.org/10.3102/0013189X211004138

Roeser, R. W. (2016). Processes of teaching, learning and transfer in mindfulness-based interventions for teachers: A contemplative educational perspective. In *Handbook of mindfulness in education* (pp.149–170). Springer.

Ryan, R. M., & Deci, E. L. (2001). On happiness and human potentials: A review of research on hedonic and eudaimonic wellbeing. In S. Fiske (Ed.), *Annual review of psychology* (pp. 141–166). Annual Reviews.

Safiye, T., & Vukčević, B. (2020). Dimensions of general psychological distress and age as the predictors of procrastination in university students. *Psihološka Istraživanja., 24*, 187–200. https://doi.org/10.5937/PSISTRA23-27810

Salari, N., Hosseinian-Far, A., Jalali, R., & Mohammadi, M. (2020). Prevalence of stress, anxiety, depression among the general population during the COVID-19 pandemic: A systematic review and meta-analysis. *Globalization and Health, 16*(1), 57. https://doi.org/10.1186/s12992-020-00589-w

Schonert-Reichl, K. A., Kitil, M. J., & Hanson-Peterson, J. (2017). *To reach the students, teach the teachers: A national scan of teacher preparation and social and emotional learning*. A report prepared for the Collaborative for Academic, Social, and Emotional Learning (CASEL). University of British Columbia.

Schwarzer, N. H., Nolte, T., Fonagy, P., Griem, J., Kieschke, U., & Gingelmaier, S. (2021). The relationship between global distress, mentalizing and wellbeing in a German teacher sample. *Current Psychology*, 1–10. https://doi.org/10.1007/s12144-021-01467-3

Serafini, G., Parmigiani, B., Amerio, A., Aguglia, A., Sher, L., & Amore, M. (2020). The psychological impact of COVID-19 on the mental health in the general population. *QJM, 113*, 531–537. https://doi.org/10.1093/qjmed/hcaa201

Shelemy, L., Harvey, K., & Waite, P. (2019). Supporting students' mental health in schools: What do teachers want and need? *Emotional and Behavioural Difficulties, 24*(1), 1–116. https://doi.org/10.1080/13632752.2019.1582742

Shoshani, A., & Slone, M. (2013). Middle school transition from the strengths perspective: Young adolescents' character strengths, subjective wellbeing, and school adjustment. *Journal of Happiness Studies, 14*, 1163–1181.

Sisask, M., Varnik, P., Varnik, A., Apter, A., Balazs, J., & Balint, M. (2014). Teacher satisfaction with school and psychological wellbeing affects their readiness to help children with mental health problems. *Health Education Journal, 73*(4), 382–393.

Sokal, L., & Eblie Trudel, L. (2020). *How to prevent teacher burnout during the coronavirus pandemic*. The Conversation. https://theconversation.com/how-to-prevent-teacher-burnout-during-the-coronavirus-pandemic-139353

Suldo, S. M., Riley, K. N., & Shaffer, E. J. (2006). Academic correlates of children and adolescents' life satisfaction. *School Psychology International, 27*(5), 567–582.

Triliva, S., Anagnostopoulou, T., & Vleioras, G. (2014). Sensitizing children to the social and emotional mechanisms involved in racism: A program evaluation. *International Journal of Emotional Education, 6*(2), 3–20.

Trinidad, J. E. (2021). Equity, engagement, and health: school organizational issues and priorities during COVID-19. *Journal of Educational Administration and History, 53*(1), 67–80. https://doi.org/10.1080/00220620.2020.1858764

UK Department of Health and Education. (2017). *Transforming children and young people's mental health provision: A Green Paper*.

Van de Sande, M. C., Fekkes, M., Kocken, P. L., Diekstra, R. F. W., Reis, R., & Gravestejin, C. (2019). Do universal social and emotional learning programs for secondary school students enhance the competencies they address? A systematic review. *Psychology in the Schools, 56*(10), 1545–1567. https://doi.org/10.1002/pits.22

Velavan, T. P., & Meyer, C. G. (2020). The COVID-19 epidemic. *Tropical Medicine and International Health, 25*, 278–280. https://doi.org/10.1111/tmi.13383

Vujčić, I., Safiye, T., Milikić, B., & Dubljanin, E. (2021). Coronavirus disease 2019 (COVID-19) epidemic and mental health status in the general adult population of Serbia: A cross-sectional study. *International Journal of Environmental Research and Public Health, 18*, 1957. https://doi.org/10.3390/ijerph18041957

Wald, J., Taylor, S., Asmundson, G. J., Jang, K. L., & Stapleton, J. (2006). *Literature review of concepts: Psychological Resiliency*. British Columbia University.

Wang, Z., Pang, H., Zhou, J., Ma, Y., & Wang, Z. (2021). What if…it never ends? Examining challenges in primary teachers' experience during the wholly online teaching. *Journal of Educational Research, 114*(1), 89–103. https://doi.org/10.1080/00220671.2021.1884823

Wang, C., Pan, R., Wan, X., Tan, Y., Xu, L., & Ho, C. S. (2020). Immediate psychological responses and associated factors during the initial stage of the 2019 coronavirus disease (COVID-19) epidemic among the general population in China. *International Journal of Environmental Research and Public Health, 17*, 1729. https://doi.org/10.3390/ijerph17051729

Wells, M., Avers, D., & Brooks, G. (2001). Resilience, physical performance measures, and self-perceived physical and mental health in older Catholic nuns. *Journal of Geriatric Physical Therapy, 2012*(35), 126–131. https://doi.org/10.1519/JPT.0b013e318237103f

Wodon, Q. (2020). COVID-19 crisis, impacts on catholic schools and potential responses part1: Developed countries with focus on the United States. *Journal of Catholic Education, 23*(1), 13–50.

World Health Organization (WHO). (2005). *Promoting mental health: Concepts, emerging evidence, practice: Summary report*. World Health Organization.

World Health Organization (WHO). (2007). *What is health promoting school?* https://www.who.int/school_youth_health/gshi/hps/en/index.html

World Health Organization (WHO). (2015). *First WHO report on suicide prevention*. https://www.who.int/mediacentre/news/releases/2014/suicide-prevention-report/en

Xiong, J., Lipsitz, O., Nasri, F., McIntyre, R. S. (2020). Impact of COVID-19 pandemic on mental health in the general population: A systematic review. *Journal of Affective Disorders*. https://doi.org/10.1016/j.jad.2020.08.001

Yıldırım, M., & Arslan, G. (2020). Exploring the associations between resilience, dispositional hope, preventive behaviours, subjective wellbeing, and psychological health among adults during early stage of COVID-19. *Current Psychology*, 1–11. https://doi.org/10.1007/s12144-020-01177-2

Yıldırım, M., & Solmaz, F. (2022). COVID-19 burnout, COVID-19 stress and resilience: Initial psychometric properties of COVID-19 burnout scale. *Death Studies, 46*, 524–532. https://doi.org/10.1080/07481187.2020.1818885

Zagkas, D. G., Chrousos, G. P., Bacopoulou, F., Kanaka-Gantenbein, C., Vlachakis, D., Tzelepi, I., and Darviri, C. (2023). Stress and wellbeing of Greek primary school educators: A cross-sectional study. *International Journal of Environmental Research and Public Health*. https://doi.org/10.3390/ijerph20075390

Chapter 9
Wellbeing in the Education System of the Republic of Moldova: Conceptualization, Promotion and Assurance

Antoci Diana and Mislitchi Valentina

9.1 Introduction

In the context of the continuous evolution of research in the psychological and pedagogical field, new horizons are emerging in the conceptualization and structuring of wellbeing. Wellbeing, defined as a complex and multifactorial dimension of human existence, is becoming more and more relevant in contemporary psychopedagogical approaches. By exploring this expanding topic, researchers and practitioners in psychology and pedagogy aim to identify and understand new dimensions that contribute to understanding and improving personality wellbeing.

This study focuses on exploring innovative aspects of wellbeing integrated into a psychological and pedagogical framework. By approaching this topic, we aim to bring to attention emerging models and theories, to highlight the mutual influences between the educational environment and wellbeing, as well as to identify effective psychopedagogical practices and interventions to promote an optimal state of the subjects involved in the teaching-learning-evaluation process.

Through the study carried out in this chapter, we aim not only to expand existing knowledge about wellbeing, but also to create a new conceptualization of wellbeing from a psychological and pedagogical perspective with subsequent applicability in the field of Educational Sciences. By exploring new dimensions, we want to contribute to the development of innovative educational strategies and programs, oriented toward the cultivation of a sustainable and progressive state of wellbeing.

A. Diana (✉) · M. Valentina
"Ion Creanga" State Pedagogical University of Chisinau, Chişinău, Republic of Moldova
e-mail: antoci.diana@upsc.md

M. Valentina
e-mail: mislitchi.valentina@upsc.md

A. A. Colomeischi (ed.), *Wellbeing in Schools of Southeastern Europe*, Human Well-Being Research and Policy Making, https://doi.org/10.1007/978-3-032-10525-7_9

Therefore, these contents are addressed to both researchers and theoreticians in the field of educational and psychopedagogical sciences, as well as to specialists, practitioners involved in the learning and development processes of individuals. In an ever-changing social and educational climate, understanding and managing well-being becomes imperative to promote truly comprehensive and tailored education and training.

Theoretical-experimental research on wellbeing has elucidated the *contradictions* between: the value of wellbeing in the formation of the integral personality and ensuring the quality of life linked to socio-educational policy, on the one hand, and the uncertainty of scientific opinions regarding the essential structural components and the context of establishment of wellbeing, on the other hand.

The identification of the ways of solving the existing contradictions determined *research problem*: what are the theoretical-praxiological benchmarks for ensuring the wellbeing of educational actors in various psycho-socio-pedagogical contexts?

The *purpose* of the conducted research was foundation and elaboration of the Pedagogical Model for ensuring the wellbeing of educational actors.

The theoretical approach to the problem allows the exploration and expansion of fundamental studies on the nature, essence, structural components, dimensions of wellbeing, factors and contexts that contribute to the establishment of wellbeing of the personality, which are reflected in the Pedagogical Model of ensuring wellbeing, providing, at the same time, a solid conceptual basis for future research.

The applicative value of the study consists in providing the theoretical-praxiological support for the development of psychological and pedagogical intervention programs to ensure wellbeing, psychoprophylaxis programs aimed at warning the emergence of disturbances in the cognitive, affective, behavioral sphere of the personality. The research creates contexts for the implementation of education policies, guiding the development of effective programs to promote wellbeing.

Therefore, the theoretical-applicative value of the given study consists in the multi-aspectual approach to wellbeing and the development of effective strategies that support a healthier, balanced and fulfilled life for the human being and society as a whole.

9.2 Wellbeing Through the Prism of Theoretical Approaches and Education Policy Documents in the Republic of Moldova

The exploration of theoretical approaches in the conceptualization of wellbeing in the Republic of Moldova and internationally is essential to understand the complexity of this subject. The study and comparison of the various theoretical perspectives attested in the Republic of Moldova with those from around the world can provide a comprehensive picture of the defining aspects of the concept of "wellbeing".

At the national level, the presence of some theoretical-analytical studies of wellbeing from the psychological and pedagogical perspective is mostly attested, in which concepts, theories and models existing at the international level are examined (Csikszentmihalyi, 1990; Peterson & Park, 2011; Ryff & Singer, 2008; Seligman, 2011 etc.), highlighted various scientific opinions regarding structural components (Allardt, 1989; Bradburn, 1969; Deci & Ryan, 2008; Konu & Rimpela, 2002; Ryff, 1989 etc.), established the limits of wellbeing (Kagan, 1992), analyzed possible correlations with personality traits, wellbeing among teachers, professional satisfaction (Colomeischi, 2017, 2019; Negură, 2014; Rusnac, 2017; Rusu & Colomeischi, 2020 etc.), emphasized the value of teachers' wellbeing in increasing the quality of pedagogical activity (Goraş-Postică & Vartic, 2022 etc.), established the correlation between academic stress and wellbeing (Suman et al., 2023 etc.), identified the perspectives of quality education by ensuring the parents and children' wellbeing (Colomeischi, 2019; Straistari-Lungu, 2016 etc.), adapted the wellbeing research tool based on five components (the feeling of being happy, self-acceptance, control over the environment, the capacity for autonomy, positive relationships with others, the purpose and meaning of life), the correlation with anxiety (Rusnac, 2017), significance and implications of the wellbeing from psychological perspective (Turchină et al., 2012), psychological wellbeing in the educational environment (Batog, 2021), etc. The deepening of research in areas such as mental health, social inclusion and equity in access to resources and services becomes crucial to develop appropriate strategies to improve the wellbeing of the population of the Republic of Moldova.

Researchers from the Republic of Moldova capitalize on the scientific results obtained at the international level in their domestic studies by referring to definitions, models, theories, evaluation tools, strategies for ensuring wellbeing, etc. and, therefore, come up with new findings, additions, opinions, clarifications, significance that anticipate future trends and ensure the implementation of progressive and innovative strategies to support the wellbeing of subjects necessary to adapt to the flow of changes at global and community level.

It also critically examines the notion of wellbeing as it has evolved over time, particularly in light of technological change, migration and social and cultural diversity.

The analysis of the term wellbeing allowed highlighting the semantic area that encompasses all the meanings, connotations and associations that the respective concept attests in the Romanian language. The concept of wellbeing, often translated into Romanian as "psychological wellbeing", "psychological health" or "subjective wellbeing", is a broad notion that reflects the way people live, feel their lives through experiences, emotions, judgments, behaviors and attitudes. Although there is no exact equivalent for this concept in Romanian, translations approximate it with terms such as "welfare" or "state of wellbeing", thus approaching its original and much more complex meaning, which involves a holistic feeling of wellbeing, comfort and individual happiness.

Approaching the concept of wellbeing, specific to the English language, translated into Romanian as "state of wellbeing" or "wellbeing" allows us to find synonymy in their application, the more frequent use of the term "welfare" in policy documents in the Republic of Moldova. The use of the term "welfare" and the recent studies initiated by some local researchers (Scutaru, 2022, 2023) concerned with the valorization of the intersectoral partnership in ensuring the wellbeing of the child are also attested.

In the territory of the Republic of Moldova, both concepts, *wellbeing* and *welfare*, are reflected in education policy documents.

In the Constitution of the Republic of Moldova (2016, p. 48) issued in 29.07.1994, in art. 47 The right to assistance and social protection, point (1) it is mentioned that "the state is obliged to take measures for every person to have a decent standard of living, which ensure the health and welfare of them and their family, including food, clothing, housing, medical care, as well as the necessary social services". The breakdown of the factors underlying this welfare is material and service ones and reflects the use of the term in financial, material contexts.

The Government of the Republic of Moldova adopted on 12.02.2018 Government Decision no. 143 (2018) regarding the intersectoral cooperation mechanism for the primary prevention of risks regarding the child's wellbeing.

In Government Decision no 143/2018, the instruction on the intersectoral cooperation mechanism for the primary prevention of risks regarding child wellbeing (Guvernul Republicii Moldova, 2018) the term child wellbeing is defined as "the satisfaction of the child's needs in all areas important for his harmonious growth and development, which ensures a good start in the first years of life and preparation for life-long achievements".

According to Government Decision no. 143 (2018) the areas of child welfare are: (a) safety—protection from violence, neglect, exploitation and harm at home, in the educational institution or in the community; (b) health—support in adopting a healthy way of life and access to medical assistance to achieve physical and mental health standards; (c) achievement—support and guidance in the process of learning and developing skills, confidence and self-respect at home, in the educational institution and in the community, in accordance with the child's age and potential; (d) care with affection—ensuring a growth and development environment that offers love, support and encouragement and that meets the child's needs; (e) activism—creating opportunities and encouraging participation in various activities in accordance with the child's interests, age and potential that contribute to harmonious growth and development; (f) respect—recognition of the importance and ensuring the right of every child to be treated with respect and dignity at any time, regardless of age, gender or origin, regardless of what he did or failed to do; at the same time, respect implies ensuring the necessary conditions for the child to be heard and participate in the decision-making that concerns him, in accordance with his age and potential; (g) responsibility—encouragement and support in assuming tasks and active roles at home, in the educational institution and the community, self-control capacity, understanding and compliance with moral and social norms, in accordance with the child's age and potential; (h) inclusion—acceptance of each child, without any differentiation, as a person who can make a valuable contribution to the family and community, the elimination of social, educational, physical and economic inequalities and acceptance as an active member of the community in which he lives and learns, in accordance with the child's age and potential.

A reference document of major importance in the planning and elaboration of policies, the permanent monitoring of the implementation progress, at the national level, is considered the European Moldova 2030 National Development Strategy (2023). In identifying the major trends for the development of the Republic of Moldova (Objective 1), an analysis of the current situation of the population is carried out and "the low level of education and mental welfare of the elderly population" is noted (51.1% and 62%, respectively). In Objective 3. *Ensuring relevant and quality education for all throughout life*, it specifies: "The holistic development of children in early education, for lifelong learning and welfare". In Objective 5. *Improving the state of physical and mental health of the population through the active contribution of a modern and efficient health system*, which meets "the needs of each individual, the need to ensure health is highlighted - a critical element that influences the quality of people's lives, being characterized not only by the absence disease, but also through physical, mental and social welfare".

The analysis of education policy documents in the Republic of Moldova allows us to find that the term "welfare" is used in a broad sense, covering various dimensions of life, such as psychological, social, physical and material ones. This suggests a holistic approach to the concept of welfare in educational policies, given that welfare is not limited to aspects such as mental health or material situation, but is seen in a wider context that includes multiple aspects of our lives. The dominant use of the term "welfare" probably reflects the concern of the authorities to ensure an educational environment that supports the overall development of subjects, including their psychological, social, educational and material aspects.

The Education Code of the Republic of Moldova (2014), in Chapter II. The mission, the ideal and the fundamental principles of education, *Article 5. The mission of education*, states that the mission of education is: b) the development of human potential to ensure the quality of life, the sustainable growth of the economy and welfare of the people. In *Article 135. Obligations of teaching, scientific-teaching, scientific and management staff*, "(1) Teaching, scientific-teaching, scientific and management staff have the following obligations: k) to discuss with children and students, individually and in groups, about their emotional and physical safety/ welfare at home/in the family and in the institution, as well as in other places they frequent".

The concept of wellbeing is totally related to the fundamental principles of education, stipulated in Article 7 of the Education Code of the Republic of Moldova (2014): the principle of equity—based on which access to learning is achieved without discrimination; the principle of quality—on the basis of which the educational activities are related to the national reference standards and to the good national and international practices; the principle of relevance—based on which education meets the needs of personal and social-economic development; the principle of centering education on its beneficiaries; the principle of social inclusion; the principle of unity and integrity of the educational space.

The Reference Framework of Early Education from the Republic of Moldova (2018, p. 23) specifies: "Early education is conditioned by the child's wellbeing and the educational environment".

The exploitation and development of the child's potential are possible by ensuring the child's wellbeing, by satisfying the basic needs: the need for security, understanding and affection, social recognition and the feeling of belonging to the group, to feel capable, intelligent and valuable, physical needs. This means: ensuring optimal conditions for growth, learning and development—the child can enjoy the company of other children and educators, feel joy and freedom of action in a calm, attractive and safe atmosphere. Under these conditions, he can direct his energy toward play, learning and daily activities with an appropriate level of challenge; encouraging functional capacities—the child feels that he is appreciated and accepted, that he is heard and noticed, thus developing his self-respect, confidence in his own strengths and in his success, tending to acquire social abilities. Moreover, each child is treated according to individual and gender needs, personality and family culture, being aware that they are treated fairly, regardless of sex, social background, culture or ethnicity.

The wellbeing and comfort of children in the activities of early education services are promoted by establishing effective, friendly and warm relationships between them—parents, educators or other children—which give the child the feeling of belonging to the peer group (Reference Framework of Early Education from the Republic of Moldova, 2018, p. 24).

The Curriculum for Early Education (2019, p. 8) uses the term "wellbeing" in a related context with other key notions: early education, holistic approach to the child, competence-centered curriculum, correlation of areas of development with areas of activity, the joy and pleasure of learning through play, secure educational environment and socio-educational partnership.

The Standards for Child Learning and Development from Birth to 7 Years (2019, p. 8) highlight the need to comply with various requirements with reference to their implementation: (1) the standards must be used in such a way that they respect the wellbeing of children and their families.

In conclusion, we specify that in educational policy documents the presence of both terms is attested: *welfare* and *wellbeing*. The use of the concept of welfare prevails. The explanation for the use of both terms, welfare and wellbeing, in educational policy documents may be related to the fact that these terms, although they may have semantic overlaps, may also have distinct nuances in certain contexts. "Welfare" is applied to refer to a wider perspective, which includes economic, social and material aspects, but the term "wellbeing" is used to highlight more subjective aspects, related to psychological state, happiness and personal satisfaction. Also, the use of both terms reflects the diversity and complexity of psycho-socio-cultural approaches and perspectives.

9.3 Psychological and Pedagogical Dimensions in the Conceptualization and Structuring of Wellbeing

Currently, psychological wellbeing is a current subject in multiple scientific researches, approached from the positions of positive psychology, a paradigm that was launched at the end of the last century (it is considered that the year of the launch of positive psychology is 1998, when Seligman (2011) as President of the Association American Psychological Association (APA) in its inaugural address stated that the purpose of psychology is to study what makes people happy), presenting an alternative approach to the problems of humanity in the social, educational, health and economic sciences through the lens of difficulties that man faces. The initiators of positive psychology Seligman and Czikszentmihalyi (2000), Peterson and Park (2011) "wanting health to be of greater interest than the absence of disease" oriented twenty-first-century psychology in the direction of researching the conditions that make people happy and turn.

Czikszentmihalyi (1990) and Peterson and Park (2011) presented positive psychology, which before the positive orientation "was focused on the model of human functioning deficiencies, focusing predominantly on the influence of pathology on the functioning of the subject within a prosperous society". The objective of positive psychology is to catalyze change by reorienting attention from fixing negative aspects of life to strengthening positive qualities. In the context of social psychology at the individual level, the focus is on capitalizing on personal experiences, such as wellbeing, satisfaction (regarding the past), hope and optimism (for the future), prosperity and happiness (present). "At the individual level, it refers to subjective experiences such as the capacity to love and relax, courage, interpersonal competences, aesthetic sensitivity, perseverance, dedication, originality, openness to the future, spirituality, talent and dedication. At the group level, civic virtues, social institutions that contribute to better citizenship, responsibility, naturalness, altruism, civility, tolerance, moderation and ethical principles are considered".

Therefore, psychology turns from concerns related to pathology to aspects related to happiness and wellbeing, with the aim of identifying the conditions that contribute to increasing subjective wellbeing, in order to ensure optimal individual and social functioning for humans. Various schools and currents in psychology and philosophy have provided theoretical explanations of subjective wellbeing, including hedonistic paradigms, which emphasize the feeling of wellbeing, comfort and general pleasure, or eudemonic paradigms, which consider the achievement of personal satisfaction as the result of growth, aspiration toward happiness and the achievement of life goals (Bošković & Šendulajengić, 2008). More and more specialists are focusing on the psychological aspects of emotional welfare or wellbeing. Apart from material prosperity, the perception of the quality of one's own life results from a "filtering" of lived experiences through the prism of schemes or value judgments regarding what life satisfaction and happiness mean.

Wellbeing is a concept often used, but with an inconsistent definition. A systematic review of the literature reveals the variability of its definitions. It has been investigated across disciplines, age groups, cultures, communities and countries, generating a considerable diversity of interpretations, which complicates comparisons between conclusions.

Happiness is a fundamental emotional state, known, accessible and felt by everyone, but it has often been neglected by researchers. A 2000 study found that negative emotions were researched dozens of times more often than positive ones. In the last two decades, there has been a significant increase in interest in identifying the factors responsible for maintaining psychological wellbeing (Seligman, 2011). After the pandemic period and at the stage of the two-year extension of the war in Ukraine, each person focuses on the search for happiness and the factors that contribute to its achievement.

In psychological research with reference to wellbeing, two paradigms have been recognized, which, from a general perspective, seem to be different, but, nevertheless, in certain aspects they are interconnected (Deci & Ryan, 2008). The hedonistic approach to wellbeing supports the identification with pleasure and happiness (Kahneman et al., 1999).

On the other hand, the eudaimonist perspective conceptualizes wellbeing in terms of developing personal resources to achieve superior performance, acting in accordance with the potential and experience of achieving purpose or meaning in life (Bošković & Šendulajengić, 2008). The difference between hedonic and eudaimonistic approaches lies in the use of subjective versus objective criteria for assessing psychological wellbeing. While hedonism focuses on subjectively determined positive experiences, the eudaimonist perspective highlights the experiences of developing and actualizing human potential, considered an essential objective for wellbeing (Deci & Ryan, 2008).

Rusnac (2017, 2018) highlights a diversity of approaches to wellbeing from a theoretical-empirical perspective, presenting them in a grouped format and some models.

For our study, the "3P" (Present, Past, and Prospect (Future)) model of Duryappah (2011, p. 683), which characterizes the subjective wellbeing of prosperous people with high levels of wellbeing, is of interest psychological, emotional and social. The present refers to the positive emotions experienced at the moment, to the current experience, the past refers to the positive reminiscence, accompanied by gratitude and the attribution of meaning to the events and experiences of the past, and the perspective (future) is projected to optimism or positive anticipation and to the goal that orients toward the future.

Duryappah (2011) considers the 3P Model to be a dynamic explanation of subjective wellbeing, arguing that the three modalities of temporal orientation interact. Subjects rate their subjective wellbeing differently at various stages of life: in childhood, the focus falls on present experience, youth orients to goals and the future, and adults seek coherence in the life story and the past. The model indicates that revisiting the past (through reminiscence and reframing) and pre-experiencing the future (anticipating the good) contribute to improved wellbeing and prevent negative judgments that affect it.

In the work entitled "Happiness: Unlocking the Mysteries of Psychological Wealth", Diener and Biswas-Diener (2008), also known as Dr. Happiness, summarizes the results of research carried out over 25 years, highlighting four components of happiness: (a) psychological wellbeing, like attitudes, goals and work engagement, matters more than money; (b) happiness is not only a state of wellbeing, but also a beneficial condition for relationships, work and health; (c) realistic expectations of happiness are useful because no one can be happy all the time; (d) an important aspect for happiness is thinking, attention, interpretation and memory, which help people improve their psychological wellbeing.

Although defining the term wellbeing is challenging, there is consensus on its multidimensional nature, which includes cognitive, emotional, social, physical and spiritual aspects. The concept of wellbeing refers to the individual's subjective perception of psychological health and quality of life, from both a cognitive and an affective perspective. Therefore, the cognitive dimension focuses on the personal meaning attributed to mental health and life satisfaction, while the affective dimension encompasses personal emotional experience, whether positive or negative.

According to the opinion of Bradburn (1969), a person with an increased level of positive emotions compared to negative ones will experience a high psychological wellbeing and vice versa. Wellbeing, also known as quality of life, is associated with functionality and health in physical, mental, emotional and social aspects. It is a dynamic state, susceptible to improvement by achieving personal and social goals, adopting healthy behaviors and developing beneficial habits. Wellbeing is expressed through two dimensions: an objective one (which includes socio-economic status, educational resources and health status) and a subjective one (related to happiness, perception of quality of life and life satisfaction).

According to Ryff (1989), mental health is not just the absence of mental illness. Positive mental health involves a state of mental wellbeing, accompanied by a healthy sense of wellbeing. Furthermore, psychological wellbeing motivates active participation in the face of various existential challenges. It is a subjective evaluation of one's life, expressed through a state of wellbeing or happiness.

Positive psychology pointed out that, for a significant period, researchers have focused mainly on deficit aspects, psychological vulnerability and pathology, neglecting to study the factors that contribute to the maintenance of psychological wellbeing. Investigating the meanings of mental wellbeing, Ryff (1989) identified six distinct dimensions: (1) self-acceptance: positive evaluation of one's own person and previous experiences; (2) environmental mastery: the ability to manage one's own life and adapt to the environment; (3) autonomy: the capacity for self-determination and resistance to social pressures, as well as the ability to think and act independently; (4) positive relationships: harmonious interpersonal relationships, which reflect the willingness to take into account the needs of others; (5) personal growth: openness to new experiences, highlighting the need for self-development; (6) purpose/meaning in life: awareness of the significance of the purpose and meaning of one's life.

Research by Ryff and Singer (2008) revealed that high levels of subjective wellbeing correlate with better neuroendocrine circulation, reduced cardiovascular risks and immune function optimum.

Seligman and Csikszentmihalyi (2000) specify that people end up in a state of wellbeing (have a high level of personal and professional fulfillment) if there are the following 5 basic elements, structured in the so-called P.E.R.M.A. model, developed by M. Seligman and named as the English acronym of the descriptive theoretical model of wellbeing. According to the model, there are 5 components that lead to psychological wellbeing and a flourishing life: "P" comes from "positive emotion" or positive emotions, probably the most obvious component connected to happiness. It refers to emotions such as joy, gratitude, forgiveness, hope, optimism and enjoying the moment. More than that, it refers to a positive outlook on life and looking for inspiration in everyday life. The "E" comes from "engagement" or engagement in activities that give us pleasure. Engagement, or full involvement in the activities we do, helps us learn and develop beautifully. Ideally, we should find those activities that completely absorb us and make us forget about ourselves. The "R" comes from "relationships" or the relationships and connections we have with others: either life partner, children, relatives, friends or the boss at work and work colleagues. Healthy relationships with loved ones make us feel loved and supported in difficult times. In addition, it helps physical health, extending our life by several years. But be careful, their quality matters, not quantity. "M" stands for "meaning" or meaning in life. Finding purpose in our lives is a crucial element of wellbeing. By understanding what we live for, we become more willing to achieve our goals and face difficulties not anyway, but with all the enthusiasm and energy we have. "A" comes from "achievement" and refers to those moments when we have achieved our goals and are victorious, starting from realistic goals. The successes achieved increase the motivation to achieve and the satisfaction of living life with meaning.

It is important to mention that wellbeing is closely related to the emotional quotient that stimulates the quality of a person's life in terms of health, material condition, access to quality education and social services, degree of life satisfaction, development potential, mental health and the quality of social relations. Thus, increasing wellbeing is ensured by shaping the lifestyle to achieve happiness, positive social relations, satisfying work, pleasant activities in free time, sufficient financial resources, quality education, etc.

Therefore, wellbeing has been defined in terms of both individual characteristics of an inherently positive state (happiness) and an existential continuum from negative to positive.

The components of wellbeing (according to Băban, 2011) are the following: (a) self-acceptance: positive attitude toward one's own person, acceptance of personal qualities and flaws, positive perception of experiences and the future; (b) positive relationships with others: trust in people, sociability, need to receive and give affection, empathetic, open and warm attitude; (c) autonomy: independent, determined, resistant to group pressures, evaluates oneself according to personal standards, is not overly concerned with the expectations and evaluations of others; (d) control: a sense of competence and personal control over tasks, creates opportunities for the valorization of personal needs, makes choices consistent with one's own values; (e) meaning and purpose in life: directed by medium and long-term goals, the positive experience of the past, the joy of the present and the relevance of the future, the conviction that it is worth getting involved, curiosity; (f) personal development: openness to new experiences, feeling of valuing one's own potential, capacity for self-reflection, perception of positive self-changes, efficiency, flexibility, creativity, need for challenges and rejection of routine.

It is certain that wellbeing is only partially influenced by the past and physical factors. The other aspects depend on the way we think and manage certain aspects of our life, but also the emotions and the feelings that influence relationships with those around us.

In essence, wellbeing is the expression of the personality's lifestyle, subjectively appreciated by him and understood as rewarding from a psychological and social point of view; it is the happiness that individuals live through the prism of their own experience and evaluate it as optimal or not.

Wellbeing is closely related to the concept of happiness. Recent measures of wellbeing, proposed by the American psychologist Lazarus (2011), refer to a global assessment of personality, related to how the achievement of existential goals bring happiness.

Also, most researchers have highlighted two types of wellbeing: subjective and objective. Subjective wellbeing is a notion frequently addressed in the social and human sciences, tangential to other terms such as "quality of life", "life satisfaction" and "psychological wellbeing".

Wellbeing is also defined by Landen and Wang (2010) as the personality's subjective perception of psychological health and quality of life on a cognitive and affective level. Researchers Bradburn (1969) and Diener and Biswas-Diener (2008) argued in their work that the cognitive component refers to the personal meaning on mental health and life satisfaction, and the affective dimension includes the personal emotional experience that can be positive or negative. It should be emphasized that the wellbeing of a subject can be determined only in the context of existing norms and value orientations, significant for a person.

Wellbeing research is an object closely related to the entire personality structure, which directly affects other components of the personal sphere involved in additional investigations. One of the central elements is the value system, which was examined in relation to wellbeing by Sagiv et al. (2015), Schwartz (1992) and Schwartz and Sortheix (2018). The researchers noted three mechanisms by which values and wellbeing may be linked. The first relates to the realization of healthy values leading to perceptions (e.g., people are kind), attitudes (e.g., tolerance) or behaviors (e.g., offering help) which in turn enhance wellbeing. Conversely, the realization of unhealthy values leads to perceptions (people threaten), attitudes (intolerance) or behaviors (avoid others) that in turn undermine wellbeing.

The second seeks to achieve healthy values which lead directly to wellbeing because it satisfies intrinsic, self-actualizing needs. In contrast, the pursuit of unhealthy values does not satisfy intrinsic needs and may require stressful ego-protective activity. The first two mechanisms argue that the pursuit of particular values influences occasional wellbeing.

The third mechanism presents the reverse occasional direction, that is, the level of wellbeing influences value priorities [idem]. For example, people who feel secure and satisfied with life have the emotional and cognitive resources to pursue autonomy (self-direction) and enthusiasm (stimulation) and care for the wellbeing of loved ones (benevolence) or society, and nature (universalism). Conversely, people who feel insecure and threatened are preoccupied with their own problems and lack the resources to pursue these values. They emphasize values whose realization promises greater safety, certainty and anxiety reduction (security, conformity, tradition and power).

According to Veugelers and Vedder (2003) who mention the scientific opinion of Berkowitz (cited by Veugelers & Vedder, 2003) regarding the development of moral judgments which does not require a complex set of values, but it is enough to have central values, among which justice and human wellbeing stand out. This approach suggests that these two fundamental values can form the necessary moral basis to guide ethical behavior and decision-making. Thus, Berkowitz (cited by Veugelers & Vedder, 2003) seems to argue that despite the diversity of moral concepts, certain key values can serve as the foundation for the development of a system of moral values and judgments. Justice, understood as fair and just treatment, and human wellbeing, which presupposes the good mood and wellbeing of the subject, are identified as essential elements in building a robust moral framework.

Narayan's (2000) poverty-based model of human values focused on the study of human needs to understand the basic values of the poor and less fortunate, realizing that survival that it is not sufficient to develop one's full potential human being (cited Antoci, 2022). The research was conducted by Narayan's (2000) in 60 countries, involving more than 60,000 people who were primarily poor, illiterate and, in some cases, remote respondents. The results of Narayan et al.'s investigation became the basis for the World Bank's understanding of poverty from the perspective of poor people, how people move from poverty to prosperity, and how they can fall back into poverty. Among the basic values of poor people Narayan et al. (2000) identified: material wellbeing (food, assets and work); bodily wellbeing (being and appearing well, health aspects and the physical environment); social welfare (child rearing and marriage); security (peace, safe environment, personal physical security, legality, security in old age and confidence in the future); freedom of choice and action; psychological wellbeing (peace of mind and happiness); harmony (spiritual life).

Another element in the sphere of personality researched in correlation to wellbeing was emotional intelligence. This, in the broadest sense, is a recognition in oneself and others of both positive and negative feelings, the ability to separate one's own feelings from empty facts, as well as the ability to sense mood, temperament, intonation and intention in communicating with other people, whether you know them or you are seeing them for the first time. "Wellbeing" is closely related to the emotional quotient that stimulates the quality of a person's life in terms of health, material condition, access to quality education or social services, people's degree of satisfaction with their lives, development potential, mental health of them, the quality of social relations (Evaluarea stării de bine a copilului în şcoală, 2019).

Goleman et al. (2019) in the book "Emotional Intelligence in Leadership" recorded that: "…the positive mood of employees has direct implications on business results. Moods influence how efficiently people work; optimistic moods stimulate cooperation, honesty and business performance".

Mîslițchi and Cimbriciuc (2020) examined the problem of the development of the educators' emotional intelligence in the institution of preschool education. They highlighted that educators' involvement in a program for the development of emotional intelligence, focused on the development of the structural components of emotional intelligence (self-regulation; self-awareness; motivation; empathy; social abilities), containing various relevant methodological activities (seminars, round tables, individual and group consultations, workshops, trainings, methodical meetings and classes, psychopedagogical advice, book exhibitions, etc.) increases the level of the educators' emotional intelligence in preschool education.

Emotional intelligence favors the stimulation and establishment of wellbeing, thanks to which we can always avoid negative thoughts, think positively and monitor the way in which the lifestyle or the events that influence the mood (Antoci & Rusu, 2021). Thus, emotional intelligence closely related to wellbeing generates conditions that stimulate self-confidence, favor autonomy and independence, emphasize uniqueness and favor everyday joys and pleasures.

9.4 The Valence of Wellbeing in the Education System

The valence of wellbeing in the education system is a particularly relevant and complex topic, to which we also pay special attention in this study. The concept of wellbeing is not only limited to the personal domain, but has significant implications within the educational process. We will explore how wellbeing can influence the attitude, performance and involvement of educational actors in the formal, non-formal and informal environment, bringing into discussion aspects related to personal development and learning success. This aspect becomes crucial in the current context of education, highlighting the connections between the psychological wellbeing of the personality and the quality of the educational experience.

In our daily activity, we are guided by the fact that "the main purpose of education is the formation of an integral character and the development of a system of competences that includes knowledge, abilities, attitudes and values that allow the active participation of the individual in social and economic life" (Codul Educației, 2014). To achieve the stated objectives, it is essential to cultivate and develop children's social competence, giving them abilities that allow them to manage their own behavior and correctly understand the behavior of those around them. Developing social competence requires attention and interaction, based on abilities such as empathy and effective communication (Curriculum Național. Învățământul primar, 2018).

In the current period, wellbeing is a central concern in educational policies. It is obvious that the wellbeing of teachers is closely related to that of children, these two components being interconnected and influencing each other. A beneficial learning environment should give equal attention to both aspects essential for the effective functioning of the education system. However, the changes and pressures to which the teaching staff is subjected negatively affect their wellbeing, having consequences for the learners. To build authentic relationships between teachers and children, key elements are needed, such as: willingness to listen, authority, mutual acceptance, reflection and sharing, respect for rules and, dedication of meaningful time. There is a general trend, still timid and difficult to implement, to promote a complex approach in education, rather than focusing exclusively on risk factors (such as distress, stress or school boredom), including addressing the transition from school dropout to perseverance. A relevant quote in this context is that of the World Health Organization from 1948 (World Health Organization, 1998) and Constitution of the World Health Organization (2005): "Health is a state of complete physical, mental and social wellbeing and does not consist merely in the absence of disease or infirmity".

Over time, sociologists and pedagogues have tried to define and integrate the concept of wellbeing within the education system, suggesting that it is essential to consider the various aspects of the individual's life and environment in order to improve the daily quality of existence. However, wellbeing is subjective and relative and cannot be treated as an absolute measure. Each participant in the educational process perceives this paradigmatic change differently, and the associated methods are based on a reflexive, future-oriented approach that brings significant benefits to the wellbeing of individuals.

Positive education challenges traditional educational paradigms globally and aims to promote wellbeing and happiness from a holistic perspective, both in and out of the classroom. This contemporary educational approach is grounded in positive psychology, a scientific field dedicated to the study of human flourishing and optimal functioning, focusing on the strengths and virtues that contribute to the success of individuals, communities and organizations. Positive psychology explores the conditions and processes that lead to or contribute to the optimal functioning of individuals, groups and institutions, with the goal of building a flourishing life and preventing the pathologies caused by meaninglessness.

In essence, the definition of positive psychology extends on three levels: (1) relative to the axis of time, it has at its center valuable subjective experiences: wellbeing, gratitude and satisfaction—past; hope and optimism—future; state of flow and happiness—present; (2) on an individual level, it refers to a series of positive characteristics such as: the ability to love, to have a vocation, courage, interpersonal abilities, aesthetic sense, perseverance, ability to forgive, originality, spirituality and talent, wisdom; (3) at the group/social level, it targets virtues such as: responsibility, altruism, care for others, moderation, tolerance and ethical conduct (Seligman & Csikszentmihalyi, 2000).

Currently, there are a number of attempts to apply alternatives to the traditional education system. The school curriculum includes mandatory hours of personal development for the preparatory class, primary classes and secondary school, but the question arises to what extent this limited time (one hour per week) is sufficient for sustainable improvement of non-cognitive abilities and wellbeing, more chosen in the context in which the other courses take place normally.

Positive education refers to empirically validated interventions and programs, extracted from positive psychology, which have an effect on the wellbeing of pupils or students (UNESCO, 2016).

Education aims at both traditional abilities and happiness, school being an environment where pupils/students have the opportunity to develop and train not only their minds, but also a series of character strengths, virtues and competences on which wellbeing is based (Seligman & Csikszentmihalyi, 2000). An essential principle of positive education is that wellbeing and effective learning are symbiotic. That's why wellbeing should be cultivated in school not only as an antidote to depression or as a way to increase satisfaction with life, but also to improve learning and foster creative thinking [idem]. But this focus on wellbeing does not refer to the promotion of feel-good experiences (which only raise the emotional tone), but, through the prism of scientific foundation, arms individuals with long-term beneficial strategies and abilities (UNESCO, 2016).

Positive education can be defined more broadly as an intertwining of the science of positive psychology with the best teaching-learning practices, with the aim of encouraging and supporting individuals and educational institutions to flourish within the community they belong to. Thus, positive education stands out as a possible solution for combating/reducing pressing problems of education and current society—the learning crisis and the prevalence and high incidence of depressive symptoms, which I mentioned earlier. Positive psychology applied in school, in general, can be found in the form (UNESCO, 2016): (1) scientifically validated intervention programs, to increase wellbeing; (2) scientifically supported proactive strategies, applied in programs aimed at the mental health of the entire school; (3) lessons about virtues or values as part of character education or value-based learning.

More specifically, the use of positive psychology in education follows two main directions: (a) support for positive development and the promotion of positive mental health (cultivation of positive emotions, behaviors and cognitions) among all actors involved in education (both students and people who take care of their development); b) the inclusion of the concepts and principles of positive psychology in the school curriculum. Positive education has already been implemented on various social groups in several schools in the USA, Australia and Great Britain.

The model of Konu and Rimpela (2002) (cited Tîrcă, 2022, pp. 14–16), considered in various countries of the world, divides the wellbeing of a school into four categories: (a) working conditions: the physical environment school, food, medical assistance services, counseling activities, etc.; (b) relationships of all kinds between members of the educational community: teachers-students/students-students/teachers-parents, etc.; (c) the means of personal achievement and the way in which they receive feedback and encouragement; (d) the state of physical and mental health.

By Allardt (1989) a model was developed where school conditions are under the umbrella of "having", social relationships are patronized by "loving", and the means of personal development and achievement are in the area of "to be". If Allardt (1989) placed health in the category of needs of the type "to have", Konu and Rimpella

(2002) turned it into a separate category, because they considered that, although it is affected by external conditions, it is a state personal.

Since wellbeing can be improved through character and behaviors formed in childhood and adolescence, the school has a crucial role in inculcating healthy behaviors through the school culture and interpersonal relationships built in this environment. The UNESCO Happy School project, implemented in Bangkok in 2016, with the aim of promoting happiness in educational institutions, by improving the wellbeing and holistic development of students, concluded that the relationships between educational actors; the learning process, free and interactive; the warm and friendly environment are the values that define the "happy school" (UNESCO, 2016). The survey conducted among teaching and managerial staff, students and parents revealed three key elements that distinguish schools where students are happy to go: people, process and place.

Within the UNESCO project, interpersonal relationships were identified as the most important factor behind a happy school. These schools promote interaction and friendships between students of different ages and encourage parental involvement and activities that train community representatives. Students cannot achieve results if they feel unsafe in school or are bullied online. We can't expect them to reach their full potential if they suffer from mental health problems and don't get the support they need. They cannot give their best if they are not provided with tools, if they are not motivated to adopt a healthy and active lifestyle in and out of school (Lyubomirsky & Lepper, 1999).

The survey participants mentioned that the teacher's attitude and qualities—kindness, empathy, enthusiasm, integrity, fairness—serve as inspirational models for students. Additionally, positive collaborative values and practices are very important in creating a happy school, including love, compassion, acceptance, respect and tolerance. For example, the object of positive education at the Australian Geelong Grammar School is to build healthy relationships between teachers and students, as well as to encourage students to "engage" in the educational process.

In the context of the growing imbalance between study time and free time, schools that care about the student's wellbeing will take care of the dosage of his workload. Also, the freedom, creativity and commitment of the educated will be a priority. Thus, happy schools must allow students to express their opinions and learn freely without fear of making mistakes, because mistakes are inherent in learning, as neuroscience research proves. For the student to be actively engaged in learning, the content will be useful, relevant and engaging, reflect meaningful and contemporary realities, and teachers will always consult them to adapt the content to their needs and interests.

The school environment, as a learning context, plays an important role in the student's social, emotional and behavioral wellbeing. A safe, non-bullying, friendly environment ranked second in the list of characteristics of a happy school. Among the responses of the respondents (UNESCO project) are: a greater emphasis on smiles, greetings, music in school; creating more open and colorful spaces; posters that contribute to the establishment of a more benevolent atmosphere, etc. The survey identified strategies involving shared games that allow students to interact and understand each other better, preventing and reducing conflicts and tensions (Draguța, 2018).

In this context, it is certain that social and emotional development has a profound impact on academic performance and subsequent success in adult life. Precisely for this reason, in the Republic of Moldova, national and institutional policies aim to ensure a friendly school environment and the development of social-behavioral competences.

It is very important that, despite all the challenges, we train today's children in social competences, so that they become integrated aspects of their natural behavior. Students' wellbeing influences their ability to reach their full academic potential. The quality of the relationships that children have with each other, and that they have with adults, as well as the quality of the learning environment, fundamentally influences their school progress. To ensure wellbeing, qualitative communication, interactivity, encouragement and motivation are considered indispensable, there have been changes in the way the learning system is viewed and approached.

The school environment, the world in which children grow and learn, continues to change. For children in the Republic of Moldova, schools are not only a place for academic education, but also for training social and emotional competences, interaction and social support. The pandemic has deeply affected education. The closure of schools not only disrupted the education process, but also children's access to school meals, welfare support and the provision of basic medical and social services. In the current crisis, it has been shown that the shift to digital technologies has left teachers, students and parents feeling overwhelmed, confused and stressed, which can lead to increased health problems. It is certain that in the conditions of the COVID-19 pandemic, it is necessary to understand what we need to do to promote wellbeing and how it can become a powerful force in the learning and development process of students.

9.5 The Wellbeing of Educational Actors: Current Research and Reflections

The wellbeing research was carried out by us in the Republic of Moldova in the urban and rural environments between February and March 2023. To measure wellbeing, we applied the synthesized questionnaire (Psychological Wellbeing Scale, developed by Ryff (1989), and Subjective Happiness Scale, developed by Lyubomirsky & Lepper, 1999) developed by Rusnac (2017), consisting of 30 items, 5 for each of the six dimensions that measure wellbeing: *the feeling of happiness, self-acceptance, control over the environment, the capacity for autonomy, positive relationships with others, the purpose and meaning of life* (Seligman, 2011, pp. 89–93). The Likert response scale is also in 7 steps—from −3 to 3 (−3—never, not at all; −2—very rarely; −

1—rarely; 0—when and how; 1—frequently; 2—very frequently; 3—always, to the greatest extent).

To measure "the feeling of happiness", we applied with modifications the Subjective Happiness Scale, developed by Lyubomirsky and Lepper (1999). The scale contains 5 items. The maximum score is 3. The average score of the subjective feeling of happiness is about −0.5 to 1.0. Scores lower than −0.5 denote sharing the feeling of unhappiness, higher than 1.0—happiness. The higher the scores, the higher the subjective assessment of happiness. The following dimensions were suggested by the Psychological Wellbeing Scale (PWBS), elaborated by Ryff in 1989, developed in 1995. Scores are calculated in the same way as previously reported.

For the "self-acceptance" scale, scores lower than −0.5 indicate low rates: non-recognition of merits, positive qualities, capacities and skills, dissatisfaction and self-disregard; greater than 1.0—high self-acceptance.

On the scale that measures the "*control over the environment*", scores lower than −0.5 indicate an inability to monitor affective states, behavior in various circumstances, the mood of those around, the course of communication, higher than 1, 0—ability to monitor the social environment and circumstances according to one's own intentions and the expectations of those around.

Just as in the previous measurements, the scores that illustrate "*the capacity for autonomy*" are also calculated: low scores denote a lack of autonomy, self-confidence and assertiveness, traits that limit a person's actions, high scores—the ability to express oneself authentically, to show initiative, to be actively involved in various projects and activities.

Calculations for the block of items with reference to measuring *positive relationships with others* (it reflects the capacity to build positive relationships with others) in the case of low scores characterize a person with insufficient communication and social relationship capacity, for high scores—sufficient potential to adapt to new environments and people, sociability, the aptitude of establishing and maintaining positive relationships with others.

High scores in the dimension "*the purpose and meaning of life*" are accumulated by people who recognize and accept the experience of the past, control their present and look optimistically at the future, see the meaning of life and personal existence. Low-scoring people lack meaning in life, have little or no goals or objectives, and see no meaning in past experiences, the present and prospects. The overall average indicates the subjective assessment of psychological wellbeing.

Sample description. The questionnaire was applied to a sample of 101 students: 51 students from rural areas and 50 students from the urban environment. Sample characteristics by sex: 17 boys (33.33%) and 34 girls (66.67%) from rural areas and 21 boys (21%) and 29 girls (58%); by age: between 12 and 14 years.

Research results. To begin with, we illustrate the wellbeing of preadolescents in rural areas (Fig. 9.1). In order to measure the wellbeing of preadolescents from rural areas, 51 students, aged between 12 and 14 years, were selected. The results of the questionnaire are presented in Fig. 9.1 and illustrating the wellbeing of a sample of 51 students from rural areas, with medium and high values. The overall subjective average being 1.14 points.

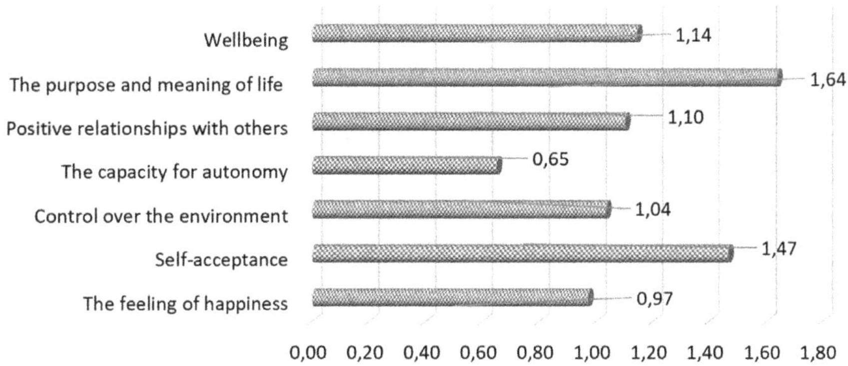

Fig. 9.1 Results of the wellbeing of preadolescents in rural areas (points)

The results obtained fall within the limits of high and medium scores. The overall wellbeing data is 1.14 points and the high and medium parameters are integrated. Thus, for the entire sample, high averages were recorded for self-acceptance (1.47), the ability to control the environment (1.04), to build positive relationships with those around (1.10), having a purpose and meaning of life (1.64). The average level was recorded in the dimension—the subjective feeling of happiness (0.97). The data shown in Fig. 9.1 is the major reference point for the experience of wellbeing.

When people are asked what a happy, rewarding and meaningful life means, they cite goals, desires and dreams for the future. Happiness is most often a by-product of participating in worthwhile projects and activities. Psychological well-being was defined by Lawton (1996, p. 328) as "the level of self-assessment of personal competence and the self, presented in terms of a personal hierarchy of objectives".

Of course, the goals and the meaning for the future are the domain of a harmonious personality, that is why in our research there are other high scores: self-acceptance—possessing a positive attitude toward oneself, recognizing and agreeing with various manifestations of the self, both of the qualities as well as defects; building positive relationships with others—based on understanding and trust, empathy and affection.

Results within the limits of the average norm were recorded for the spirit of autonomy, the ability to monitor the social environment and the subjective feeling of happiness.

Regarding the psychological wellbeing of preadolescents in the urban environment (Fig. 9.2), we note the presence of high and very high values. The overall average being 1.87p.

The results denote high scores. Thus, the highest scores were recorded for dimensions of psychological wellbeing, such as having purpose and meaning in life (2.26), self-acceptance (2.42) and subjective feeling of happiness. Also, at a fairly high level, scores were recorded for dimensions such as: the ability to monitor the social environment (1.25) and the ability to build positive relationships with others. The score for the general assessment of psychological wellbeing is 1.87, above average.

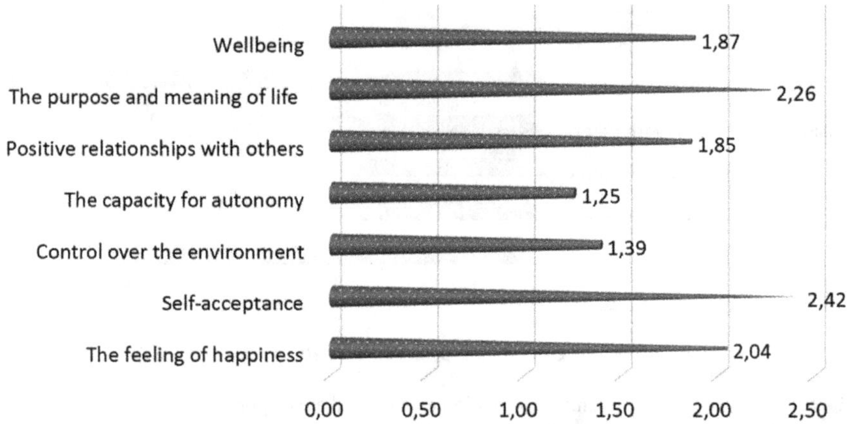

Fig. 9.2 Results of the wellbeing of preadolescents in urban areas (points)

Self-acceptance is in this case the major reference point for the experience of wellbeing.

Through the following calculations, we intended to identify if there is a significant difference between the dimensions of wellbeing in rural and urban preadolescents. Analyzing Figs. 9.1 and 9.2 we found that the values attributed to wellbeing are much higher in the urban environment than in the rural one. The significant differences that can be seen in the dimensions of psychological wellbeing are the following: the subjective feeling of happiness −1.07; self-acceptance −0.95; the ability to monitor the social environment −0.35; spiritual autonomy −0.6; the ability to build positive relationships with others −0.75, and having the purpose and meaning of life −0.62. Depending on these results, we can say that the biggest gaps are recorded in the dimensions of psychological wellbeing such as: subjective feeling of happiness and self-acceptance. Regarding the psychological wellbeing, the score for rural students is 1.14, and for urban students the score is 1.87. Thus, we can register a difference of −0.73.

The obtained results indicate significant differences in the general assessment of psychological wellbeing between preadolescents from urban and rural environments. The higher score recorded in urban students suggests a more pronounced psychological wellbeing in this group compared to preadolescents in rural areas.

These findings can be interpreted in the context of differences in environment and life experiences between urban and rural environments. The urban environment brings with it a number of advantages and opportunities that can contribute to individual wellbeing, such as easier access to educational resources, cultural and recreational facilities, and a greater diversity of social interactions.

On the other hand, preadolescents from rural areas may experience a different set of living conditions, with limited resources and a narrower social setting. These aspects can influence their stress level, personal satisfaction and, implicitly, psychological wellbeing.

It is important to note that these observations only provide a general perspective and that each individual may react uniquely to the influences of their environment. Interpretation of these results should be made with the complexity and variability of factors contributing to psychological wellbeing in mind.

Thus, for students from both living environments, the highest scores were recorded in such dimensions of psychological wellbeing as: having purpose and meaning in life, self-acceptance and the ability to build positive relationships with others. The score for the general assessment of psychological wellbeing is 1.14 for students from rural areas, slightly below average, and 1.87 for students from urban areas.

Concerned with solving the problem of ensuring the wellbeing of the beneficiaries of the education system, in the period August-October 2023, we carried out a study focused on the assessment of the wellbeing of teaching staff.

The purpose of the study carried out by us in 2023 aimed to evaluate the wellbeing of preschool teachers. In this sense, the Questionnaire "Evaluation of wellbeing at the school level" proposed by Tîrcă (2022, p. 87) was applied, which scored defining aspects of the wellbeing of teaching staff in various contexts: work as a staff member didactic; the objectives and purpose of the early childhood education institution; the relationship with the manager of the institution and colleagues; learning and development opportunities; inclusion and fair treatment in the preschool educational institution; resources and workload; pay and benefits; leadership and change management; employee involvement; organizational culture; etc.

The sample of subjects involved in the study carried out by us constituted 350 preschool teachers (Fig. 9.3), both from the urban environment (144 educators, 41.1%) and from the rural environment (206 educators, 58.9%), with the age aged between 20 and over 60 (Fig. 9.4): 20–30 years—51 educators (14.6%); 30–40 years old—126 educators (36%); 40–50 years old—97 educators (27.7%); 50–60 years old—68 educators (19.4%); over 60 years old—8 educators (2.3%).

The professional experience of the pedagogues involved in the study we carried out focused on the assessment of the wellbeing of preschool teachers (Fig. 9.5): 0–2 years—28 educators (8%); 2–5 years—35 educators (10%); 5–10 years—66 educators (18.9%); 10–15 years—54 educators (15.4%); 15–20 years—65 educators (18.6%); over 20 years—102 educators (29.1%).

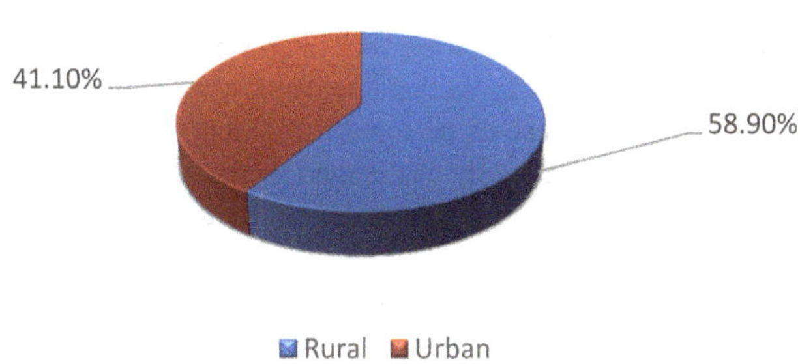

Fig. 9.3 Characteristics of the sample according to the criterion of rural/urban environment

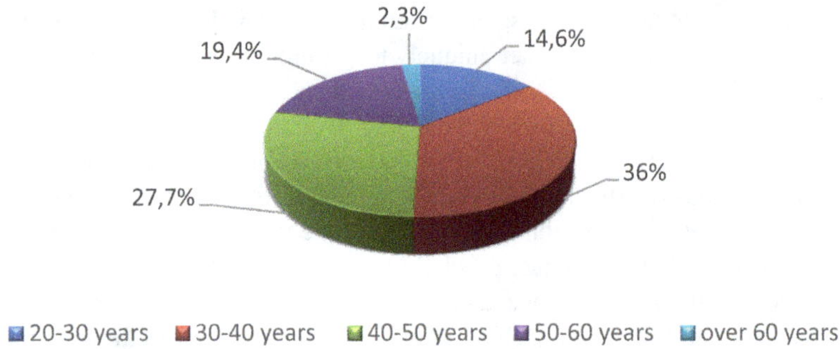

Fig. 9.4 Characteristics of the sample according to the age criterion (%)

Fig. 9.5 Characteristics of the sample according to the criterion of professional experience

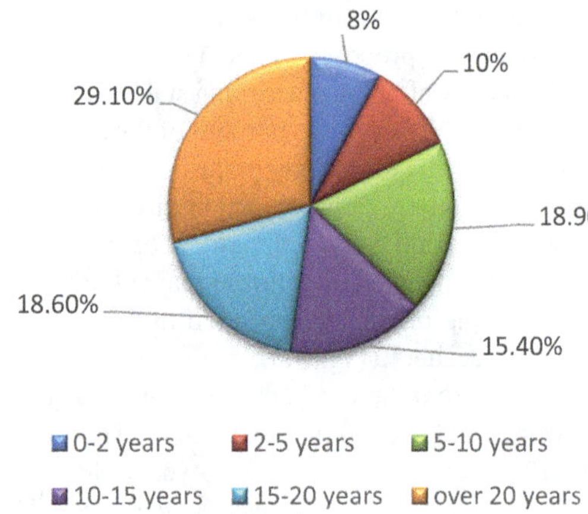

The wellbeing of educators ensured by the professional activity carried out in the early education institution concerned the following aspects: interest in the profession; the challenge provided by the work; the sense of personal achievement provided by work; involvement in decisions affecting work; making work-related decisions (Fig. 9.6).

58.3% of educators claim that they are very interested in the professional activity they carry out as a teacher; 40% agree that interest in work promotes wellbeing, and work implicitly provides a sense of personal fulfillment (43.1%). Educators highlighted the fact that they are intensely challenged by the work done in the preschool educational institution (33.4%), and they make efforts to face the challenges of the job of educator (56.3%).

At the same time, it is noted the need for teachers to be equal partners in making decisions that affect their work (on average 43.3%), recording an average of 4.5% who claim that they are not or insignificantly involved in making decisions that it directly affects their professional activity. The possibility of educators to be co-opted in deliberating on the ways of carrying out the activity was confirmed at a high level

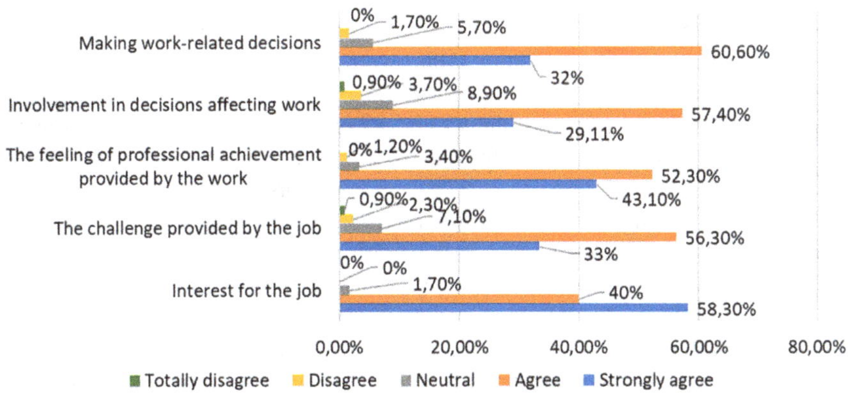

Fig. 9.6 Educators' opinion regarding the satisfaction generated by the work of an educator (%)

by 32% of the surveyed respondents, and on average 3.7% claimed that they are not offered this opportunity in the institution where they work.

With reference to the objectives and purpose of the early education institution (Fig. 9.7), on average between 35.1 and 40.3% of educators attest to a clear understanding of the purpose and objectives of the institution, as opposed to approximately more than 2% who claimed that they were confused in the explicit specification of the purpose and the objectives of the institution in which they operate. The exact understanding of their own contribution to the achievement of the objectives of the preschool education institution was assigned to 40% of the surveyed pedagogues.

The processing and interpretation of the study data (Table 9.1) allowed highlighting the fact that the wellbeing of educators is also influenced by the subordinate-manager relationship, highlighted by factors such as: the motivation of subordinates to ensure professional performance (45.7%), the attention given by the director to certain aspects related to the personal sphere, important for the educator (18.9%),

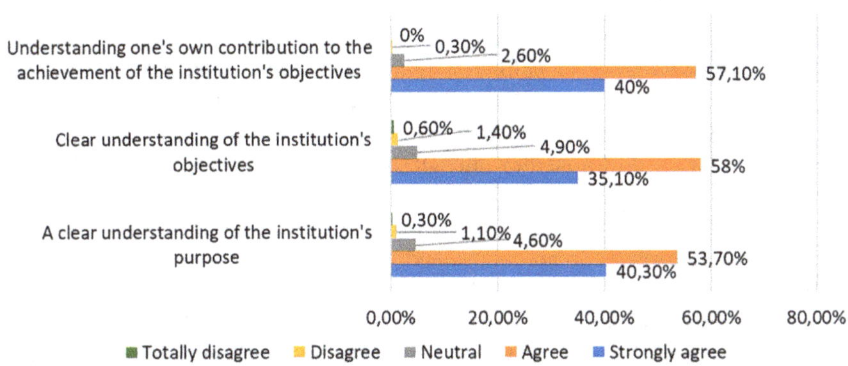

Fig. 9.7 Educators' opinion regarding the wellbeing generated by understanding the purpose and objectives of the institution where they work (%)

the manager's openness and acceptance of ideas proposed by subordinates (32.9%), advising educators on understanding their own contribution to the achievement of the institution's objectives (36.9%), educators' trust in the decisions taken by the manager (31.1%), recognition of the merits and professional value of subordinates (37.1%) and providing systematic feedback on how the educator fulfills the obligations of the position (27.1%). Also, 27.1% of educators stated that they regularly receive feedback on how they perform their tasks; 34% confirmed that the feedback they receive always helps them improve their performance; on average 42.3% believe that their performance is evaluated correctly; 14% stated that the low performance of educators is effectively addressed by the manager.

The study offered the possibility of identifying the vision of educators regarding ensuring wellbeing in the context of capitalizing on positive interpersonal relationships with colleagues in the institution where they work (Fig. 9.8). In this sense, 32% of the number of respondents specified the permanent support they benefit from in case they face certain problems; on average, 42.6% of educators stated that teaching and managerial staff are strengthening their efforts to identify ways to improve the services provided by the institution; in general, the permanent encouragement of educators to propose ideas and solutions to increase the quality of the educational and managerial process (35.1%); on average, 5% of the educators specified that the wellbeing is distorted by the difficulties of interrelationship with work colleagues, the lack of mutual support in moments of crisis, the low level of motivation of educators to cooperate in ensuring the quality education of the young generation.

The processing of the study data allowed the identification of the teachers' opinion regarding the provision of wellbeing generated by learning and development opportunities (Fig. 9.9). In this sense, 36.9% of educators specified that they permanently capitalize on learning and development opportunities related to their own needs; the learning and development activities they participated in during the last 12 months contributed to improving their own performance (46.3%); on average 40% of respondents stated that the institution where they work offers career development opportunities; learning and development activities completed in the institution are directly proportional to professional progress (38.3%).

The study carried out by us highlighted the opinion of teaching staff toward another factor generating the wellbeing of educators: the correct and fair approach to employees at work (Fig. 9.10). In this sense, teaching staff fully highlight the fairness with which they are treated at work (30.9%), specify the manifestation of respect from those with whom they interact (on average 43.15%), state that they feel valued for their work who provide it (total—25.2%; partially—55.4%), believe that the institution respects and values individual differences (on average 44.3%). On average, 6% of educators do not feel valued, respected and treated correctly at all.

Regarding the wellbeing favored by the program, the conditions, the workload, the technical-material base of the kindergarten where they work (Table 9.2), the total agreement of the educators regarding the following aspects is attested: the clarity of the environment's expectations regarding the status of the educator (48%); timely obtaining relevant information for professional activity (41.7%); the clarity of the objectives that need to be achieved (40.9%); possessing a high level of professional

Table 9.1 Educators' opinion regarding the actions of the manager of the preschool education institution aimed at ensuring the wellbeing of employees (educators no., %)

No	Statement	Strongly agree	Agree	Neutral	Disagree	Totally disagree
1	My manager motivates me to be more effective in my profession	160 45,7%	134 38,3%	35 10%	8 2,3%	13 3,7%
2	My manager is paying attention to my life outside of work	66 18,9%	150 42,9%	90 25,7%	22 6,3%	22 6,3%
3	My manager is open to my ideas	115 32,9%	177 50,6%	38 10,9%	7 2%	13 3,7%
4	My manager helps me to understand how I can contribute to the achievement of my institution's objectives	129 36,9%	167 47,7%	33 9,4%	13 3,7%	8 2,3%
5	Overall, I trust the decisions made by my manager	109 31,1%	189 54%	33 9,4%	10 2,9%	9 2,6%
6	My manager recognizes when I perform my tasks well	130 37,1%	180 51,4%	24 6,9%	11 3,2%	5 1,4%
7	I receive regular feedback on how I perform my tasks	95 27,1%	198 56,6%	41 11,8%	11 3,1%	5 1,4%
8	The feedback I get helps me improve my performance	119 34%	189 54%	26 7,4%	11 3,2%	5 1,4%
9	I believe that my performance is evaluated correctly	106 30,3%	193 55,2%	32 9,1%	14 4%	5 1,4%
10	Poor performance is addressed effectively	49 14%	215 61,4%	69 19,7%	15 4,3%	2 0,6%

competences (36.6%); capitalizing on the various educational means available to the institution for the effective implementation of the proposed activities (23.1%); optimal dosing of workloads (28.3%); ensuring the balance between professional and private life (20.9%).

With reference to the educators' opinion regarding the wellbeing generated by the payment and the benefits offered by the workplace (Fig. 9.11), we found the following situation: only 13% of the educators fully support the idea that the salary obtained adequately reflects the professional performance; only 10.9% of educators

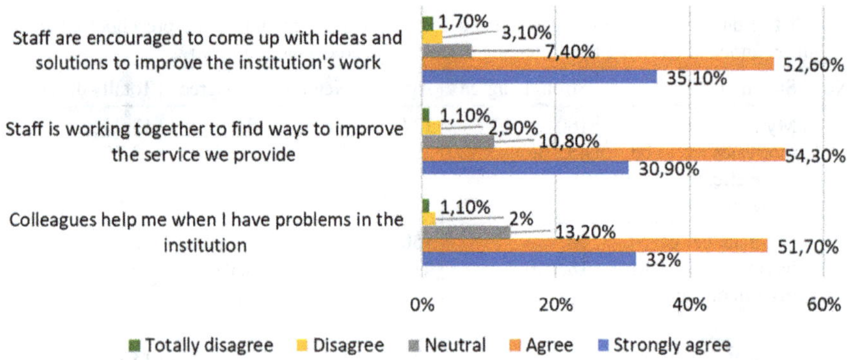

Fig. 9.8 Opinion of teaching staff regarding ensuring wellbeing in the context of capitalizing on effective interpersonal relationships with colleagues in the institution where they work (%)

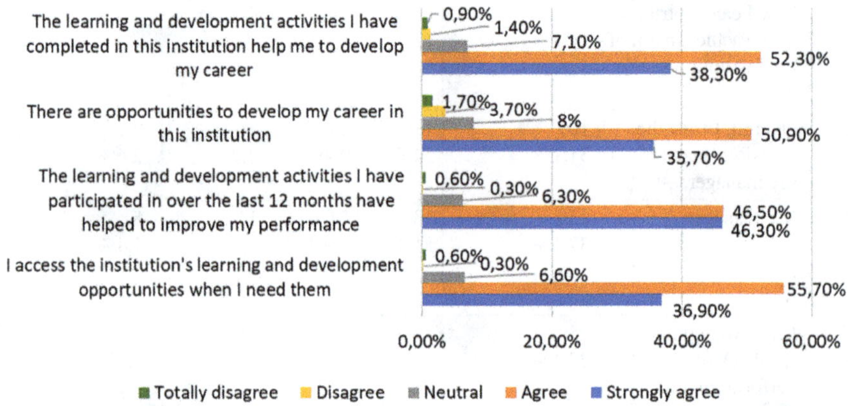
The learning and development activities I have completed in this institution help me to develop my career
0,90%
1,40%
7,10%
52,30%
38,30%
There are opportunities to develop my career in this institution
1,70%
3,70%
8%
50,90%
35,70%
The learning and development activities I have participated in over the last 12 months have helped to improve my performance
0,60%
0,30%
6,30%
46,50%
46,30%
I access the institution's learning and development opportunities when I need them
0,60%
0,30%
6,60%
55,70%
36,90%
0,00%
20,00%
40,00%
60,00%
Totally disagree
Disagree
Neutral
Agree
Strongly agree

Fig. 9.9 Educators' opinion regarding the provision of wellbeing generated by learning and development opportunities (%)

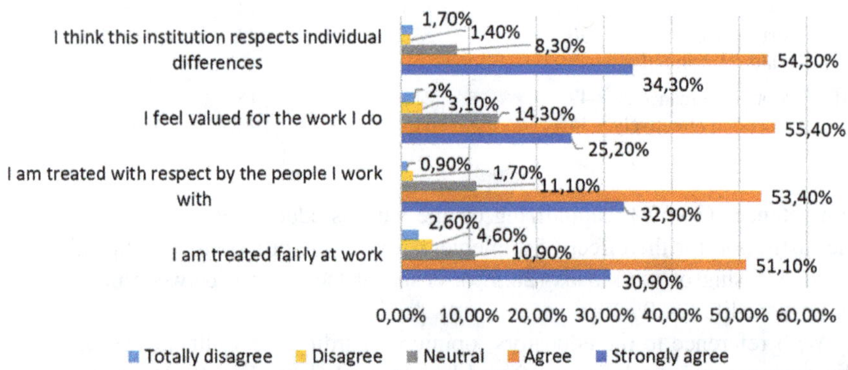

Fig. 9.10 Educators' opinion regarding the wellbeing ensured by inclusion and fair treatment at the workplace (%)

Table 9.2 Preschool teachers' opinion regarding the wellbeing favored by the resources and workload in the institution where they work (educators no./%)

No	Statement	Strongly agree	Agree	Neutral	Disagree	Totally disagree
1	As a teacher, I know clearly what is expected of me	168 48%	170 48,6%	12 3,4%	0 0%	0 0%
2	I get the information I need to do my job well	146 41,7%	181 51,7%	15 4,3%	4 1,1%	4 1,1%
3	I have clear work objectives	143 40,9%	196 56%	8 2,3%	2 0,6%	1 0,3%
4	I possess the competences I need to do my job effectively	128 36,6%	205 58,5%	13 3,7%	3 0,9%	1 0,3%
5	I have the necessary tools to carry out my activities effectively	81 23,1%	210 60%	47 13,4%	9 2,6%	3 0,9%
6	I have acceptable workloads	99 28,3%	221 63,1%	20 5,7%	8 2,3%	2 0,6%
7	I achieve a good work-life balance	73 20,9%	188 53,7%	58 16,5%	23 6,6%	8 2,3%

are satisfied with the package of benefits offered by the teaching staff in preschool education; only 7.7% of educators think that their salary is reasonable.

The state of wellbeing generated by the effective monitoring of changes can be seen on average in 27% of preschool teachers, who believe that the institution in which they work, as a whole, is well managed, implicitly in the context of ongoing

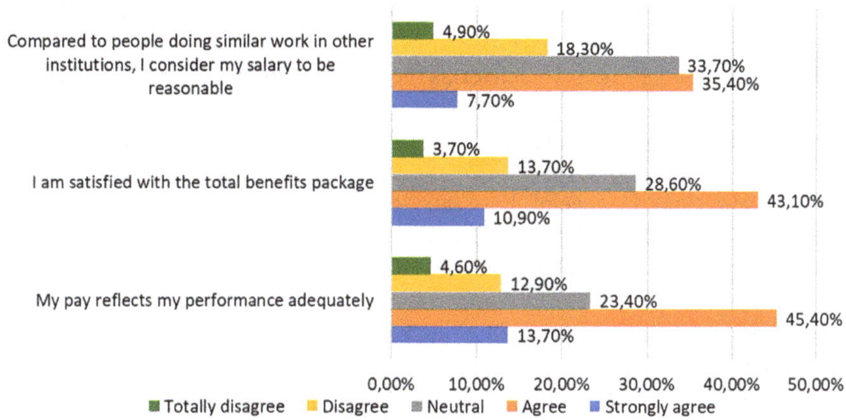

Fig. 9.11 Educators' opinion regarding the wellbeing generated by the payment and benefits offered by the workplace (%)

transformations and reforms in the education system, the team management has a clear vision of the institution's future, and the interventions and decisions taken are in line with the institution's values, change is well managed in the institution where they work, educators being involved in the decision-making process, a fact that favors the establishment of wellbeing in among employees (Table 9.3). The results of the survey of pedagogues highlight the fact that on average 6% of educators are skeptical about the interventions carried out in the kindergarten to ensure wellbeing in the context of the changes that have occurred; on average 2% of educators express their total disagreement with reference to the management of changes in the institution where they work.

The processing of the data obtained from the survey allowed the elucidation of the opinion of the pedagogues regarding the wellbeing generated by the involvement at work (Fig. 9.12), 36.3% of the educators specifying the fact that they are strongly attached personally and professionally to the institution where they work, they express satisfaction that they are part of the group of teaching staff of the respective institution that they recommend as a successful one (39.1%), the kindergarten is the environment that inspires the teaching staff to attest to high performance in the profession of educator (40%) and motivates them to get fully involved in achieving the proposed objectives (36%).

In relation to the state of wellbeing generated by the organizational culture of the institution where they work (Fig. 9.13), the total agreement of the educators is confirmed for the following aspects: the provision of quality educational services (38.6%); supporting new ideas and initiatives (28.3%); strong group membership (36%); establishing friendships among colleagues (32%).

Analyzing the Fig. 9.14, we can mention that 64 educators (18.3%) believe that they have a high level of anxiety; to a small extent, 197 educators (56.3%) attest to anxiety, and 89 educators (25.4%) claim that they are not anxious.

The processing and interpretation of the data (Fig. 9.15) allowed the highlighting of 307 educators (87.7%) who consider that the things they do in life are largely relevant; 42 educators (12%) highlight their value to a small extent, and 1 educator (0.3%) claims that the things he does in his life are not valuable.

The data from the Fig. 9.16 deliver us the following information: 222 educators (63.4%) state that they are happy to a great extent, 117 educators (33.4%) assess the level of happiness as being attested to a small extent; 11 educators (3.1%) consider themselves unhappy.

To the question "In general, how satisfied are you with your life at present?" (Fig. 9.17), the teaching staff gave the following answers: to a great extent—276 educators (78.9%); to a small extent—70 educators (20%); not at all—4 educators (1.1%).

Study focused on the assessment of the wellbeing of preschool teachers allowed the highlighting of the contexts that generate balance, harmony of educators with themselves and those around them, but also the situations that lead to imbalance and difficulties in performing professional activity at a high level of quality.

Educators specified the value in generating wellbeing of the belief that the things they achieve in life are largely relevant (87.7%).

Table 9.3 Educators' opinion regarding the wellbeing generated by leadership and change management (%)

No	Statement	Strongly agree	Agree	Neutral	Disagree	Totally disagree
1	I feel that the institution where I work, as a whole, is well managed	27,7%	50,9%	14%	5,4%	2%
2	The management team in my institution is sufficiently visible	30%	53,7%	10,3%	4,3%	1,7%
3	I believe the actions of the management team are consistent with the values of my institution	26,6%	56,9%	11,4%	4%	1,1%
4	I think the management team has a clear vision for the future of the institution	30,9%	54,3%	10%	3,1%	1,7%
5	Overall, I trust the decisions made by the management team	28%	54,3%	13,4%	2,9%	1,4%
6	I feel that change is well managed in the institution where I work	28,3%	55,7%	12%	2,6%	1,4%
7	When changes are made in the institution, they are usually for the better	29,7%	52%	15,1%	2,3%	0,9%
8	I am informed about the issues that affect me	20,9%	62,9%	11,4%	4%	0,9%
9	I have the opportunity to express my views before making decisions that affect me	22%	59,2%	13,4%	3,7%	1,7%

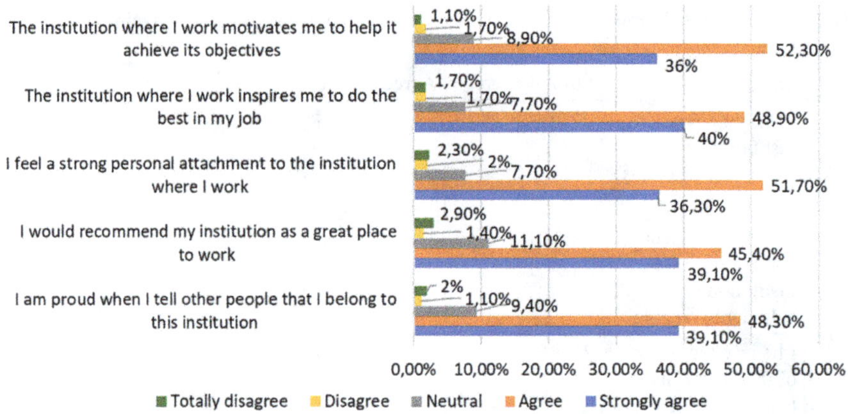

Fig. 9.12 Preschool teachers' opinion regarding the wellbeing generated by employee involvement at work (%)

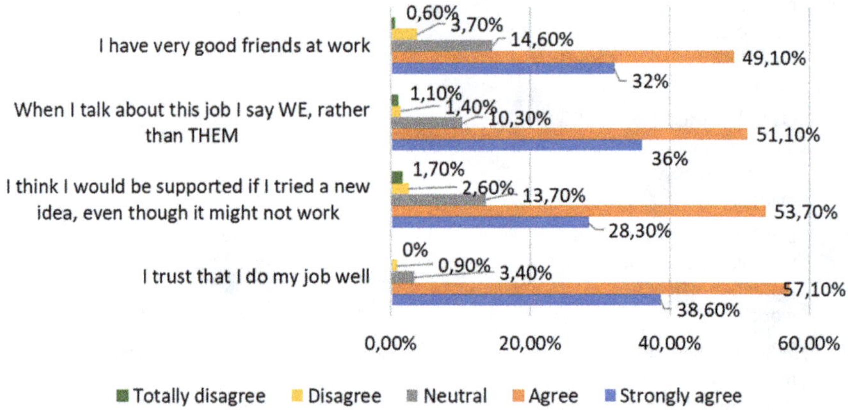

Fig. 9.13 Preschool teachers' opinion regarding the wellbeing generated by the organizational culture of the institution where they work (%)

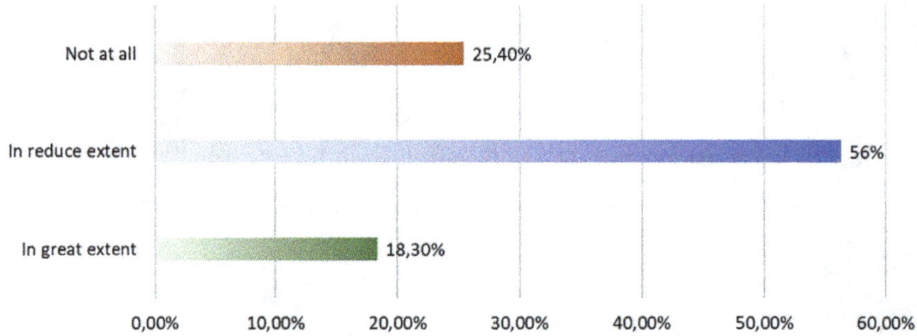

Fig. 9.14 Preschool teachers' opinion regarding their own level of anxiety at the time of the assessment (%)

Fig. 9.15 Preschool teachers' opinion regarding the extent to which they consider the things they achieve in life to be valuable (%)

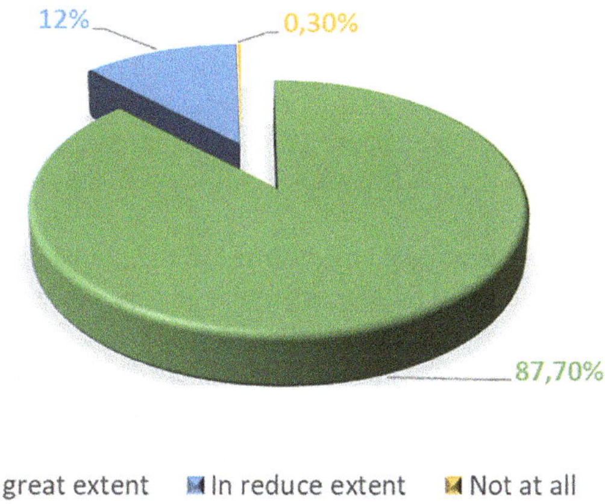

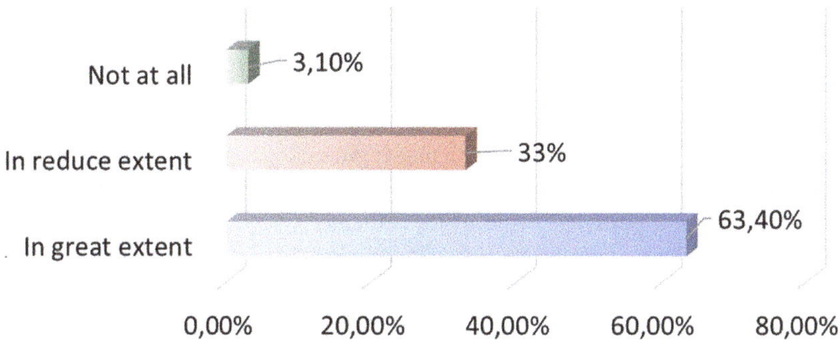

Fig. 9.16 Preschool teachers' opinion regarding the level of happiness at the time of the evaluation (%)

Fig. 9.17 Preschool teachers' opinion regarding the level of life satisfaction (%)

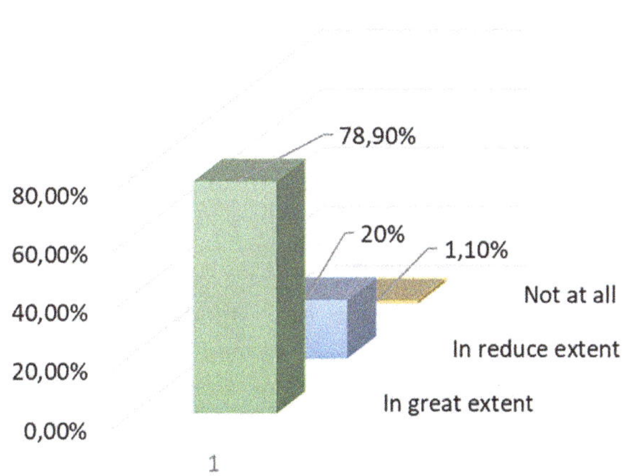

Among the determining factors that currently ensure the wellbeing of preschool teachers are: interest in the profession of educator (58.3%); increasing professional performance thanks to the learning and development activities they participated in during the last 12 months (46.3%); the feeling of personal achievement ensured by the work in the kindergarten (43%); possession of relevant information with reference to professional activity (41.7%); the clarity of the objectives that need to be achieved in the educational environment in the kindergarten (40.9%); clear understanding of the purpose of the kindergarten and personal involvement in achieving the objectives of the preschool educational institution (40%).

For the most part, the educators highlighted the support they receive from their colleagues (41.9% on average) and the manager of the institution (45.7%); they noted the satisfaction generated by belonging to the group of teaching staff (on average 43.7%) and the strong personal attachment to the institution where they work (36.3%).

The research also allowed the highlighting of the most significant factors that, according to the educators' opinion, diminish the wellbeing of preschool teachers: the salary and the demotivating benefits package offered by the early education institution (payment for the provision of educational services being appreciated as motivating only by 13.7% of pedagogues, very satisfied with the benefits of the job, being only 10.9%; firm supporters that their salary is reasonable compared to people who perform a similar activity, attesting to only 7.7%); low appreciation of the professional and personal value of the educator (only 25.2% of educators feel highly valued at their workplace); the reduced possibilities of involvement offered to educators in making decisions with reference to professional activity (29.11% of educators highlight the high level of involvement in decisions that affect their work; 32% claim that they chose to decide how they carry out their work; only 29, 7% of educators believe that changes in the preschool institution are usually to the benefit of the beneficiaries); the limited resources available to the kindergarten for the efficient implementation of the multiple activities specific to the preschool institution (only 23.1% of educators attest to the possibility of high-level utilization of the various educational means); the large volume of work, the multitude and diversity of tasks specific to the position of educator (only 28.3% claim that the optimal dosage of work tasks is ensured); difficulties in providing effective feedback by the management team of the institution regarding the performance certified by educators (only 27.1% attest to regular feedback on how they perform their tasks; 30.3% believe that their performance is evaluated correctly and for only 14% it seems that poor performance is effectively addressed in the institution in which it operates).

We specify the fact that, despite the difficulties they face in their professional activity, although only 20.9% of educators manage to ensure a high level of balance between professional life and private life, the majority of educators claim that they are happy to a large extent (63.4%), as they are largely satisfied with their current life (78.9%), a fact that ensures balance and harmony in the relationship with the actors of the educational process, pedagogues becoming life examples worthy of following.

9.6 The Foundation and Development of the Pedagogical Model for Ensuring the Wellbeing

The development of the Pedagogical Model for ensuring wellbeing is an essential approach from the perspective of the field of education, integrating effective practice and strategies for promoting wellbeing among the learners involved in the educational process. This model not only aims to provide a solid conceptual framework, but also to provide practical tools for facilitating an atmosphere conducive to personal and academic development.

The foundation of the Pedagogical Model is based on the deep understanding of the factors that influence the wellbeing of learners in the educational environment, elucidating multiple dimensions, designating various theories of wellbeing and highlighting relevant educational research findings. Thus, it is proposed to build a holistic framework, adapted to the specifics of the pedagogical context, which outlines effective directions for optimizing the educational experience.

The main objective of the developed Pedagogical Model is to create an environment conducive to the cognitive, emotional and social development of the subject. It integrates personalized strategies, teaching techniques adapted to the needs of students and innovative ways of assessment, considering that wellbeing is not just about cognitive aspects, but also includes emotional and relational dimensions.

Through this initiative, it is aimed not only to identify the influencing factors on wellbeing, but also to offer practical solutions and concrete guidelines for teachers, practitioners, specialists in the field in order to effectively implement this model within the educational process. Thus, the foundation and elaboration of this Pedagogical Model for ensuring wellbeing represent a significant step toward building a healthy educational environment conducive to the holistic development of the personality.

In order to strengthen the development process and effectively support the functionality of the Pedagogical Model in Wellbeing Ensuring, it is essential that the structure guarantees that it is based on solid theoretical content. Such a foundation can be achieved by establishing the conceptual framework of wellbeing from the perspective of multiple triadic interactions (Antoci & Mîsliţchi, 2024a), which brings a nuanced understanding of the dynamic interrelationships between the main structural components, environments and contexts that contribute to the efficiency of the educational ecosystem. Moreover, the proposed approach offers educational providers the necessary premises to identify strategic points of intervention and support in order to optimize the wellbeing of subjects, sensitive to individual and contextual differences. Thus, this theoretical construction of the conceptual framework regarding wellbeing increases effectiveness.

The meaning of the phrase "conceptual framework of wellbeing" (Fig. 9.18) refers to the set of organized and interconnected elements that form the basic structure of wellbeing from the perspective of multiple triadic interactions. Conceptual framework is a support for the development and organization of the central components and specific contents of the respective entity. It is a fundamental structure that provides direction and coherence to the whole approach of the integrative and dynamic process of ensuring wellbeing with the implications of intra- and interpersonal contexts.

The contextual importance of the quality of interpersonal and intrapersonal life for the wellbeing of the personality derives from the complexity of external influences (social, cultural, historical) and the condition of the internal determinants (self-identity, psychological, physiological) that ensure the presence of the corresponding wellbeing. The quality of interpersonal life, referring to relationships and interactions with others, and the quality of intrapersonal life, focused on aspects such as the way of thinking particularly exposed in the mentality, self-evaluation, management of emotions, are two interconnected dimensions that contribute substantially to the wellbeing of a people.

In an interpersonal context, positive and supportive relationships that create a benevolent atmosphere have a significant impact on wellbeing. Healthy social connections, emotional support and positive interactions with those around us can directly influence our level of personal happiness and satisfaction. A supportive social environment can provide a support network during difficult times, thus contributing to higher psychological wellbeing.

On the other hand, intrapersonal quality of life refers to how the individual perceives himself and manages aspects such as self-esteem, self-acceptance and emotion management. Positive self-evaluation and emotional awareness can contribute to overall wellbeing. The ability to cope with stress, improve your mood and guide your own personal development are key aspects in building a good intrapersonal balance.

The quality of intrapersonal life is ensured not only from a psychological perspective, but also from a physiological one through the optimal functioning of nervous,

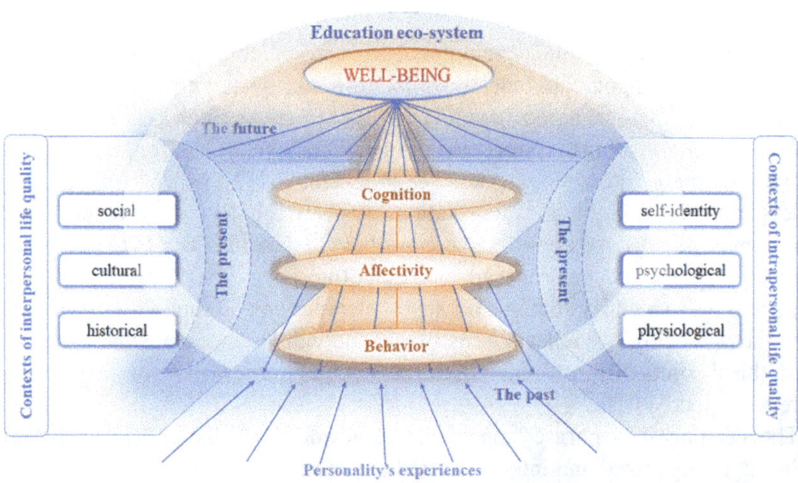

Fig. 9.18 Conceptual framework of wellbeing from the perspective of multiple triadic interactions (Antoci & Mîslițchi, 2024a)

endocrine, cardiovascular, etc., systems, which directly influence wellbeing. For example, a balanced level of neurotransmitters (such as serotonin and dopamine) supports a positive emotional state and contributes to positive self-evaluation. Hormonal regulation (for example, cortisol and the stress hormone) is decisive for coping with stress and maintaining emotional balance.

Physical activity has a significant impact on wellbeing, with physical exercise improving mood by releasing endorphins, which is a prerequisite for strengthening a positive self-image. Quality sleep is important for physiological regeneration and cognitive efficiency, constituting the basis of intrapersonal balance.

Therefore, understanding the intra- and interpersonal context in which a person develops and interacts is essential to create effective strategies to promote wellbeing. The holistic approach, which integrates both social and individual aspects, is crucial for building a comprehensive framework for promoting psychological wellbeing among individuals.

The past, present and future construction of wellbeing refers to how subjects construct and experience their wellbeing according to events and perceptions related to these three temporal dimensions.

The past. Past experiences, memories and past events can strongly influence a person's wellbeing. Successes, obstacles overcome and past relationships contribute to the formation of identity and the way the individual relates to himself. Also, past traumas or negative events can emotionally influence wellbeing.

The present. Wellbeing is obviously related to the subject's present experiences and circumstances. The quality of social relationships, success in daily activities, health and level of satisfaction with current life are all important aspects of wellbeing today.

The future. Anticipating and planning for the future can also influence wellbeing. Goal setting, having a positive outlook and optimism about the future direction, can contribute to higher wellbeing. On the other hand, anxiety about the future and worries about insecurity can negatively affect wellbeing.

By analyzing and understanding these temporal dimensions, subjects can develop a deeper awareness of the factors that influence their wellbeing and adopt strategies to improve that state in each of these time dimensions.

The structural components of wellbeing are represented by: behaviors, affectivity and cognition. These elements reflect the different dimensions of the human experience and contribute to the complex understanding of wellbeing.

Behaviors refer to the observable actions and external manifestations of personality. These include how a person interacts with his environment, engaging in activities, relating to others, manifesting internal states, etc. Healthy behaviors, being proactive and engaging in enjoyable activities can contribute significantly to wellbeing.

Affectivity refers to the emotional aspects of wellbeing. We include here a varied palette of emotions, moods, feelings such as: happiness, sadness, joy and anxiety. Understanding and managing positive and negative emotions is essential to a person's emotional wellbeing.

Cognition involves the processes of thinking, perceiving, evaluating and interpreting information, events and experiences in external reality. This can include beliefs, attitudes, perceptions of life and oneself. Healthy cognition can involve a positive evaluation of one's life, personal abilities and available resources.

These three components interact and influence each other. For example, positive thinking (cognition) can contribute to a better affective state (affect), and this, in turn, is externalized through positive behaviors. The holistic approach to these dimensions allows for a more complete understanding of wellbeing and provides a basis for developing and maintaining a balanced and fulfilling life.

Synthesizing the perspectives outlined above and linking them to wellbeing, we can propose the concept of an Education Ecosystem, where wellbeing takes center stage. This concept views education as a dynamic, interconnected system, emphasizing the interactions among its key components—students, teachers, parents, school administration, the community and the environment. These interactions, both direct and indirect, shape the learning process and the wellbeing of all participants in the educational landscape.

Within this framework, wellbeing in the education ecosystem represents a healthy, balanced environment where every participant—students, teachers, support staff and parents—feels safe, valued and motivated. This collective sense of wellbeing fosters the realization of individual potential and drives the overall success of the education system.

The concept of wellbeing within the Education Ecosystem goes beyond merely addressing the absence of problems or conflicts. It emphasizes fostering a positive and inclusive environment within educational institutions, one that supports the physical, emotional, social and academic growth of both students and staff.

In this context, wellbeing is reflected in the quality of interpersonal relationships, the satisfaction and active participation of students and staff in school activities, and the level of support and collaboration among all members of the school community. It also encompasses the presence of policies and practices that uphold respect, celebrate diversity and ensure equity.

In the current educational landscape, wellbeing is no longer viewed as a peripheral concern, but as a central dimension of effective pedagogy and holistic human development. A Pedagogical Model for ensuring wellbeing (PMEW) presented in the Fig. 9.19 designed to ensure wellbeing must therefore transcend traditional instructional frameworks and integrate emotional, social, cognitive and ethical dimensions of the learner's experience.

Scientific foundations regarding wellbeing represent a complex intersection of multiple scientific fields, highlighting significant connections from a physiological, pedagogical, psychological, social, etc., perspective. These scientific foundations provide a comprehensive perspective on the factors, contexts that contribute to the wellbeing of the subject.

Physiological aspects of wellbeing include the analysis of bio-chemical and neurological reactions of the whole organism. Endorphins, neurotransmitters and hormonal responses are involved in regulation in managing stressful situations, ensuring wellbeing.

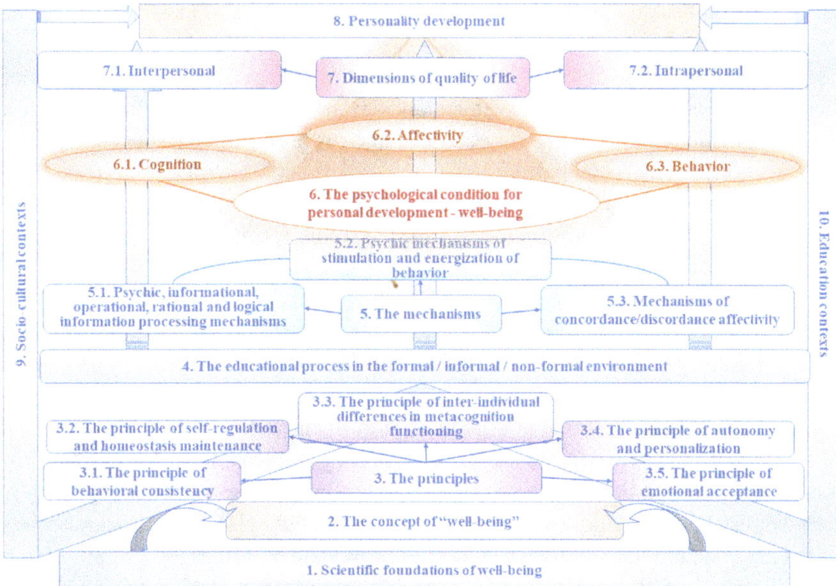

Fig. 9.19 Pedagogical Model for ensuring wellbeing by Antoci and Mîslițchi

The state of wellbeing, from the psychological, pedagogical and social perspectives, is supported by a series of scientific foundations that reveal the importance of the educational environment in the formation of the personality and in establishing its state of wellbeing.

Psychology brings into discussion aspects such as the subjective perception of life, personal satisfaction and emotional development. A. Maslow's theory of the hierarchy of needs (cited by Antoci, 2022) and Seligman's studies (identifying and promoting factors that contribute to psychological wellbeing and living a fulfilled life) provide conceptual frameworks for understanding the reasons and psychological dimensions of the state of good (Seligman, 2011). These theories are included in the field of positive psychology or humanistic psychology. Positive psychology brings to the discussion concepts such as happiness, satisfaction and personal development. In the educational environment, this translates into an emphasis on cultivating personal resources, developing socio-emotional abilities and encouraging subjects to reach their maximum potential.

Social learning theory of Bandura (cited by Antoci, 2022) claims that individuals shape their behaviors and attitudes based on observing and interacting with others in their environment (Antoci, 2022). In formal, informal, non-formal educational contexts, positive interpersonal relationships, cooperation and mutual support contribute to the wellbeing of subjects.

According to Self-Determination Theory (SDT), developed by Deci and Ryan (2008), individual satisfaction and wellbeing are closely related to a sense of autonomy, competence and social connectedness. In an educational environment that promotes these elements, subjects feel more engaged and experience a higher level of wellbeing.

Human personality development, viewed from the perspective of Ecosystem Theory, established by Bronfenbrenner and Evans (2000), is also referred to as development in context or human ecology. The proposed model suggests that the development of the human being is influenced by the interactions with its environment, including the educational environment. The resources and support available in the school, family and community contribute to the formation of a well-balanced state.

Research in the Neuroscience of Education (Fischer & Bidell, 2006) developed the Dynamic Skill Theory, which examines how cognitive skills develop over time, has highlighted the links between cognitive, emotional processes and wellbeing. Educational strategies that stimulate cognitive and emotional development, as well as stress management, can have a positive impact on wellbeing (Fisher & Bidell, 2006). Educational neuroscientist Immordino-Yang and Damasio (2007) states how emotions and personal experiences influence learning and development.

Flow theory, originally developed by Csikszentmihaly (1990), examines optimal experiences and the state of flow in activities. Flow state describes the overall psychological experience that we usually have when we are completely absorbed in an activity that demands the maximum of our abilities, that involves us to such an extent that we often lose track of time, but in which we have the feeling of full control of the situation, of efficient use of the resources at our disposal, accompanied by the satisfaction that certified performance gives us.

Overall, the wellbeing education perspective integrates these theories and concepts, highlighting the essential role of the educational environment in shaping personality and promoting sustainable wellbeing.

Sociology examines the connections between the subject and society, highlighting the importance of social relationships, community cohesion and social support in determining wellbeing. Cultural factors and social context contribute significantly to how people experience wellbeing.

These interconnected perspectives reveal the complexity of the concept of wellbeing, highlighting the influence of various domains on individual experience. The integration of these scientific foundations provides a holistic framework for research and interventions aimed at improving the wellbeing of subjects.

The analysis of scientific theories and models from the scientific literature led us to the reconceptualization of wellbeing, especially valuing the physiological, psychological, pedagogical, social aspects, being transposed into the Pedagogical Model of ensuring wellbeing:

> **Wellbeing** represents a complex system of holistically organized contents from a cognitive-affective-behavioral perspective, in interpersonal (social, cultural, historical) and intrapersonal (personal identity, psychological, physiological) contexts being transposed in the present with a focus on the experiences from past and designing in the future to increase the quality of life. (Antoci & Mîsliţchi, 2024b)

In the context of wellbeing, the application and observance of sound principles contribute to the development of a positive outlook for ensuring the quality of life. Respecting the principles for the establishment of wellbeing in the educational process contributes to the orientation of the personality toward a balanced and satisfying life.

The principle of behavioral consistency refers to the tendency of individuals to maintain their behavior and actions consistently in various situations and contexts. This principle is based on the idea that people have a natural predisposition to act in a way consistent with their own values, beliefs, norms, regardless of the circumstances. Internal consistency is evidenced by subjects' tendency to act in accordance with their own beliefs and values, adapting behavior according to what they believe to be right or appropriate according to their own standards. Behavioral stability highlights how the subject behaves in a situation, having the probability of exhibiting the same behavior in similar situations in the future. Subjects with behavioral consistency are often perceived as genuine and credible because their behavior is consistent with what they really feel and believe. We emphasize that these individuals demonstrate resistance to external influences, which makes them less susceptible to external pressures or social influences when it comes to changing their fundamental behavior. The principle of behavioral consistency highlights the importance of consistency and authenticity in human interactions, having significant effects on social relations and individual perception in the community.

The principle of self-regulation and maintenance of homeostasis aims at the manifestation of an organism's ability to adjust and maintain a constant internal balance despite changes in the external environment. The triggering of internal mechanisms allows the regulation of functions automatically, stimulates the ability to detect changes in the environment and initiate appropriate responses to maintain optimal internal conditions. The principle of self-regulation and maintenance of homeostasis are essential for the adaptability and survival of the human being in variable and constantly changing environments. The ability to maintain constant internal balance is the result of the activation of complex and interconnected mechanisms that ensure the optimal functioning of the entire bio-psycho-socio-cultural system of the personality.

The principle of inter-individual differences in the functioning of metacognition consists in the fact that the subject is aware of the way in which he or other people perceive and treat information; it also refers to what the subject knows about the differences between people focused on the particularities of information processing, starting from the knowledge of variations in one's own cognitive functioning, respectively, to the knowledge of the differences between oneself and others regarding cognitive functioning. Cognitive knowledge includes awareness of the tasks and requirements related to the characteristics of available information; it also aims at what the subject knows about the cognitive procedures that he can apply, according to his cognitive capacities, in order to achieve the proposed goals. Metacognitive experiences are the result of the feeling triggered by the effort felt and the yield obtained in the process of learning or solving a cognitive task. Metacognitive experience (found in the scientific literature as "metacognitive control" and "self-regulatory strategy") refers to both the subject's cognitive and affective experiences.

The principle of autonomy and personalization reveals the independence of the subject in the learning process focused on the personalized planning of actions through the development of the plan/scheme for acquiring the material, internalizing it, projecting it in future situations in an individualized way, emerging from the particularities of the learner.

The principle of emotional acceptance is promoted by humanistic education through the free expression, identification and acceptance of the diversity of emotional states, being important for the formation and development of the personality. Ensuring emotional expressiveness is necessary for the progress of the human being and responsible for the state of balance, the state of wellbeing.

The educational process in the formal, informal and non-formal environment differs according to the context and characteristics of each environment. *Formal education* takes place within officially recognized educational institutions such as schools, colleges and universities. The educational process is well organized and structured, based on defined academic programs, well-systematized teaching-learning-evaluation. The teachers are professionals with academic qualifications, and the students follow standardized curricula.

Informal education takes place outside the structured framework, through everyday experiences, social interactions, expanding learning contexts, etc. The educational process does not have a clear structure and is not rigorously planned as in a formal way. Learning occurs spontaneously, giving each subject, including family members, friends, the community, etc., opportunities for abilities training in a free and informal way.

Non-formal education comprises organized and intentional activities that are not integrated into a formal setting, but are planned and conducted intentionally. Education is purposefully organized but lacks the rigidity of the formal environment. Activities include workshops, trainings, projects, internships, etc. Participants are of various age groups and of various educational levels, participating voluntarily and in an organized manner. The development of competences is carried out in a flexible and friendly way, connected to the requests, personal and professional interests of the beneficiaries. Thus, the educational process differs depending on the environment in which it takes place, whether it is formal, informal or non-formal, each having distinct goals and characteristics that ensure the establishment of wellbeing.

The mechanisms that influence wellbeing are key elements in understanding and managing the psychological balance of the subject and need to be considered when modeling wellbeing. Among them we highlight the informational-operational psychic mechanisms of primary information processing that are based on sensations, perceptions and mental representations. By means of them, the information regarding the variations of the various characteristics of the environmental stimuli is processed, provided that these variations have meaning for the organism. By virtue of the principle of the interaction of psychic processes in the personality system, these mechanisms relate the various sensory information received with those stored in the memory plane.

Psychic mechanisms of rational-logical processing of information: thinking, memory and imagination. These psychic mechanisms achieve a superior type of coordination of behaviors, because they process information by means of logical-rational operations. Among these, thinking holds a central place, providing categorical and determinative information, through processing of generalization and abstraction, interacting with all other mental processes.

Psychic mechanisms of stimulation and energization of behavior: motivation and affectivity. Through these mechanisms, the body's energy is restructured and redistributed, its tension or relaxation. The motivational mechanisms signal the states of necessity, innate and acquired, primary and secondary of the subject, selecting and activating the appropriate behaviors according to their anticipated consequences. In this sense, motives represent neuro-psychic mechanisms that stimulate, trigger and energize behaviors.

Affectivity mechanisms provide information in the form of specific subjective experiences regarding the concordance/discordance ratio between the dynamics of motivational events and the dynamics of external demands. Thus, affectivity becomes a signaling mechanism and awareness of anticipated consequences, of motivational satisfaction.

Wellbeing is the psychological condition relevant to personal development, a fundamental aspect that influences the evolution and progress of the personality in multiple areas of life. Psychological wellbeing represents balance and harmony at the mental and emotional level, having an essential role in facilitating personal development.

By maintaining a state of wellbeing, the subject becomes more receptive to the process of learning and personal growth. This psychological condition favors positive attitudes toward change, promotes adaptability and stimulates motivation to explore new opportunities for acquiring new knowledge and forming skills and attitudes.

The dimensions of interpersonal and intrapersonal quality of life have a significant contribution in improving the wellbeing of the personality, influencing important aspects of psychological and social life.

The quality of interpersonal life is represented by positive social relationships: healthy and harmonious interactions with others, based on trust, empathy and mutual support, have a significant impact on wellbeing. Positive social connections contribute to a sense of belonging by providing emotional and social support. Effective communication, a valuable condition of the quality of interpersonal life, gives the subject the opportunity to express his needs, thoughts and emotions in interpersonal relationships, increases mutual understanding and creates a favorable environment for building and maintaining healthy relationships. The presence of quality relationships, characterized by harmony, mutual respect and collaboration, contributes to a sense of fulfillment and satisfaction in interpersonal life.

On the intrapersonal quality of life dimension, self-acceptance is significant. Positive self-evaluation, acceptance of qualities and shortcomings, together with a positive perception of past experiences, are key aspects that contribute to building a healthy self-image. The ability to make autonomous decisions and manage one's own life, resistance to social pressures and self-determination are essential elements of autonomy that support wellbeing. Awareness of the meaning of life, setting goals and directing toward them gives life a deep meaning, positively influencing wellbeing.

By capitalizing on these dimensions, the subject maintains and improves the quality of life and stimulates wellbeing, reflected in a positive perception of the world and of one's own personality.

9.7 General Conclusions

The study carried out regarding the provision of wellbeing highlights the existing contexts in the Republic of Moldova by highlighting especially the educational, psychological and social ones. The results of the study led to the formulation of the following general conclusions:

Wellbeing within the education system of the Republic of Moldova is a complex phenomenon, influenced by multiple dimensions such as pedagogical, psychological, social, physiological and material.

Theories and representative models of researchers like Ryff, Bradburn, Deci, Ryan, Konu, Rimpela, Allardt, Seligman, Csikszentmihaly, Fischer, Immordino-Yang, Colomeischi, Rusnac, etc., constituted essential foundations for the conceptualization and interpretation of personality wellbeing in various educational contexts.

The wellbeing of teachers in the early childhood education institution is generated, in particular, by the conviction that the things they achieve in life are relevant to a large extent, the interest in the job of educator, the performances certified in the professional activity, the feeling of personal achievement ensured by working in the kindergarten, support from colleagues and the manager of the institution, the satisfaction generated by belonging to the group of teaching staff and the strong personal attachment to the institution where they work.

The low level of wellbeing of preschool teachers is conditioned by various factors, among which stand out: the low appreciation of the professional and personal value of the educator; the demotivating salary and benefits package offered by the early childhood education institution; the large volume of work, the multitude and diversity of tasks specific to the position of educator; the limited resources available to the kindergarten for the efficient implementation of the multiple activities specific to the preschool institution; difficulties in providing effective feedback by the management team of the institution regarding the performance certified by the educators.

The Pedagogical Model for ensuring wellbeing by Antoci and Mîslițchi represents a functional ideational construct that highlights the synergy between multiple and interconnected components: scientific foundations (physiological, psychological, pedagogical, social), principles (behavioral consistency, self-regulation and maintenance of homeostasis, respect for inter-individual differences in the functioning of metacognition, autonomy and personalization, emotional acceptance), mechanisms (informational-operational, rational-logical processing of information, stimulation and energization of behavior, mechanisms of affectivity), structural system (cognition, affectivity, behavior), the defining contexts (socio-cultural, educational), the educational process (in the formal, informal and non-formal environment), the dimensions of the quality of life (intrapersonal, interpersonal) and the finality (personality development).

The establishment of the wellbeing of the personality is promoted by the integrality and interconditioning of the following principles: principle of behavioral consistency, principle of self-regulation and maintenance of homeostasis, principle of inter-individual differences in the functioning of metacognition, principle of autonomy and personalization, principle of emotional acceptance.

The study highlights the continued importance of wellbeing research in the education system, emphasizing the need for flexible and adaptable approaches to social and educational changes.

These conclusions provide a deeper understanding of wellbeing in the educational context of the Republic of Moldova, supporting the need for effective educational and social interventions to improve the quality of students' and teachers' lives.

Competing Interests The authors have no conflicts of interest to declare that are relevant to the content of this chapter.

References

Allardt, E. (1989). An indicator system: „Having, Loving, Being" (Working Papers).

Antoci, D. (2022). *Teoria și metodologia formării orientărilor valorice la adolescenți și tineri. Teza de doctor habilitat*. Universitatea de Stat din Tiraspol.

Antoci, D., & Rusu, R. (2021). Inteligența emoțională și starea de bine. *Pedagogie în învățământul preșcolar și primar* (pp. 21–29). Tipografia Universității de Stat din Tiraspol.

Antoci, D., & Mîslițchi, V. (2024a). Prospects in wellbeing approach for ensuring learning eco environment. In ВІСНИК Національного університету «Чернігівський колегіум» імені Т. Г. Шевченка, Серія: Педагогічні Науки. Випуск 26 (182), 151–157. https://doi.org/10.58407/visnik.242627. ISSN 2663-9114.

Antoci, D., & Mîslițchi, V. (2024b). Starea de bine: transferul inovativ în ecosistemul educațional. In „Research – Innovation – Innovative Entrepreneurship": International Congress, Ed. Ediția 2, 17–18 mai 2024 (Ediția 2, pp. 20–30). Chişinău. CEP UPSC. ISBN 978-9975-46-964-7. https://doi.org/10.46727/c.17-18-05-2024.p20-30

Batog, M. (2021). Starea psihologică de bine în mediul educațional. In *Institutul de Ştiințe ale Educației: ascensiune, performanțe, personalități* (pp. 188–193). Print-Caro SRL.

Băban, A. (2011). Consiliere educațională. Ghid metodologic pentru orele de dirigenție şi consiliere. Ed. a III-a. ASCR.

Bošković, M., & Šendulajengić, V. (2008). Mental health as eudaimonic wellbeing. *Psychiatria Danubina, 20*(4), 452–455.

Bradburn, N. M. (1969). *The structure of psychological wellbeing*. Aldine.

Bronfenbrenner, U., & Evans, G. (2000). Developmental science in the 21st century: Emending questions, theoretical model, research designs and empirical findings. *Social Development, 9*(1), 115–125. https://doi.org/10.1111/1467-9507.00114

Cadrul de referință al Educației timpurii din Republica Moldova. (2018). Lyceum.

Codul Educației al Republicii Moldova. Nr. 152 din 17 July 2014. In *Monitorul Oficial al Republicii Moldova*, 24 October 2014, Nr. 319–324 (634). http://lex.justice.md/index.php?action=viewandview=docandlang=1andid=355156

Colomeischi, A. A. (2017). Teachers' life satisfaction and wellbeing: Engagement Influences. In O. Clipa (Ed.), *Studies and current trends in science of education* (1st ed.; Vol. 2; pp. 139–150). Lumen. https://doi.org/10.18662/lumproc.icsed2017.16

Colomeischi, A. A. (2019). Starea de bine psihologică. In *Construind poduri: promovarea stării de bine în familie. Manual pentru părinți* (pp. 43–57). Lumen.

Constituția Republicii Moldova Nr. 1 din 29–07–1994, publicat: 29 March 2016. In Monitorul Oficial Nr. 78 art. 140. https://www.legis.md/cautare/getResults?doc_id=136130andlang=ro

Constitution of the World Health Organization. (2005). In *World Health Organization: Basic documents* (45th ed.). World Health Organization.

Csikszentmihalyi, M. (1990). *Flow: The psychology of optimal experience.* Harper and Row.

Curriculum Național. Învățământul primar. (2018). Lyceum.

Curriculum pentru educație timpurie. (2019). Lyceum.

Deci, E. L., & Ryan, R. M. (2008). Hedonia, eudaimonia, and wellbeing: An introduction. *Journal of Happiness Studies, 9*, 1–11.

Diener, E., & Biswas-Diener, R. (2008). *Happiness: Unlocking the mysteries of psychological wealth.* Wiley-Blackwell.

Draguța, O. (2018). Starea de bine a elevului de azi – succesul și sănătatea adultului de bine. *Revista Didactica Pro..., revistă de teorie și practică educațională, 4–5*(110–111), 80–85.

Durayappah, A. (2011). The 3P model: A general theory of subjective wellbeing. *Journal of Happiness Studies: An Interdisciplinary Forum on Subjective Wellbeing, 12*(4), 681–716. https://doi.org/10.1007/s10902-010-9223-9

Evaluarea stării de bine a copilului în școală. (2019). Coord. S. Irimie. Cluj-Napoca: Centrul Regional de Sănătate Publică Cluj. https://insp.gov.ro/download/cnepss/stare-de-sanatate/rapoarte_si_studii_despre_starea_de_sanatate/sanatatea_copiilor/rapoarte_tematice/2018/Sinteza-%E2%80%93-Stare-de-bine-in-scoala-2018.pdf

Fischer, K. W., & Bidell, T. R. (2006). Dynamic development of action and thought. In R. M. Lerner (Ed.), *Handbook of child psychology. Vol 1: Theoretical models of human development* (6th ed., pp. 313–399). Wiley.

Goleman, D., Richard, B., & Mckee, A. (2019). *Inteligența emoțională în leadership.* Ediția a III-a. Curtea Veche Publishing.

Goraș-Postică, V., & Vartic, A. (2022). Starea de bine a cadrelor didactice – condiție pentru calitatea activității pedagogice. In *Managementul educațional. Pedagogia școlii superioare* (pp. 194–200; Vol. 6). Tipografia Universității de Stat din Tiraspol.

Guvernul Republicii Moldova. (2018). HG 143/2018 din 12.02.2018 pentru aprobarea Instrucțiunii cu privire la mecanismul de cooperare intersectorială pentru prevenirea primară a riscurilor privind bunăstarea copilului. In Monitorul Oficial Nr. 48–57 art. 168, 16 February 2018. https://www.legis.md/cautare/downloadpdf/102076

Immordino-Yang, M. H., & Damasio, A. (2007). We feel, therefore we learn: The relevance of affective and social neuroscience to education. *Mind, Brain and Education, 1*(1), 3–10. https://doi.org/10.1111/j.1751-228X.2007.00004.x

Kagan, S. (1992). The limits of wellbeing. In E. F. Paul, F. D. Miller, Jr., & J. Paul (Eds.), *The good life and the human good* (pp.169–189). Cambridge University Press.

Kahneman, D., Diener, E., & Schwarz, N. (1999). *Wellbeing: The foundations of hedonic psychology.* Russell-Sage.

Landen, S. M., & Wang, C.-C.D.C. (2010). Adult attachment, work cohesion, coping, and psychological wellbeing of firefighters. *Counselling Psychology Quarterly, 23*(2), 143–162. https://doi.org/10.1080/09515071003776028

Lawton, M. P. (1996). Quality of life and affect in later life. In C. Magaiand & S. H. McFadden (Eds.), *Handbook of emotion, adult development, andaging* (pp. 327–348). Academic Press.

Lazarus, R. (2011). *Emoție și adaptare. O abordare cognitivă a proceselor afective.* Editura Trei.

Lyubomirsky, S., & Lepper, H. (1999). A measure of subjective happiness: Preliminary reliability and construct validation. *Social Indicators Research, 46*, 137–155.

Mîslițchi, V., & Cimbriciuc, A. (2020). Development of the educators' emotional intelligence in the institution of preschool education. International Forum for Education. *Challenges of Modern Education: Educatioan-Teacher-Learner, 13*, 107–130.
Negură, I. (2014). Optimizarea stării de bine ca problemă psihologică. In *Formarea competențelor de rezolvare a problemelor psihologice în procesul instruirii inițiale și continue a psihologilor* (pp.14–56). UPS „I. Creangă".
Peterson, C., & Park, N. (2011). Character strengths and virtues: Their role in wellbeing. In S. I. Donaldson, M. Csikszentmihalyi, & J. Nakamura (Eds.), *Applied positive psychology: Improving everyday life, health, schools, work, and society* (pp. 49–62). Routledge/Taylor and Francis Group.
Rusnac, S. (2017). Cercetarea stării de bine psihologic: Metodologie și rezultate. *Psihologia socială în secolul XXI: Provocări, tendințe, perspective* (pp. 101–115). Universitatea Liberă Internațională din Moldova.
Rusnac, S. (2018). Condiții profesionale pentru realizarea stării de bine psihologic: abordare teoretico - conceptuală și experimentală. In *Prolegomene din istoria psihologiei în Republica Moldova* (pp. 89–106). Pan Europe.
Rusu, P. P., & Colomeischi, A. A. (2020). Positivity ratio and wellbeing among teachers. The mediating role of work engagement. *Frontiers in Psychology, 11*(1608), 1–10. https://doi.org/10.3389/fpsyg.2020.01608
Ryff, C. D. (1989). Happiness is everything, or is it? Explorations on the meaning of psychological wellbeing. *Journal of Personality and Social Psychology, 57*(6), 1069–1081. https://doi.org/10.1037/0022-3514.57.6.1069
Ryff, C. D., & Singer, B. H. (2008). Knowthy self and become what you are. A eudaimonic approach to psychological wellbeing. *Journal of Happiness Studies, 9*, 13–39. https://doi.org/10.1007/s10902-006-9019-0
Sagiv, L., Roccas, S., & Oppenheim, S. (2015). Values and wellbeing. In S. Joseph (Ed.), *Positive Psychology in Practice* (pp. 103–121; 2nd ed.). Wiley.
Schwartz, S. H. (1992). Universals in the content and structure of values: Theory and empirical tests in 20 countries. In *Advances in experimental social psychology* (pp.1–65; Vol. 25). Academic Press.
Schwartz, S. H., & Sortheix, F. M. (2018). Values and subjective wellbeing. In E. Diener, S. Oishi, & L. Tay (Eds.), *Handbook of wellbeing* (pp. 833–847). DEF Publishers.
Scutaru, A. (2023). Paradigma holistică – reper metodologic în interpretarea conceptului: bunăstarea copilului. In *Cercetarea, dezvoltarea și inovarea din perspectiva eticii globale* (pp. 176–184). Tehnica-UTM.
Scutaru, A. (2022). Mecanisme funcționale de implementare a parteneriatului intersectorial axat pe asigurarea bunăstării copilului. In *Dialog intercultural polono-moldovenesc* (pp. 31–37). Tipografia UST.
Seligman, M., & Csikszentmihalyi, M. (2000). An introduction to positive psychology. *American Psychologist, 55*(1), 5–14. https://doi.org/10.1037/0003-066X.55.1.5
Seligman, M. E. P. (2011). *Flourish: A visionary new understanding of happiness and wellbeing.* Atria Books.
Standarde de învățare și dezvoltare a copilului de la naștere până la 7 ani. (2019). Lyceum.
Straistari-Lungu, C. (2016). Starea de bine a copilului – perspectivă spre o educație de calitate. In *Tehnologii didactice moderne* (pp. 133–137). Cavaioli.
Strategia Națională de Dezvoltare „Moldova Europeană 2030". (2023). [citat 16 November 2023]. https://gov.md/ro/moldova2030
Suman, M., Goriuc, P., & Serbulenco, A. (2023). Corelația dintre stresul academic și starea de bine printre studenții mediciniști. In *One health and risk management* (p. 95). USMF „Nicolae Testemițanu".
Tîrcă, A. (2022). Hai cu starea de bine în școală!: ghid pentru profesori, directori și părinți. Ed. a 2-a. Corint Internațional.

Turchină, T., Bolea, Z., & Platon, C. (2012). Starea subiectivă de bine – semnificaţii şi implicaţii. *Studia Universitatis Moldaviae (Seria Ştiinţe ale Educaţiei), 5*(55), 115–118.

UNESCO. (2016). *Happy schools: A framework for learner wellbeing in the Asia-Pacific*. UNESCO;/Bankok: UNESCO Asia and Pacific Regional Bureau for Education. Disponibil. http://unesdoc.unesco.org/images/0024/002441/244140e.pdf

Veugelers, W., & Vedder, P. (2003). Values in teaching. *Teachers and Teaching: Theory and Practice, 9*(4), 377–389. https://doi.org/10.1080/1354060032000097262

World Health Organization. (1998). The role of the pharmacist in self-care and self-medication. World Health Organization. [citat 20 August 2023]. https://apps.who.int/iris/handle/10665/65860

Chapter 10
Wellbeing and Mental Health Promotion at School. The Case of Romania

Aurora Adina Colomeischi

10.1 Introduction

Wellbeing in school settings is a multifaceted construct that has been explored through different theoretical models, each contributing to a holistic understanding of the factors that promote and sustain students' wellbeing. Our chapter on wellbeing in Romanian schools aims to provide an overview based on integrative insights from prominent models of wellbeing and resilience to conceptualize wellbeing in educational contexts.

We used four theoretical and practical models that present wellbeing as a psychological dimension of human development (Kern, 2022; Seligman, 2011) or as an asset derived from the combination of resources within school settings embedded in the wider social context, and resilience as a universal capacity that enables a person, group or community to prevent, minimize or overcome the harmful effects of adversity (Grotberg, 1995a, 1995b).

Seligman's PERMA model is foundational in this realm, positing that wellbeing is comprised of five core elements: Positive Emotion, Engagement, Relationships, Meaning, and Achievement (Seligman, 2011). These components suggest that for students to thrive, schools must cultivate environments where positive emotions are nurtured, engagement with learning is profound, relationships are supportive, a sense of meaning is developed, and achievements are recognized and celebrated. Seligman's PERMA gives also an intervention model, since school could design and implement specific projects and programs to support the holistic development of children.

A. A. Colomeischi (✉)
Faculty of Psychology and Scienes of Education, "Ştefan cel Mare", University of Suceava, Suceava, Romania
e-mail: adina.colomeischi@usm.ro
URL: https://usv.ro/

A. A. Colomeischi (ed.), *Wellbeing in Schools of Southeastern Europe*, Human Well-Being Research and Policy Making,
https://doi.org/10.1007/978-3-032-10525-7_10

Building on Seligman's work, Kern's PERMA-H model adds a crucial dimension of health, emphasizing the role of physical and mental wellbeing as intrinsic to overall wellbeing (Kern, 2022). In the school context, this translates to the importance of physical activity, nutrition, and sleep, alongside mental health support, considering a healthy mind and a healthy body as pivotal for children to thrive within educational context.

Konu and Rimpelä's model of Wellbeing at School is developed upon the Allrdt's model of wellbeing and it broadens the scope by incorporating the school environment's structural and social elements, emphasizing that student wellbeing is influenced by school conditions (having), social relationships (loving), means for self-fulfillment (being), and health status (health) (Konu & Rimpelä, 2002, p. 84). So school gives a child a sense of belonging, a supportive community, a space for personal growth and self-expression and the safe place for growth and development. It suggests that the school's culture, resources, and practices are pivotal in shaping the experiences that contribute to a student's sense of wellbeing. This model points to the significance of supportive structures and a positive climate as essential ingredients for nurturing student wellbeing.

The Grotberg's resilience model provides a framework for understanding how children overcome adversity, positing that resilience is fostered through a combination of personal strengths and external support, summarized as "I Have," "I Am," and "I Can" (Grotberg, 1995a, 1995b). Within schools, this model underscores the importance of building students' capacities for resilience through supportive relationships, fostering positive self-identities, and equipping them with coping skills. This paradigm delineates the external support systems, internal personal strengths, and social and interpersonal skills that equip students to cope with challenges and adversities. It emphasizes that resilience is not just the ability to bounce back but also the capacity to endure and adapt, which is crucial for maintaining wellbeing in the dynamic and sometimes stressful school environment.

Integrating these models, wellbeing in schools can be understood as a dynamic state wherein students' emotional, social, and physical needs are met in a supportive and engaging environment that enables them to overcome challenges and achieve personal and academic growth.

Our aim was to integrate the concepts of school wellbeing, subjective wellbeing, and resilience into a coherent model of school wellbeing and resilience. In the figure below, we have integrated the key elements derived from each model in a way that highlights their interconnectedness and their role in promoting a positive educational environment.

This model aims to promote an understanding that wellbeing and resilience in a school setting are multidimensional, encompassing emotional, social, and physical domains, and are developed within the wider social context of family and community.

Fig. 10.1 presents a conceptual model that integrates the constructs of school wellbeing and resilience. Here's an interpretation of the diagram:

Outer layers: present the community and the family as social actors that play a fundamental role in a student's wellbeing and resilience, forming the environmental

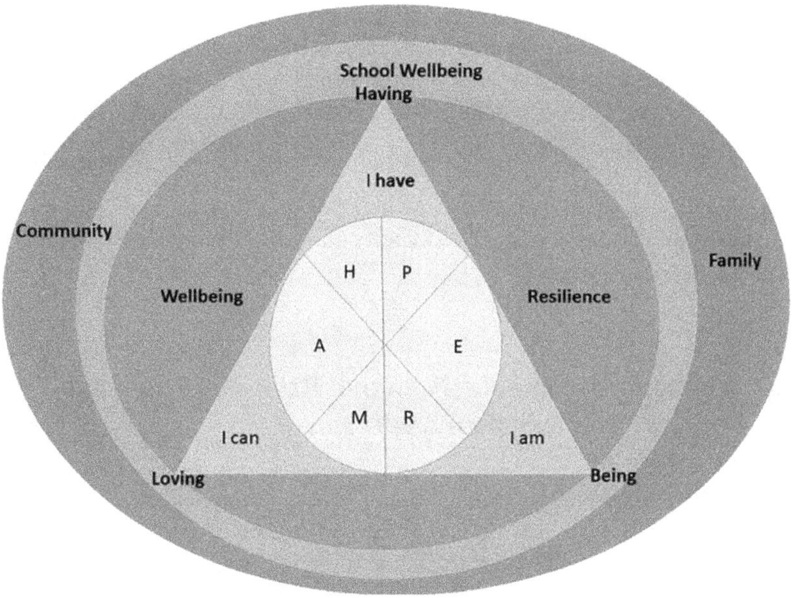

Fig. 10.1 Integrated model of school wellbeing and resilience (author)

context in which school wellbeing is promoted. Here are the values of both family and community that influence children's development.

The middle layers represent the school as an institution that fosters the wellbeing of pupils and is likely to be shaped by the surrounding influences of community and family.

The triangle should be seen from two perspectives: an external one and an internal one.

The external perspective leads us to understand the three central components of school wellbeing that have been identified as the vertices of the triangle: *Loving, Having, Being*. *Loving* could refer to the relationships and emotional connections that students develop during their school life; *Having* could refer to the school climate, school conditions, policies, and measures, all the resources and support available to students at this level; *Being* represents students' sense of self and personal growth within the school environment.

The inner triangle includes the three pillars of resilience, which are also linked to the three dimensions of school wellbeing. *I have* refers to the external support, resources, help that a pupil could get; *I can* refers to the social skills or abilities to solve problems, to cope; *I am* considers the internal resources of a pupil, such as self-esteem, values, and strengths.

The central circle, inscribed to the triangle, represents the dimensions of subjective wellbeing promoted by the PERMA-H model (positive emotions, engagement, positive relationships, achievement, and health).

The model suggests a multi-layered approach to understanding school wellbeing and resilience, where individual student factors of wellbeing and resilience are supported and enhanced by broader environmental factors such as school, family, and community. This model emphasizes the interconnectedness of various components that contribute to a student's ability to thrive and be resilient in the school environment.

Our chapter will provide an overview upon the school wellbeing within Romanian educational system, following to identify elements that are consonant with our theoretical model proposal.

10.2 Wellbeing at School—National, Regional, and School Policies, Whole School Approach

Since September 2023 Romania has new laws for education, one for the pre-university level and another one for the university education. The Pre-University Education Law No. 198 of 2023 heralds significant transformations, striving toward a brighter future for all children and adolescents in Romania. According to the Report regarding the pre-university education system (decembre 2023) concepts such as equity, performance, investment, respect, and safety have been translated into concrete and foreseeable actions by this law. These measures, tailored to the needs of educational beneficiaries, establish a unified and structured framework for addressing prevailing issues within the national pre-university education system and effectively catering to students' educational needs at every stage of their journey. By implementing a range of integrated measures, including scholarships, competency-focused curriculum, personalized teaching approaches, remedial education programs, financial support for rural teachers, targeted investment in education, and desegregation efforts, the law ensures that every student is empowered to realize their full potential.

A number of measures have already been taken to improve the wellbeing of children and teachers at school. There is great interest in expanding counselling and guidance services by increasing the number of school counsellors in accordance with the provisions of (Education Ministry Order) EMO No. 3.642/2023. The Ministry of Education has allocated 1,200 new school counsellor positions nationwide, bringing the national average to approximately one counsellor per 800 students. According to the Ministry of Education's report, there are currently 2,288 counsellors employed in psycho-educational support offices, covering a total of 2,751,233 students and preschool children in the entire public education system nationwide. The increase in the number of school counsellors will lead to an improvement in the access of pupils and preschool children to psycho-educational support services, school and career guidance, as well as to information, counselling, and support activities for pupils at risk of school exclusion and for their families. This measure will also lead to the expansion of the network of school psycho-educational support services and the intensification of violence prevention activities in schools.

The Romanian Agency for Quality Assurance in Pre-University Education proposes a guide for internal and external evaluation of wellbeing at school since at the end of 2020, new quality standards were approved by Government Decision No. 994/2020.

According to Decision No. 631 of 11 May 2022 (see Table 10.1), which amends the Annex to Government Decision No. 994/2020 on the Approval of the Standards for Provisional Operating License and the Standards for Accreditation and Periodic External Evaluation in Pre-University Education, there are specific emphases related to the issue of promoting wellbeing at school. In the following table, we point out some specific requirements included in this decision that should be found at the school level.

The wellbeing is one of the major factors that are required in order one school to be authorized or accredited by external evaluation. So, in order to improve participation and learning outcomes, the educational institution must also enhance the wellbeing of children/youth in all learning-related activities, whether conducted at school, at home or in other learning contexts and situations. The wellbeing concept is explained, considering the most important aspects, underlining that it is not about a continuous happiness or a joyful state of the learner, but also, according to the contemporary models of wellbeing it is about order and predictability (based on rules), discipline (including punctuality), and perseverance and effort (including the fears and frustrations associated with a learning journey filled with obstacles). In the same time, the formative role of negative emotions is emphasized, since it could be associated with change. The authors of the guide propose a definition of wellbeing at school based on the scientific literature such as "Wellbeing is obviously a multidimensional concept, encompassing elements related, among many others, to the physical, psychological, and emotional development of children (identity and confidence, self-management, initiative, resilience), social behavior (empathy, self-care, and respect for oneself and others, civic engagement), relationships (friendship, fairness, prosocial attitudes, respect), or the learning environment's ability to be friendly, supportive, promote collaboration, diversity, or readiness for development. Therefore, to improve participation and learning outcomes, educational institutions must enhance the wellbeing of children/youth in all learning-associated activities, conducted at school, home, or in other learning contexts and situations" (Nedelcu et al., 2018). Taking into account this context, "wellbeing in school" is defined as the predominantly positive attitude of children/youth toward learning, school, teachers, and peers, determined and influenced by individual, familial, school, and community factors. The guide makes an inventory of these factors, to which it associates actions carried out at the level of the educational institution for: understanding the attitude of children/youth toward learning, school, teachers, and peers; understanding the positive or negative factors that influence this attitude, for each child/student individually; improving wellbeing through actions at the level of factors that influence (positively or negatively) this attitude.

In the Table 10.2, we present the main dimensions and factors of wellbeing considered by the Romanian Agency for Quality Assurance in Pre-University Education

Table 10.1 Wellbeing integrated within criteria and indicators for external evaluation of schools

Area: A. Institutional Capacity Criterion: a) Institutional, Administrative, and Managerial Structures Indicator 1. Existence, structure, and content of project documents: development plan and managerial plan	
Requirements for the provisional operating authorization standard	Requirements for the accreditation standard and periodic external evaluation
A.2. Defining within the PDI/PAS of strategic targets and programs that explicitly address the improvement of participation in education, learning outcomes, and the wellbeing of preschoolers, preschoolers/students in general, and for preschoolers, preschoolers/students belonging to disadvantaged/vulnerable categories existing at the level of the educational unit	B.3. The evidence and presentation of results obtained in the implementation of the PDI/PAS regarding the improvement of participation in education, learning outcomes, and the wellbeing of preschoolers, preschoolers/students in general, and, if applicable, for disadvantaged/vulnerable groups of preschoolers, preschoolers/students existing at the level of the school unit
Domain: B. Educational Effectiveness Criterion: a) Content of study programs Indicator 10. Curriculum design and planning of learning activities	
Requirements for the provisional operating authorization standard	Requirements for the accreditation standard and periodic external evaluation
	B.55. Designing learning activities for developing key competencies, enhancing literacy and numeracy, and promoting the wellbeing of preschoolers/preschoolers/students
Domain: B. Educational effectiveness Criterion: a) Content of study programs Indicator 11. Implementation of learning activities, ensuring participation and achieving wellbeing	

(continued)

Table 10.1 (continued)

Requirements for the accreditation standard and periodic external evaluation	Requirements for the reference standard
B.76. Systematic assessment of wellbeing for each nursery student/preschooler/student. Existence of evidence regarding the improvement of wellbeing	C.77. Carrying out learning activities (within the core subjects/activities, school-based curriculum, and/or through extracurricular activities) that address the improvement of learning outcomes and wellbeing of nursery students/preschoolers/students belonging to disadvantaged/vulnerable groups existing in the school C.104. Reviewing the educational offerings and programmatic documents based on the assessment of progress achieved in learning outcomes and wellbeing for preschoolers, preschoolers/students belonging to disadvantaged/vulnerable groups, and those talented and/or capable of high performance, or identifying measures to improve the highlighted aspects

Table 10.2 Dimensions and factors of wellbeing in Romanian school (adapted from ARACIP (2021). Internal and external assessment of wellbeing)

Individual	Health and Safety	Health level: health condition, possible illnesses, healthcare Health-related behaviors: nutrition (quantity/quality), sleep, smoking, alcohol/drug consumption, obesity, etc.; physical exercise/sports Personal safety behaviors within the school and neighborhood: "running," "climbing," crossing public streets, etc.
	School Participation and Learning Outcomes	Participation in education and school attendance Attained qualifications—diplomas and certificates School results in key and specific competencies Level of "life skills": decision-making, financial management, household activities Self-perception of school results and own abilities and competencies Critical thinking Career-related knowledge and behaviors—potential schools and qualifications, their requirements, salary and development opportunities, etc. Engagement in school life—cognitive, emotional, and behavioral levels Personal viewpoints on identified issues Positive attitude toward learning—curiosity, engagement in the learning process, motivation for results Interactive, ethical, and safe use of technologies—Internet, social networks, etc. Creativity: interests and artistic results
	Psychological and Emotional Development	"Happiness"/"positive wellbeing," life satisfaction Self-management: autonomy level (age-dependent), emotional control, perseverance, time management Initiative: planning personal activities, identifying resources to achieve personal goals, positive risk-taking, motivation Confidence: positive self-identity and self-confidence, including as part of a social and natural whole Optimism and resilience: positive approach and constructive adaptation to adversity
	Social Development and Behavior	Moral dimension: integrity, ethical behavior Civic awareness and behaviors: motivation and concern for the community, civic knowledge, self-civic image, and conscious involvement Manifested prosocial values: care for others, empathy Environment-related behavior Social learning: communication, cooperation, conflict resolution skills Cultural understanding: understanding of other cultures and cross-cultural communication

(continued)

Table 10.2 (continued)

At the Relationships Level	Family Relationships	Positive relationships with parents: warmth, closeness, communication, support, positive appreciation Positive relationships with siblings and extended family: warmth, closeness, communication, support, positive appreciation
	Peer Relationships/ Peer Group	Friendship: mutual support, positive (appreciative) behaviors, the possibility of meeting friends/peers or inviting them home
	School Relationships	Positive relationships with school staff (especially teachers): students' opinions about the support received Positive engagement and close bonds: participation in school life and extracurricular activities; the sense of belonging to school and acceptance by peers
	Community Relationships and at the Macro-social Level	Sense of community belonging and engagement in community institution activities—including through recreational activities Civic engagement: current or past participation in organizations (e.g., human rights organizations, youth clubs, religious organizations); intentions regarding future political and civic participation as adults (e.g., voting, participating in electoral events, volunteering, etc.) Community work/volunteering Relationships in the virtual environment: the number of hours spent in virtual interactions Positive group identity: positive relating to one's own group membership, without discriminating against other groups/people
At the Context Level	Family	Resources: stable employment, adequate income, education level, number of adults in the household, existence of health services, existence of cognitive/educational resources (books, phone, Internet, magazines, newspapers, etc.) Safe housing: good condition, absence of dampness and smoke, etc. Family communication, role models, time spent with children, discussions with children, structuring and monitoring children's activities, high expectations Learning and complementary support activities (enrichment: parents read books to children, go to the library together, go out (to town, for a walk, to events, etc.) with children) Quantity and quality of social, familial, and professional networks parents are involved in (friend/co-worker group)

(continued)

Table 10.2 (continued)

	Peers/Friends	The peer group does not engage in risky behaviors and has good school results
	School	Access to good schools: parents are satisfied with the school or, conversely, want to transfer their children (show interest in quality education) Safe school: protection against harassment, discrimination, delinquency
	Community and Macro-social Systems	Safe neighborhood: absence of violence, delinquency or a "toxic" environment (predominantly perceived as generating negative emotions and "ill-being") Positive social norms: promoted values support diversity, tolerance, work, family, etc. Cultures/subcultures: social values, lifestyles, spending patterns Belief systems: spiritual, philosophical, political, economic, etc. Community activities: positive physical environment, sufficient spaces, and recreational facilities, adequate staff Community institutions/organizations: active environmental, religious, social, political, civic institutions/organizations Social services, public health, employment, economic services, etc., adequate

System in order an educational setting to get the authorization or accreditation by external evaluation.

10.2.1 National Programs and Projects

There are some specific measures issued by the Ministry of Education regarding the consolidation of the social package for education, targeting students from at-risk groups. We could mention the implementation of annual national social programs: Euro 200, Hot Meal, School Supplies, High School Allowance, Scholarships, Student Transportation, School Program, Material Support for Children with SEN and/or Disabilities, Social Vouchers. All these programs are dedicated to enhance the life quality of the students and to sustain their wellbeing.

The "Euro 200" Program, with its main objective being the implementation of measures to incentivize the purchase of computers, by providing financial aid determined based on social criteria, aims to develop students' and pupils' skills in using computing technology.

The "Hot Meal" initiative plays a role in decreasing school dropout rates and ensuring fair and unbiased access to education for all preschoolers and students across Romania. For example, in the academic year 2022–2023, 178,000 preschoolers and students enrolled in public pre-university education received either a complimentary hot meal or a food package, per day. The students belonged to educational institutions considered socio-economic and geographical disadvantages, as well as the financial constraints preventing many families from supporting their children's engagement in school activities.

The "School Supplies" program provides free school supplies to students in need, at every school year beginning. In correlation with this program, families with poor incomes benefit from educational vouchers.

The new Education Law 198/2023 established that students receive scholarships according to their learning results, and these have the role of motivating them to achieve higher results and performance.

Starting with 2020 the Ministry of Education implements the National Pilot Program "After-School" Program—as a national initiative to foster the remedial activities for primary and low-secondary schools in Romania. Within the project, a national framework was established through which pre-university educational institutions organized remedial activities, starting from the second semester of the 2020–2021 school year. The main objectives of the project consist in preventing early school leaving through systemic measures to increase students' access to learning experiences in primary and secondary pre-university education by participation in remedial learning activities.

Within the "Relevant Curriculum, Open Education for All—CRED" project there were conducted learning activities tailored to the specific needs of vulnerable students.

The outcomes from testing supplementary interventions aimed at assisting students from vulnerable demographics have revealed the significant impact of the Ministry of Education's initiative in curbing early school dropout rates. These efforts conducted within the 25 selected school units can serve as exemplary models for educators nationwide to replicate or modify, aiming for comparable achievements. At the primary level, educational initiatives encompassed overseeing homework completion, providing guidance, and conducting remedial sessions tailored to students facing learning challenges. The array of support and personal development initiatives for students encompasses diverse interventions, including remedial support for those struggling with emotional or linguistic disorders, counseling sessions, and other specialized activities. These include fostering independent reading habits, fostering self-awareness, facilitating interpersonal interactions for emotional and social growth, engaging in hands-on activities across various domains (arts, sciences, technologies), exploring thematic projects suggested by students, parents, or teachers, and promoting physical activity. For lower secondary education, an extensive package of complementary educational activities was rolled out, aligning with support and personal development initiatives for students. These encompassed aiding with homework and providing remedial sessions. The support and personal development program also covered a range of interventions, including psychopedagogical support to bridge learning gaps, psychological counseling, career guidance, activities to enhance learning and performance (particularly for vulnerable student groups), preparing students for school competitions, sports and artistic events, international recognition contests, organizing festivals and exhibitions, creating school publications, participating in European collaborative initiatives, and preparing students for life beyond school. These activities aimed at self-awareness, fostering an active mindset, social integration, instilling responsible environmental attitudes, promoting sustainable development, enhancing communication and critical thinking skills, advocating a healthy lifestyle, preventing violent and risky behaviors, and engaging in physical activities.

The Ministry of Education in partnership with Ministry of Labor and Social Solidarity and with Ministry of Health implemented the project *Creation and Implementation of Integrated Community Services to Reduce Poverty and Social Exclusion,* co-financed by the European Social Fund through the Human Capital Operational Program. The aim of this project is to enhance social inclusion and combat poverty by developing and testing integrated community services in 139 rural and small urban communities with high levels of social marginalization, both moderate and severe. According to the Report of ME in the educational field, the aim is to increase the level of education, reduce school dropout rates and low school participation, improve academic performance, access to informal education programs, and access to school counseling and career guidance services (https://mmuncii.ro/j33/index.php/ro/proiecte-programe/in-curs-de-implementare/5566-fp-sci).

The Ministry of Education is executing the Grants Scheme as part of the National Program for Reducing School Dropout (PNRAS), which is funded through Romania's National Recovery and Resilience Plan. This initiative benefits of a total funding allocation of 543 million euros and it is approved by Government Decision no. 1.309/2021. PNRAS sets out to achieve several overarching objectives, including reducing the incidence of school dropout by at least 25% across participating educational institutions from 2021 to 2026, thereby lowering their risk categorization. Additionally, it strives to enhance student performance in national assessments, increase the proportion of students successfully completing lower secondary education, encourage greater participation of lower secondary education graduates in the National Evaluation for 8th grade graduates, and facilitate a higher transition rate from lower secondary to upper secondary education (https://www.edu.ro/PNRAS).

The Ministry of Education has continued to execute grants under the Secondary Education Project (ROSE), which facilitates the transition of students from upper secondary education to tertiary education. This project employs a decentralized approach by providing individual grants to high schools. The primary objectives of these grants include reducing the dropout rate in high schools, increasing graduation rates, and enhancing performance on the baccalaureate exam. High schools are engaged in various activities aimed at achieving these goals, such as remedial sessions, counseling, career guidance, coaching, personal development initiatives, and the cultivation of socio-emotional skills. Additionally, they organize extracurricular and informational events, as well as undertake minor renovation projects, interior refurbishments, and procurement of necessary resources (https://www.rose-edu.ro/).

As a specific measure proposed for 2024 the Ministry of Education report mentions ensuring resilience through: "developing resilience mechanisms at the pre-university education institutions to support students in adapting to uncertainties and crisis situations; preparing students to cope with perpetually changing social dynamics through disciplines aligned with the needs of democratic society; educating children in the spirit of safeguarding their physical and emotional integrity, emphasizing health awareness and proper self-care; combating bullying in all its forms; enhancing student safety by promoting among children, parents, and other stakeholders (teachers, state authorities, community, etc.) the tools and information necessary to recognize and effectively combat bullying phenomena; developing, through the common national action plan for increasing student and teaching staff safety, integrated measures and specific actions to expand partnerships on legal issues and combating acts of violence in schools, themes that facilitate students' awareness of their rights, obligations, and the consequences of their actions" (Ministry of Education, 2023, p. 135).

Starting with November 2023 the Ministry of Education promote the national program entitled "Together We Take Courage"—School Violence and Crime Prevention Program as a measure to mitigate the prevalence of school violence. According to the program outline its purpose is the prevention and reduction of violence and crime in the school environment and it is operationalized by five objectives: creating a safe, welcoming, and supportive climate for all involved beneficiaries (preschoolers, students, staff, and parents) at the level of educational units; improving the relationships/cohesion between school staff, families, and preschoolers/students, including their collaboration to support victims in managing traumatic situations and to encourage perpetrators to improve their behavior; empowering preschoolers/students to report acts of violence and witnesses to adopt strategies to support victims and discourage violent behavior by perpetrators; improving the social and emotional skills of preschoolers/students, including their ability to identify, interpret, express, and self-regulate emotions in a constructive manner toward themselves and others; Raising awareness of the consequences associated with committing acts of violence and crimes. “Together We Take Courage” is going to be implemented by Regional Centers of Educational Assistance and Resources during the school year 2023–2024, fostering the wellbeing for both students and teachers within school settings (https://edu.ro/anti_violenta).

10.2.2 National Curriculum and Frameworks for Promoting Wellbeing

In Romania, according the Education Law no 198/2023 (art.13 (1)) the compulsory education includes preschool education, primary education, lower secondary education and upper secondary education (high school); the children with ages from 3 to 18 are to be involved in formal educational activities during their personal development (see Fig. 10.2).

There are educational policies that sustain the promoting wellbeing through school, both through regular curriculum and the optional one.

Our presentation is focused on the identification of the modalities for wellbeing promotion for the educational cycles (preschool, primary, lower secondary, upper secondary) both at the curriculum level and at the extracurricular activities.

The educational system from pre-university level encompasses a specific service regarding the psychological and pedagogical assistance for students, teachers, and

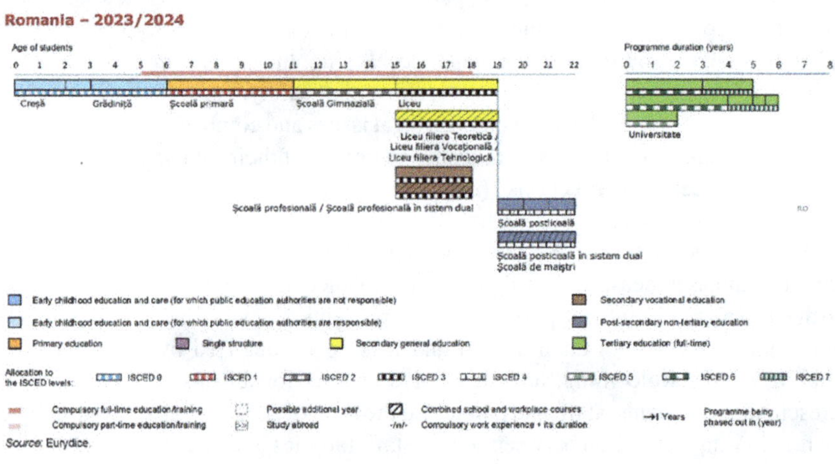

Fig. 10.2 Romanian educational system (Eurydice, 2023)

parents. The County Center for Educational Resources and Assistance, as an educational institution, is specialized in providing, coordinating, and monitoring specific educational services with the goal of ensuring access for all stakeholders in education to quality support, counseling, and educational and remedial services. The County Center for Educational Resources and Assistance is an entity related to pre-university education with legal personality, subordinate to the Ministry of Education, methodologically coordinated by the County School Inspectorate, and funded by the County Council.

Services offered include:

- Psychopedagogical assistance services for students, teachers, and parents, provided through the County Psychopedagogical Assistance Center (CJAP) and school psychopedagogical assistance offices;
- Services consisting of various speech therapy treatments, provided through Inter-School Speech Therapy Offices (CLI);
- Support and guidance services for children, students, and young people with Special Educational Needs (CES), provided through the Service for Evaluation and School and Vocational Guidance (SEOSP);
- School mediation services, provided by school mediators;
- Consultancy services for improving the quality of services for adapting students and parents to the school educational context and promoting school-family-community cooperation;
- Services aimed at aligning the educational offer with the specific requirements of the labor market and implementing modern teaching-learning-assessment and counseling strategies, through the realization of specialized studies and research;
- Services to facilitate the relationship between units and institutions of pre-university education with the community through partnerships, projects, and programs;
- Various volunteer services.
- Wellbeing for Early Childhood Education and Care Settings.

The early childhood education and care (ECEC) (for children from birth to the age of 6 years) is part of educational system and includes, according to the National Education Law, ante-preschool education (for children aged 0–3 years) and preschool education (for children aged 3–6 years); the latter is compulsory. The preschool education is organized through kindergartens (educational settings with regular or long educational program, 5 or 10 h, respectively). In Romania ECEC is free of charge and it offers a high-quality educational service to families and communities.

The Ministerial Order No. 4694/2.09.2019 introduced a unified early childhood education and care (ECEC) curriculum for children from birth to 6 years, replacing age-specific guidelines with a comprehensive approach. This new curriculum, now in effect across all early childhood settings, outlines a pedagogical framework aimed at fostering holistic development and enabling children to achieve their full potential. It emphasizes individualized teaching strategies tailored to each child's interests, needs, and abilities. Key principles of the ECEC curriculum include:

- Child-focused education, emphasizing the recognition and respect for each child's unique qualities and needs.
- Upholding children's rights, including education and freedom of expression.
- Active learning, encouraging children's active participation and decision-making in learning activities.
- Integrated development through a multidisciplinary approach.
- Interculturalism, promoting an understanding and respect for diverse national and ethnic values.
- Equity and non-discrimination, ensuring equal developmental opportunities for all children, regardless of background.
- Viewing education as a collaborative interaction between educators and children, recognizing the significance of both parties in the educational process.

Based on these principles, the wellbeing is promoted especially at these ages, for both children and their families.

According to the Curriculum 2019, ECEC should take a holistic approach, addressing five areas of child development, such as: physical development, health and personal hygiene; socio-emotional development; cognitive development and knowledge of the world; development of language, communication, and the premises for reading and writing; learning skills and attitudes. The area of physical development, health, and personal hygiene covers a wide range of skills and abilities (from broad movements such as skipping, running, to fine movements such as drawing or modeling), but also coordination, sensory development, along with knowledge and skills related to personal care and hygiene, nutrition, other health maintenance, and personal safety practices. The area of socio-emotional development concerns the onset of the child's social life, his/her ability to establish and maintain interactions with adults and children. Social interactions mediate how children view themselves and the world around them. Emotional development is particularly concerned with children's ability to perceive and express their emotions, to understand and respond to the emotions of others, and the development of the self-concept that is crucial to this domain. Closely related to the self-concept is the development of the child's self-image, which has a decisive influence on the learning process. So, some prerequisites for wellbeing promotion are already embedded into the new curriculum.

According to the New Curriculum (2019), ***the ECEC curriculum*** is the main curricular product and the essential regulatory component of the early childhood education, the official, normative, and binding document that marks the overall organization of the teaching–learning–assessment process for each age level and type of early childhood education institution.

The document proposes in a simple form the indicators to be followed in the context of the development of early learning projects. It is systematically organized by age level, with reference to four age ranges (0–18 months, 19–36 months, 37–60 months, 61–72/84 months), and includes all the learning activities for each age group and level, specifying the number of hours per week allocated to each category of learning activity. The curriculum is compulsory for all early education institutions, thus ensuring respect for the principle of equal opportunities to education.

The age ranges (0–18 months, 19–36 months, 37–60 months and 61–72/84 months) that appear in the curriculum, as well as the categories/types and number of hours allocated for activities are the result of correlating the realities of the system with the *Fundamental Benchmarks in Early Learning and Development of Children from Birth to 7 Years* (Ionescu, 2010) and with European and global trends in the field.

The learning activities (both preschool and ante-preschool) set out in the ECEC Curriculum will lead to the achievement of outcomes that will shape the child's later competences. These learning activities integrate planned and systematic actions, constantly organized by the teacher in order to raise the level of children's skills. As a rule, in the design of learning activities, the educator will also take into account the involvement of the family, with a major emphasis on the involvement of the child, who will be put as often as possible in specific situations of exploration and practice of skills. Learning activities can be carried out individually, in small groups or with the whole group of children.

To ensure the consistent and coherent application of the Early Education Curriculum (approved by Ministerial Order No. 4694 on 2 August 2019) and the Methodology for the organization and functioning of nurseries and other early childhood education units (approved by Government Decision No. 566/2022), as well as to establish a unified, inclusive, and quality early education system as outlined in the "Educated Romania" Project initiated by the Romanian Presidency and ratified by the Romanian Parliament in 2021, annually, the Ministry of Education issues a "methodological letter" to ECEC teachers nationwide, outlining key directives and guidelines for the year. In this respect, in a constructive approach to effective communication, the cooperation and support for an inclusive, integrated education system and quality, with excellent teachers, in such methodical letters there are proposed different issues to be addressed.

For example, for 2023–2024 here are the main issues communicated to the preschool teachers from all over the country:

A. A proposal for a child-friendly approach to the transition from family environment to a new learning context;
B. Suggestions for the organization and conduct of methodological work weekly;
C. Educational counselling activity for parents;
D. Questions relating to the Early Education Curriculum which persist. Questions that have arisen in the process of integrating nurseries into the education system;
E. School regulations and documents with which we operate in education this school year;
F. Proposed themes for methodical activities and pedagogical circles;
G. Educational projects and programs being carried out this school year in early education.

(extract from Methodological Letter for 2023–2024 school year, https://www.edu.ro/educatie_timpurie

The 2023 edition highlighted the significance of easing the transition from family to kindergarten, offering strategies to ensure the wellbeing of children and families.

Based on this methodological letter, promoting a friendly approach to early education involves facilitating smooth transitions into educational programs through partnerships with parents and tailored procedures, detailed as follows: initial parent-childminder meetings, exploration and familiarization, adaptation program, interactive activities, support and benefits, continued partnership.

After enrolling in a nursery or kindergarten, teachers arrange meetings with parents to introduce themselves and explain the child's adaptation program to the educational environment. This usually occurs in the first two weeks or even before the course starts, during holidays or the last school week. The first meeting allows parents and children to explore the educational setting (classrooms, common areas, playgrounds, etc.) and meet the staff through organized tours. This program spans the first two weeks or the last week of the previous school year, requiring dedicated time daily. Activities, designed for small groups and flexible scheduling, focus on outdoor and interest-center engagement. Involving parents directly, these activities aim to build trust and familiarity. They include movement games, role-plays, finger-painting, and crafting welcome posters, emphasizing fun, self-confidence, and achievement. Parents provide emotional support, fostering a secure transition for children into the nursery or kindergarten environment. This process helps children adapt, boosts parental confidence in the childcare team, and allows teachers to assess each child's needs and adaptation pace. Beyond the initial adaptation, ongoing collaboration between teachers and parents may support socio-emotional development, with parents participating in educational activities as "second teachers" or volunteers.

This approach ensures a smooth, supportive transition from home to early educational settings, benefiting children, parents, and educators alike, contributing to the wellbeing promotion for all.

Teachers are supervised and they have the possibilities to participate at professional meeting discussing and debating different topics, suggested for the school year. One of the topics is related to the role of the early childhood education settings in child development and, implicitly, in creating the child's wellbeing. Teachers reflect on the topic, defining specific modalities to provide children wellbeing within educational interaction with children, through both curriculum and extracurricular activities.

For example, the letter for 2022–2023 defined the school year as themed "Play, Respect, and Joy," this being the most important guidance for the early education efforts. Play is emphasized as: a tool for communication and building resilience; a vehicle for development and learning; a catalyst for creativity; a method for relaxation and recuperation; an instructional strategy; and a framework for conducting educational activities. The Respect is highlighted in terms of: Self-respect; Respect for others; adherence to universal human values passed through generations, including behavioral norms in various contexts such as family, educational settings, public transportation, trips, and public spaces; appreciation of national values, including notable Romanian figures, history, geography, customs, traditions, and folklore and respect for nature and living heritage. Joy is presented as: an emotion to be experienced; a lifestyle to cultivate; a feeling to share with others; a foundation for wellbeing and growth.

Wellbeing is embedded into theories and practices at preschool educational level in Romania, is part of the extended curriculum, and addresses the particular needs of children, families, and educators.

For the academic year 2021–2022 one of the guidelines suggested to take into attention the environment created for learning and play. According to this recommendation the learning environment should be a friendly classroom that reflects diversity and that supports everyone's learning. Regarding the environment for preschoolers, it's crucial that the space is meticulously planned and designed to be a positive, inspiring, and educational setting. It should be a welcoming, attractive place where children feel at home, conveying to both the children and visitors the essence of what occurs in the world and in a standard early education service, whether it's referred to as a kindergarten or a nursery school. This space should reflect and facilitate the learning and play activities that are fundamental to early childhood development.

The Ministry of Education has consistently initiated, alongside important partners with experience in the field, educational projects dedicated to preschool/early childhood education. According to 2023 methodological letter, the following projects are to be developed during the school year 2023–2024:

"– The national educational program to stimulate interest in reading "Let's Read for the Third Millennium" (MEd, county school inspectorates, kindergartens, local communities); continues through Ovidiu Ro initiatives: Reading Workshops and the "Read Me 100 Stories" project;
– The national educational program for ecological education "EcoKindergarten" (MEd, county school inspectorates, kindergartens, local communities); continues with the "Garden of Peace, Relaxation, and Learning" project;
– The national educational program to stimulate interest in physical education and sports "Kalokagathia" (MEd, county school inspectorates, kindergartens, local communities); the project has seen numerous developments, especially in the form of local sports competitions.
– Values education project: "Play, Respect, and Joy!" (MEd, county school inspectorates); the project has developed at the county level and has generated a series of generic activities, including intergenerational community support. (https://www.edu.ro/educatie_timpurie)

Analyzing the list above it is obviously the interest of the Ministry of Education in sustaining wellbeing promotion through early childhood educational settings using different means and tools: literature and lectures, outdoor activities, sport and physical education, education for values and social-emotional development.

10.2.3 Wellbeing in Primary, Lower Secondary, and High School

According to the Law of Education (art.15), the primary education is 5 years long, comprising the preparatory grade and grades I to IV. Primary education is developed on the basis of the National Curriculum. The primary education is compulsory and all the students benefit of free of charge textbooks. There are two national assessment stages, for the second grade and for the fourth grade.

As per the regulations outlined in the National Education Law (Law 1/2011), educational institutions have the option to offer supplementary activities to their students beyond regular school hours through School After School Programs, subject to approval by the board of directors. These programs encompass educational, recreational, and leisure activities, often organized in collaboration with parent associations and public authorities. Additionally, they may include remedial learning sessions aimed at reinforcing acquired skills or accelerating learning progress. Where feasible, partnerships may be established with nongovernmental organizations specializing in these areas.

The Ministry of National Education establishes the curriculum for primary education. Aligned with the overarching goals of education, the current curriculum for primary education outlines specific objectives for this level: guaranteeing the initial phase of fundamental education for every child; fostering the development of each child's individuality, while respecting their unique pace and level of growth; ensuring that each child attains essential knowledge, skills, and attitudes conducive to meaningful and innovative engagement with both the social and natural environments, thereby facilitating further educational opportunities (https://eurydice.eacea.ec.europa.eu/ro/national-education-systems/romania/romania).

The curriculum is organized by curricular area, such as: *Language and communication*; *Mathematics and natural sciences*; *Human being and society*; *Physical education, sports and health; Arts; Technologies; Counselling and guidance.* Under the curricular area related to counseling and guidance there is a specific discipline of study entitled *Personal Development*, providing a very good frame for fostering personal and emotional wellbeing. The school offers also the possibility to develop curriculum upon school decision, and this enables teachers to design, create, and implement new optional programs, subordinated to one of the curricular area, or integrated ones. This could also be a very good opportunity to foster wellbeing through choosing specific domain for optional courses (such as emotional education, social-emotional learning, and mental health).

10.2.4 Curricular Area: Counseling and Guidance

The Counseling and Guidance activities included in the curriculum for grades preparatory through 4 are designed to assist students in finding answers to various questions related to their orientation and development (Who am I and what qualities do I have? How can I make friends at school and at home? Where can I get information or assistance? What do I need to do to learn better? What do I want to become and what do I need to do to feel fulfilled?). The content of these activities is flexible and can be adapted to meet the individual needs of students, educational institutions, as well as the community and society as a whole. In a pragmatic manner, teachers can engage in educational projects both within and outside the school setting, at national, regional, or local levels, and collaboration with specialists such as doctors, lawyers, social workers, psychologists, sociologists, police officers, and firefighters can be requested.

By participating in the activities proposed in the Counseling and Guidance curriculum, under the guidance of teachers, students are provided with opportunities to develop their motivation, self-confidence, and learning skills. As a result, they become better prepared for subsequent educational levels, can set realistic goals, actively participate in school and social life, and become more self-aware and aware of their surroundings.

During Counseling and Guidance sessions, students have the opportunity to practice effective communication, relationship-building, and efficient learning skills, and to understand how to apply these skills in various social contexts. They acquire knowledge and skills that help them become responsible members of the school community, family, and peer group, actively engaging in lifelong learning and building their own future through assuming responsibilities. Throughout each year of primary education, students will develop new skills for self-exploration, evaluating their own activities and social life, setting personal goals, and developing action plans to achieve them (according to the Annex to Minister of Education and Research Order No. 5286/09.10.2006). The framework objectives for this curricular area are: (1) developing self-awareness and a positive self-concept; (2) developing interpersonal skills in various contexts; (3) developing information utilization skills in the learning process; (4) acquiring career exploration and planning skills; (5) practicing skills for managing a high-quality lifestyle.

We easily figure out that this learning frame provides the opportunity to learn about self and others, to develop and enhance personal skills, to boost the social skills and learning to learn abilities for flourishing and wellbeing. In Table 2, we present a sequence from School Syllabus of Counseling and Guidance for the fourth grade related to the content:

Learning Contents

1. Self-awareness and personal development
   1.1 Self-awareness
   • Personal interests and abilities: individual characteristics
   1.2 Change, growth, development
   • Preparation for change and for the fifth grade
   2. Communication and social skills

2.1 Social skills

• Roles in groups

2.2. Family

• Relationships between family members. Family values and practices—critical aspects to be discussed with parents (related to growth, relationships with peers and teachers)

3. Information and learning management

3.1 Efficient learning

• Learning (in a narrow sense)—optimal conditions for efficient learning

• Efficient study skills: organizing learning content, balancing effort and relaxation/rest periods

• Learning discipline: engagement, perseverance, responsibility, task commitment

• Internal and external conditions: learning environment (space, ambiance), personal health status

• Effective learning tools: ICT

4. Career planning

4.1 Exploring priorities

• Priorities and objectives regarding personal activities (personal journal, daily, weekly activity lists)

5. Lifestyle quality

5.1 Personal life quality

• Arguments accompanying decisions to act in difficult situations (e.g., accidents in transportation, excursions, hiking, etc.)

• Problem-solving alternatives; implications

(extract from School Curriculum for the Curriculum Area Counseling and Guidance GRADES I—IV GRADES V—VIII Approved by the Minister's Order No. 5286/09.10.2006).

According to the document *Methodological Guidelines in Counseling and Guidance for the Transition from Grade VIII to Grade IX* the educational offer provided by the Counseling and Guidance curriculum yields numerous benefits, including:

- Improved academic performance and narrowing of achievement gaps among students.
- Increased student engagement in school activities, leading to a reduced dropout rate.
- Mitigation of social isolation, a common precursor to feelings of alienation and instances of violence.
- Reduction of bullying occurrences within the school environment.
- Promotion of positive self-esteem and interpersonal relationships among students.
- Encouragement of greater involvement in extracurricular pursuits.
- Heightened awareness of academic and career pathways.
- Strengthening of student–teacher relationships, fostering a conducive learning environment.
- Enhancement of students' competencies, better preparing them for future success.

– Engagement of students, along with their families or guardians, in a comprehensive counseling and guidance framework.

In lower secondary school (gymnasium), students embark on a journey of self-discovery through counseling and personal development classes. These sessions facilitate the cultivation of self-awareness, emotional intelligence, and confidence, while also nurturing decision-making, communication, and social skills. Additionally, students develop a positive outlook toward schooling and acquire effective learning strategies. Transitioning into high school, additional activities are introduced to support students in managing their personal wellbeing. This includes exploring various dimensions of life—emotional, academic, social, moral, and physical—and understanding their dynamic interplay. Furthermore, students are equipped with the necessary tools and resources to navigate information and media responsibly, promoting independence and informed decision-making.

We present in the Table 10.3 the general competences and the contents proposed for the curricular area Counseling and Guidance for middle school and for the high school in Romania.

The whole experience offered by this curriculum area is a framework for promoting wellbeing through learning experiences that lead to greater self-awareness and meaning, experience of positive emotions, acquisition of skills for developing positive relationships, increased motivation and commitment to personal learning, and an environment for experiencing success and achievement.

Although it was developed in 2006, the Counseling and Guidance School Curriculum was designed to be approached in a flexible manner. Teachers have the freedom to initiate the educational process in any class and can choose any of the specific competencies based on the students' needs. The two disciplines in the

Table 10.3 Competences and contents proposed by counselling and guidance curricular area

General competencies for middle school	General competencies for high school
1. Adopting positive attitudes toward oneself and a healthy and balanced lifestyle 2. Harmonious relationships with others in both school and extracurricular contexts 3. Reflecting on motivation and the effectiveness of learning strategies for progress 4. Making decisions regarding further studies and career paths by leveraging self-awareness, education, and occupational information	1. Exploring personal resources that influence career planning 2. Integrating interpersonal skills for personal and professional development 3. Appropriately utilizing information in one's own activities to achieve success 4. Developing a personal and professional development plan 5. Practicing skills for managing a high-quality lifestyle
Content areas middle school	**Thematic modules high school**
I. Self-awareness and healthy and balanced lifestyle; II. Socio-emotional development; III. Learning management; IV. Career management	I. Self-awareness and personal development; II. Communication and social skills; III. Information and learning management; IV. Career planning

Counseling and Guidance curriculum, namely Personal Development in Primary Education and Counseling and Personal Development in middle school, extend into the ninth grade to continue supporting the wellbeing of students, adapting to their particularities and the needs of student classes.

10.2.5 Elective Curriculum

An important part of curriculum is the optional curriculum decided by school. There are some optional programs, approved by the Ministry of Education that could be delivered in schools, especially for high schools such as: Prepared for life. Education for life and community (for middle school), the Character First (optional program for middle school), and Management of Emotions (for high school).

The curriculum for the course "*Prepared for Life: Education for Life and Community*" is founded on a set of values aimed at assisting children in preparing for and navigating life's obstacles. Within this framework, the curriculum places a strong emphasis on fostering responsibility and fostering positive social interactions across various contexts such as family, school, peer groups, local communities, and other familial environments. This elective course promotes a holistic understanding of individuals, with specific attention given to the following dimensions:

- Bio-behavioral dynamics: encompassing aspects like identity, bodily awareness, self-discipline, skill development, healthy habits, as well as organizational and self-management abilities.
- Psycho-emotional dynamics: addressing psycho-sexual and personal growth, emotions, self-awareness, self-acceptance, confidence-building, and behavioral patterns.
- Spiritual dynamics: focusing on moral development, including integrity, integration, freedom, and responsibility, alongside respect for life. It also explores spiritual growth, including one's relationship with oneself, with others, and with the broader world, while acknowledging and embracing personal vocations.
- Relational dynamics: covering the management of relationships within family, peer groups, communities/society, and other relational spheres.

Consequently, the proposed curriculum emphasizes the cultivation of character by reinforcing responsibility and fostering healthy social interactions. It aids students in comprehending the stages of physical, emotional, and intellectual development and gradually integrates age-appropriate discussions on sexuality.

The elective course *Management of Emotions* is developed within a national program and it is designed for students in grades 9 through 12, and aims to assist them in exploring their emotions amid the transitions from middle school to high school or from high school to higher education or the professional life. It focuses on adapting to new school or organizational cultures, forging connections with new groups or communities, and adjusting to new academic demands. Its primary goal is to establish a foundation for emotional wellbeing in the classroom, impacting both individuals and the overall educational environment. Additionally, it caters to adolescents' needs by helping them understand their own and others' strategies for emotional expression and regulation across various settings, including virtual platforms, given the increasing reliance on digital communication among young people. As such, this course is integral to a holistic approach to supporting mental health, fostering emotional growth, and aiding adolescents in identifying potential signs of mental health issues early on, such as anxiety, depression, or eating disorders. Recognizing and addressing these signs represents a crucial initial step in providing timely support and intervention, whether for oneself or for others.

Inclusive Education and the Development of Critical Thinking (Annex 2 to Order No. 4800/26.08.2022 issued by the Ministry of Education.), an elective subject for grades IX–X, promotes a model of learning that aims to develop individuals who are able to critically analyze their social environment, investigate its specific problems and identify and implement solutions in order to contribute to the construction of a democratic, tolerant and just society for all its members. The specific learning approach of this discipline begins with the personal experiences of each student, stemming from the family, school, or community environment. From the perspective of critical thinking promoted by this program, students learn to be attentive and considerate to the details of a social situation, to challenge social prejudices and norms, and to engage with relevant arguments in support of a viewpoint aimed at improving the social environment.

10.3 Romanian Teachers' Wellbeing

There are some studies conducted on the Romanian teachers' population figuring out different factors and variables which are correlated with wellbeing or life satisfaction or job satisfaction. Ignat and Clipa (2012) present the fact that good emotional intelligence in Romanian teachers is positively correlated with a positive attitude toward work, satisfaction with life, and job satisfaction; in a study Bota (2013) concluded that Romanian teachers show high job satisfaction compared to British secondary school teachers and other professions, despite the poor state of education in Romania. A study done on the data derived from TALIS identified that professional development and career time are the most influential factors in job satisfaction and teacher's self-efficacy in Romanian lower secondary schools (Zoller & Bacskai, 2020). Ortan et al. (2021) conducted a study on 658 K-12 (pre-university) teachers, from the North-West region of Romania with the aim to examine the relationship between teacher job satisfaction and four main categories of determinants: self-efficacy, relational aspects (colleague collaboration, student behavior, school management), work-related aspects (administrative workload, teaching tasks), and working conditions, in order to identify various implications for teachers' wellbeing. The results indicated that self-efficacy, promotion, positive student behavior, and working conditions significantly impact teacher job satisfaction and wellbeing, leading to higher levels of involvement from teachers, students, and parents.

In a study which examines the response of Romanian teachers to professional challenges amid an evolving educational landscape, Obrad and Circa (2021) seek to assess the effects of professional shifts on teaching practices in Romania from March to June 2020 and determine the key factors influencing work engagement during telework. Conducted on a representative sample of 400 Romanian teachers, spanning all levels of the nation's educational system, the research offers insights with a 5% confidence interval and a 95% confidence level. The results showed that perceived student engagement and motivation are major determinants of work engagement among teachers in the context of teleworking during the COVID-19 pandemic in Romania. Obrad (2020) brought updated information on the complex relationship between stress and resilience in the case of employees from the area of education. Among other results, this research highlighted the structure of work engagement and the mediating role of professional support in the relationship between stressors and resilience mechanisms. The main result indicated that online teaching during COVID-19 in Romania led to increased stress and resilience in teachers, with professional support playing a mediating role.

Rusu and Colomeischi (2020) in a study conducted on a sample of 1,335 teachers concluded that higher positivity ratio in teachers leads to increased work engagement, which in turn positively affects their wellbeing.

Colomeischi (2014) argued for the importance of raising the teachers‘ satisfaction to work through their personal development, at least at some level such as emotional stability, emotional intelligence, boost the happiness balance, develop the positive affectivity and pleasant feelings. Within the particular study, it appears that the emotional traits considered (emotional intelligence, emotional stability, negative mood regulation, empathy, positive affect, negative affect, pleasant feeling, unpleasant feeling, happiness balance, psychological flourishing) make a difference regarding the teachers work satisfaction.

The results of a study on 1390 Romanian teachers (Colomeischi & Ursu, 2023) suggest that perceived stress had significant negative associations with the dimensions of wellbeing and life satisfaction. Furthermore, all three dimensions of wellbeing (emotional wellbeing, social wellbeing, psychological wellbeing) were significantly positively associated with teachers' life satisfaction. Additionally, all wellbeing dimensions mediated the negative effect of perceived stress on life satisfaction. Overall, the results from this study indicate that all three dimensions of wellbeing are an important protective factor that could help us to comprehend the negative effect of teachers' perceived stress on their life satisfaction.

10.3.1 National Programs and Initiatives to Promote Teachers' Wellbeing

The national programs for the improvement of teachers' professional competences have developed frameworks for the promotion of wellbeing, because each professional development activity incorporates resources that contribute to making the profession more enjoyable, to defining a specific professional meaning, and to ensuring the promise of professional success. All these, seen in light of Seligman's PERMA wellbeing model, (Seligman, 2011) are elements that build teachers' wellbeing.

The "Relevant Curriculum, Open Education for All—CRED" project (https://www.educred.ro/eu-sunt-cred/despre-proiectul-cred/) was initiated to address the evolving roles of teachers and their need to deeply understand and effectively implement the values of the new National Curriculum, transforming them into true educators beyond their traditional roles. Its goals include: (1) ensuring a unified competency-based curriculum approach among stakeholders to guarantee equal opportunities for vulnerable and second-chance pupils. (2). Encouraging competence-focused teaching by developing and utilizing open educational resources for the new curriculum in primary and secondary education. (3) Equipping 55,000 teachers with the skills for a methodological approach that emphasizes key competencies and tailors learning to individual student needs, aiming to prevent dropouts. (4) Enhancing the quality and relevance of school activities for vulnerable groups to decrease early school leaving through innovative projects that promote key competencies in engaging learning environments for at least 2,500 students. Within this vast project there are opened experiences for teachers to become creators of education by proposing optional learning projects.

The project PROF—"Professionalization of the teaching career" (https://www.edu.ro/PROF, https://www.eprof.ro/)—is coordinated by Ministry of Education and it is developed to offer a frame for mentoring and coaching in education. By 2023, it had as an aim to establish a national framework for mentoring in pre-university teaching careers via a network-based institution. This involved providing continuous training and professional development for 28,000 educators to enhance pedagogical skills, particularly in practical classroom teaching. The training covered e-learning, inclusivity, curriculum design, assessment methods, Tele-school, anti-bullying strategies, and transdisciplinarity. It's designed to adapt teaching staff to the digitalization of education and address the needs of students from vulnerable groups, such as the Roma, children with special educational needs (SEN), hospitalized children, and those from socio-economically disadvantaged backgrounds. The teachers found themselves cared for and experienced opportunities for enhanced wellbeing.

The national program for promoting teacher's wellbeing provided by INIM Institute, a nongovernmental organization, brings out into community attention the necessity of cultivating teachers' mental health and wellbeing. The INIM Institute's mission is to enhance the skills of top-tier educators in Romania and Eastern Europe by creating responsive training programs informed by the research. These programs are tailored to meet the evolving educational and societal needs, with a strong focus on emotional intelligence, wisdom, solidarity, and resilience to address stress reduction. The core values of INIM are compassion, fairness, diversity, solidarity, and inclusion (INIM = Learning Together). INIM conducted a study aimed at screening the mental health of teachers in Romania; the "Teacher Flourishing Evaluation" from Harvard University's Human Flourishing Program was used to assess teachers' wellbeing across five dimensions: (1) happiness and life satisfaction; (2) physical and mental health; (3) purpose and meaning; (4) character and virtue; (5) close social relationships. The study sought to determine the wellbeing of teachers, with participation from 5,227 educators in Romania, predominantly women and from urban areas. Results show that only 32.5% are thriving, while 61.9% have moderate mental health. The majority feel that their work does not enhance their wellbeing, highlighting a lack of autonomy, recognition, and support from school management. Teachers emphasize the importance of discussions about mental health, recognition of their efforts, and support for developing emotional skills. (https://fundatiatransylvaniacollege.ro/wp-content/uploads/2021/11/VEZI-REZULTATELE-STUDIULUI.pdf) "Happy Teachers for Romania" provide opportunities for personal and professional development for teachers, addressing their emotional needs, reducing stress, and enhancing resilience.

10.4 Good Practices for Promoting Wellbeing at School—International Programs and Projects

The pursuit of wellbeing within educational settings has garnered significant attention worldwide, as educators and policymakers alike recognize the profound impact of mental, emotional, and social health on students' learning and development. Considering the European Educational Space, a diverse array of international programs and projects have emerged, aiming to integrate wellbeing promotion into the very fabric of school cultures. These initiatives underscore the critical role that schools play not only in imparting academic knowledge but also in fostering holistic development and resilience among students. We are trying to outline some good practices for wellbeing promotion, and to highlight the promising potential of international programs and projects designed to enhance the wellbeing of school communities within European partnerships.

Through a lens of global collaboration and innovation, we will delve into how these efforts contribute to creating supportive, inclusive, and empowering learning environments where all students can thrive.

PROMEHS—Promotion Mental Health at School is an international Erasmus+ partnership, developed to create educational policies for mental health in education. As we could learn from their presentation is the first mental health curriculum developed by researchers, policymakers and scientific associations from seven countries, promoting a whole school approach. The Erasmus+ Key Action 3 project,

Promoting Mental Health at Schools (PROMEHS), funded by the European Commission from 2019 to 2022, aims to develop, implement, and assess a mental health curriculum for schools. This initiative is a collaborative effort among researchers, policymakers, and scientific communities from seven European nations: Croatia, Greece, Italy, Latvia, Malta, Portugal, and Romania. Its goal is to forge connections between educational programs and institutions, thereby integrating research, practical applications, and policy. PROMEHS establishes a comprehensive framework for the creation and execution of a universally applicable, evidence-based mental health curriculum within schools. This includes providing high-quality training for teachers, as well as offering supervision, meetings, and creating handbooks and guidelines tailored for educators, students, parents, policymakers, and various stakeholders. The PROMEHS curriculum focuses on three key areas (two of them focused on promotion and the other one on prevention): fostering social and emotional learning, enhancing resilience, and preventing social, emotional, and behavioral issues. It adopts a comprehensive whole school approach that emphasizes the collaborative efforts of students, teachers, families, school leaders, community stakeholders, and policymakers. PROMEHS is designed as a universal program, seamlessly integrating into the school curriculum with multi-year guidance provided through seven handbooks. These handbooks cater to a wide age range of students (3 to 18 years old), their parents, and teachers, offering multi-year support. Activities for students and teachers in kindergarten through to secondary school, including home-based projects with parents, are outlined in four of these handbooks. These activities are based on the S.A.F.E. approach (Durlak et al., 2015) and aim to be part of the regular curriculum. The remaining three handbooks provide mental health promotion guidelines for teachers, parents, and policymakers. To accommodate diverse linguistic needs and cultural contexts, all handbooks are available in seven languages: Croatian, English, Greek, Italian, Latvian, Portuguese, and Romanian. Additionally, PROMEHS includes a comprehensive professional development program for teachers, comprising both initial training and ongoing support, to ensure the program's effective and consistent implementation. PROMEHS developed a validated curriculum through experimental research, proposing an evidence-based program to be implemented in schools. The evaluation of the PROMEHS program with more than 10,000 students from six different countries indicates that the program positively impacted both students' and teachers' behaviors in the experimental group compared to the waiting group (Cefai et al., 2022; Colomeischi et al., 2022). There was an improvement among students in all five areas of social and emotional learning based on teachers' evaluations (but only marginally according to parents' and students' evaluations), with the biggest increase in self-awareness and social awareness skills. Overall, there was an increase in students' social and emotional skills and prosocial behavior and a decrease in internalized and externalized difficulties (www.promehs.org).

The "*SEEVAL—Social and Emotional Education—Building inclusive schools and ownership of values*" project (ref. No 612219-EPP-1-2019-1-BG-EPPKA3-IPI-SOC-IN) is carried out with the European Commission's support through the K3 Erasmus+ program. It involves a consortium of partners from Bulgaria,

Italy, Malta, Austria, Greece, and Romania. SEEVAL is dedicated to developing a training course for educators and action protocols that adopt a comprehensive school approach to Social and Emotional Education (SEE). The project gathered and disseminated educational practices for social and emotional learning as Open Educational Resources to equip educators with the necessary pedagogical and didactic tools (Botnariuc et al., 2023). These tools aim to foster students' skills in self-management, self-awareness, social awareness, responsible decision-making, relationship building, and values. Targeting middle and early high school students (ages 10–16), the project particularly focuses on those from disadvantaged backgrounds, such as minorities, migrants, refugees, and socially disadvantaged groups, ensuring that both educators' and learners' needs are met. The project itself provides very good and high-quality opportunities for both students and teachers to enhance their wellbeing and overall functioning (https://seeval-project.eu/).

RODAWELL introduces a holistic approach to enhancing wellbeing within schools, drawing inspiration from the Danish model of school wellbeing. A key achievement of this initiative is the establishment of the *Romanian-Danish Center for Children's Wellbeing—RodaWell*, providing comprehensive services including training, support materials, and evaluative measures to refine teachers' educational methodologies. The initiative specifically addresses the needs of educational settings that cater to a significant number of at-risk children, including those facing challenges such as special educational needs, poverty, parental migration, neglect, abuse, or health concerns. Some of the projects' objectives are to: formulate and deliver targeted teacher training programs; support pilot schools and kindergartens in promoting children's wellbeing; develop and distribute resources for kindergartens and schools to address the educational requirements of at-risk children with a focus on wellbeing; offer policy recommendations to incorporate child wellbeing as a critical factor in educational programming. RodaWell champions the idea that child wellbeing can be fostered through the promotion of autonomy, meaningful relationships, and explorative learning within an inclusive environment. The project mission is concentrated on four key areas, leveraging insights from educational psychology and the successful practices of the Danish project partners (https://rodawell.fpse.unibuc.ro/).

ENRETE—Enhancing Resilience Through Teacher Education is an European Erasmus+ partnership with the primary goal to foster the establishment of educational settings that enhance the resilience and development of disadvantaged students. The project involved six partner universities from Europe, coordinated by the University of Malta, with USV, University of Rijeka (Croatia), University of Lisbon (Portugal), University of Pavia (Italy), and University of Crete (Greece) participating. The project aimed at enhancing the quality and relevance of university studies by focusing on the development of an innovative curriculum relevant to the European socio-economic context. Overall, the project sought to create learning environments through teacher training that promotes the resilience and harmonious development of marginalized children, providing them with tools, resources, and learning contexts that facilitate academic and socio-emotional learning and, therefore, foster social inclusion and the practice of active citizenship. The generous idea of the project was to develop a master's degree training program in the field of promoting resilience in school through teacher training. Key objectives include: crafting a series of modules for a master's program focused on resilience in schools, especially aimed at training educators to support the resilience of vulnerable children in early childhood and primary education; running a pilot to train educators from each participating country on module implementation; incorporating a cycle of quality assurance tests and feedback from both internal and external evaluators to refine the course content and structure; engaging with stakeholders at the national and European levels to leverage project findings, thereby influencing the European educational policy landscape; introducing a European Masters in Resilience Education, grounded in the ENRETE-developed modules, at the project's conclusion.

The *EMJM FLOURISH, an Erasmus Mundus Joint Master focusing on Resilience in Educational Contexts*, is a comprehensive two-year, full-time program designed to fulfill the educational requirements of children living in challenging and underserved environments. By concentrating on their inherent strengths and fostering their abilities within supportive settings, this program aims to offer a substantial, pertinent, and well-rounded education. Its goal is to enhance the skills of educators and professionals in developing environments that boost resilience, thereby providing children and adolescents with the essential tools and skills to successfully navigate the obstacles they encounter in their education and overall development (https://flourishproject.mt/).

In 2015, the Suceava County School Inspectorate initiated the social accountability project *R.E.S.P.E.C.T* starting from the educational needs of the child. It contributes to harmonizing the educational climate, the heart and soul of the school, fostering respect for diversity, collaboration and communication, and the wellbeing necessary for academic success. The aim of the project is to prevent aggression and violence in schools by creating a harmonious, inclusive educational environment conducive to practicing civilized behaviors and attitudes. This ensures that every student feels encouraged, motivated, and safe, able to manage their emotions responsibly through a tolerant, non-discriminatory attitude, actively communicating in an assertive and non-violent manner. The campaign components are: Responsibility, Education, Safety, Prevention, Education, Communication, Tolerance. Every school year, through formal and nonformal education, students and teachers from Suceava county develop together meaningful activities for violence prevention and wellbeing promotion. The project was awarded within national contest as "Creator of Education" project in 2020 (https://educatiafnonf.wordpress.com/).

10.5 Research Studies on Wellbeing of Students and Teachers

10.5.1 Study on Children's Wellbeing in Romania

10.5.1.1 Research Design

This research belongs to the category of cross-sectional studies, focusing on the identification of relationships between school climate, resilience, and wellbeing in the Romanian school population. Therefore, school climate was operationalized using five dimensions: teacher support, school connectedness, peer connectedness, rules clarity, and reporting and seeking help mechanisms. In addition, the study also seeks to identify the possible influences that demographic variables have on school climate and the two determinants of success: resilience and wellbeing.

10.5.1.2 Research Problem

Is there an interaction between school climate, resilience, and wellbeing in the Romanian school population? Are dimensions of school climate (teacher support, peers connectedness, school connectedness, clarity of rules in the school environment, strategies for reporting and seeking help) predictors of resilience and wellbeing? What is the role of wellbeing in the relationship between school climate and resilience?

10.5.1.3 Research Variables

Demographic variables: gender (female, male) and level of education (primary, lower secondary, high school).
Dependent variable: resilience and wellbeing;
Independent variable: teacher support, school connectedness, peer connectedness, rules clarity, and reporting and seeking help.

10.5.1.4 Research Hypotheses

Hypothesis 1: There are significant differences between children who are in different grades in terms of their perception of school climate.
Hypothesis 2: There are significant differences between children from different level of education in terms of their wellbeing.
Hypothesis 3: There is a relationship between students' resilience, wellbeing and their perception of the school climate at the school they attend.
Hypothesis 4: School climate dimensions are predictors of student resilience.

Hypothesis 5: School climate dimensions are predictors of student wellbeing.
Hypothesis 6: Wellbeing mediates the relationship between school climate and resilience.

10.5.1.5 Research Methodology

Sample: the research was carried out on a sample of 529 pupils in grades I–XII, aged between 8 and 19, with an average age of 13.7 years. Of these, 72 (13.6%) are primary school pupils, 266 (50.3%) are secondary school pupils and 191 (36.1%) are secondary school pupils. Analyzing the background, the research participants come from both urban ($N = 308$) and rural ($N = 221$) areas. In terms of gender, 42% of the subjects are male and 58% are female. 35.9% of the students who participated in the study ($N = 190$) have parents working abroad (both or at least one of them).

10.5.1.6 Data Collection Procedure

The data were collected by distributing an online questionnaire to pre-university teachers who are master students at Stefan cel Mare University in Suceava, who in turn facilitated access to a sample of students who agreed to participate in the study, who responded to the questionnaire distributed through the Google Forms platform. Prior to this, parental consent was sought by distributing a participation agreement that they signed.

10.5.1.7 Instruments

The variable *resilience* was measured using the *Child and Youth Resilience Measure (CYRM-R),* a version designed for children and youth aged 10 to 22 years, which consists of 17 items with 5 response options to the question *To what extent do the sentences below describe you?* corresponding to a Likert scale, where 1 means Not at All and 5 means A Lot. Resilience can be calculated by summing up all responses, as the instrument does not contain reversed items, which is the total score used in this research. The instrument also contains two subscales, one assessing personal resilience and one corresponding to children's resilience in relation to caregivers (Jefferies et al., 2019). The scale shows good internal consistency, as Cronbach's α value is 0.941.

To analyze the dimensions that make up the variable *school climate,* the tool "What's Happening In This School?" was used (WHITS), which consists of 6 scales corresponding to various aspects of school climate as perceived by students. The scales are: teacher support, school connectedness, peer connectedness, rules clarity, affirming diversity, and reporting and seeking help. The instrument contains 48 items formulated similar to statements to which the child has to respond on a Likert scale choosing a score between 1 and 5, where 1 represents almost never, 2 rarely, 3 sometimes, 4 often, 5 almost always. The score of a scale is found by calculating the average of the scores on the items that make up the scale, each scale consisting of 8 items (Aldridge & Ala'I, 2013). Out of the six dimensions, we have used the following in the present research: teacher support, school connectedness, peer connectedness, rules clarity, and reporting and seeking help The scale measuring students' perceived school climate shows good internal consistency (the values of Cronbach's alpha are such as: teacher support—0.907, peer connectedness—0.899, school connectedness—0.940, rule clarity—0.906, reporting and seeking help—0.885).

The variable *wellbeing* was measured using the Stirling Children's Wellbeing Scale. The Stirling Children's Wellbeing Scale (SCWBS) was initiated by the Stirling Educational Psychology Service with the aim of creating a holistic, positively worded scale to measure emotional and psychological wellbeing in children (Liddle & Carter, 2015). The SCWBS consists of 12 items measuring emotional and psychological wellbeing. All items on the scale are rated on a 5-point Likert-based scale. Children are asked to rate some statements or descriptions about how they might have felt or thought about things in the last few weeks. The Likert scale is used where 1 means *never* and 5 means *all the time.* Cronbach's α value is 0.949.

10.5.1.8 Data Analysis Strategy

We used Jamovi program and SPSS28 to perform the analyses. To test the correlational hypotheses, we applied Pearson Correlation Analysis. Hypotheses testing differences in means were tested using the independent samples t-test and the one-way ANOVA test. We also used multiple regression analysis to identify the extent to which aspects of school climate may predict students' levels of resilience and wellbeing.

10.5.1.9 Results

Descriptive statistics.

Descriptive analysis of scores on: resilience, wellbeing, teacher support, peers connectedness, school connectedness, reporting and seeking for help, and rules clarity is presented in Table 10.4.

Means differences

Hypothesis 1: There are significant differences between children who are in different grades in terms of their perception of school climate.

To test this hypothesis, we applied the one-way ANOVA in Jamovi for each dimension that makes up this variable: teacher support, peer connection, school connection, clarity of rules in the school environment, and reporting and seeking for help within the school.

Table 10.4 Descriptive analysis of scores for study variables

Descriptives							
	Resilience	Wellbeing	Teacher support	Peers Connectedness	School connectedness	Rules clarity	Reporting and seeking help
N	529	529	529	529	529	529	529
Mean	68.59	46.44	3.56	4.10	3.93	4.14	3.84
Standard deviation	12.87	9.83	0.94	0.80	0.95	0.83	0.90

The analysis showed that there were significant differences between the categories analyzed in terms of **perception of teacher support**: F(526) = 22.4, $p < 0.001$ (see Table 10.5). In order to compare the means of the categories of the variable teacher support, according to educational level, we applied the Tukey test. According to it, primary school students (M = 4.10, SD = 0.784, N = 72) have significantly higher means in terms of perception of support received from teachers than secondary school students (M = 3.65, SD = 0.939, N = 266): $t(526) = 3.73$, $p < 0.01$ and those in high school (M = 3.29, SD = 0.916, N = 191): $t(526) = 6.45$, $p < 0.01$. There were also significant differences in perceptions of teacher support between middle school (M = 3.65, SD = 0.939, N = 266) and high school (M = 3.29, SD = 0.916, N = 191) students: $t(526) = 4.18$, $p < 0.01$ (Table 10.6).

Table 10.5 One-way ANOVA test applied to school climate dimensions by grade level

One-Way ANOVA				
	F	df1	df2	p
Teacher support	22.4	2	526	< .001
School connectedness	5.41	2	526	0.005
Rules clarity	4.16	2	526	0.016

Table 10.6 Descriptive analysis of school climate dimension scores by grade level

Group descriptives					
	Level of education	*N*	Mean	SD	SE
Teacher Support	1	72	4.10	0.784	0.0924
	2	266	3.65	0.939	0.0576
	3	191	3.29	0.916	0.0663
School connectedness	1	72	4.26	0.840	0.990
	2	266	3.94	0.949	0.0582
	3	191	3.84	0.966	0.0699
Rules clarity	1	72	4.38	0.759	0.0894
	2	266	4.16	0.865	0.0530
	3	191	4.05	0.811	0.0587

No significant differences were found between the categories analyzed on the dimension of **peers connectedness.**

In terms of **school connectedness**, the analysis showed that there were significant differences between students from different educational backgrounds: F(526) = 5.41, $p = 0.005$ (see Table 10.5). In order to compare the means of the categories of the school connectedness variable by educational step, we applied the Games-Howell post hoc test. According to this test, primary school students (M = 4.26, SD = 0.840, N = 72) have significantly higher means for the school connection variable than secondary school students (M = 3.94, SD = 0.949, N = 266): t(526) = 2.85, p = 0.014 and those in secondary school (M = 3.84, SD = 0.966, N = 191): t(526) = 3.53, $p < 0.002$. There were no significant differences between the other categories analyzed (Table 10.6).

Analyzing the dimension that measures the **rules clarity in the school environment**, it is clear that there are significant differences between students from different educational backgrounds: F(526) = 4.16, $p = 0.016$ (see Table 10.5). In order to compare the means of the categories of the variable rules clarity, according to educational step, we applied the Tukey's post hoc test. According to it, primary school students (M = 4.38, SD = 0.759, N = 72) have significantly higher means for the rules clarity variable than high school students (M = 4.05, SD = 0.811, N = 191): t(526) = 2.86, $p = 0.012$. There were no significant differences between the other categories analyzed (Table 10.5).

As regards the dimension of perception of **reporting and seeking help in the school environment,** no statistically significant differences were found between the categories analyzed.

The hypothesis is partially confirmed, identifying differences in students' perceptions of school climate by grade level for three of the five dimensions analyzed: teacher support, school connectedness, and rules clarity within the school environment.

Hypothesis 2: There are significant differences between children from different level of education in terms of their wellbeing.

To test the above hypothesis, we applied the one-way ANOVA test in SPSS. The analysis showed that there were significant differences in wellbeing between the categories analyzed: F(526) = 4.025, $p = 0.018$. In order to compare the means of the categories of the wellbeing variable, according to school level, we applied the Bonferroni post hoc test (see Table 10.7). According to this test, students from high school have significantly lower means for wellbeing than students from primary school. No significant differences in wellbeing were found between other educational level (lower secondary and primary or high school) *The hypothesis is partially confirmed.*

Hypothesis 3: There is a relationship between students' resilience, wellbeing, and their perception of the school climate created at the school they attend.

Table 10.7 Post hoc Bonferroni test for differences in the wellbeing variable between the categories of educational levels analyzed (1—primary school, 2—lower secondary school, 3—high school). (*. The mean difference is significant at the 0.05 level.)

					95% Confidence Interval	
(I) school level	(J) school level	Mean Difference (I-J)	Std. Error	*p* value	Lower Bound	Upper Bound
1.00	2.00	2.97734	1.29868	.067	−.1416	6.0963
	3.00	3.82206*	1.35190	.015	.5753	7.0689
2.00	1.00	−2.97734	1.29868	.067	−6.0963	.1416
	3.00	.84472	.92715	1.000	−1.3820	3.0714
3.00	1.00	−3.82206*	1.35190	.015	−7.0689	−.5753
	2.00	−.84472	.92715	1.000	−3.0714	1.3820

We could figure out a good correlation between the variables, with rather high correlations between resilience and school climate and wellbeing and school climate.

In Table 10.8, we could see the good correlations between the variables.

Hypothesis 4: School climate dimensions are predictors of student resilience.

To test the extent to which students' perceptions of school climate predict their level of resilience, we conducted a multiple linear regression analysis in Jamovi in which we included as predictors the five aspects of school climate considered in this research: teacher support, school connectedness, peer connectedness, rules clarity, and reporting and seeking for help within the educational institution. The analysis indicated that 31% ($R^2 = 0.311$) of the variance in resilience is explained by the prediction model involving the five dimensions of school climate [$F(5, 523) = 47.3$,

Table 10.8 Results of Pearson correlation analysis of the relationships between school climate and its dimensions, resilience, and wellbeing

	1	2	3	4	5	6	7	8
1. Resilience	–							
2. Wellbeing	0.561*	–						
3. Teacher support	0.457	0.452*	–					
4. Peer_ Connectedness	0.483*	0.537*	0.499*	–				
5. School_ connectedness	0.525*	0.534*	0.678*	0.762*	–			
6. Rule_clarity	0.460*	0.460*	0.602*	0.513*	0.671*	–		
7. Reporting and seeking help	0.411*	0.438*	0.543*	0.448*	0.573*	0.655*	–	
8. School climate	0.568*	0.588*	0.817*	0.775*	0.898*	0.833*	0.785	–

Note $^*p < .001$

$p < .001$] (Table 10.9). Of the five predictors analyzed, *teacher support* ($t = 2.63$; $p = .009$) and *peer connection* ($t = 3.93$; $p < .001$) significantly predicted student resilience (Table 10.10). Thus, of the school climate dimensions, peers connectedness and teacher support are significant predictors of student resilience. The hypothesis is confirmed.

Hypothesis 5: School climate dimensions are predictors of student wellbeing.

To test the extent to which students' perceptions of school climate predict their level of wellbeing, we conducted a multiple linear regression analysis in Jamovi in which we included as predictors the five aspects of school climate considered in this research: teacher support, school connectedness, peer connectedness, rules clarity, and reporting and seeking for help within the educational institution. The analysis indicated that 36% ($R^2 = 0.362$) of the variance in wellbeing is explained by the prediction model involving the five dimensions of school climate [$F(5, 523) = 59,4$, $p < .001$] (Table 10.11). Of the five predictors analyzed, *teacher support* ($t = 2.31$; $p = .002$), *peers connectedness* ($t = 5.76$; $p < .001$) and *reporting and seeking for help* ($t = 2.66$, $p = 0.008$) significantly predicted student wellbeing (Table 10.12). The hypothesis is confirmed.

Hypothesis 6. Wellbeing mediates the relationship between school climate and resilience.

We tested the mediation role of wellbeing considering predictor the school climate and the dependent variable the resilience. As we could figure out from the diagram below there is a partial mediation role of wellbeing.

Table 10.9 Regression analysis result on the predictive power of resilience based on the dimensions that make up school climate

Model Fit Measures							
				Overall model test			
Model	R	R2	Adjusted R2	F	df1	df2	*p*
1	0.558	0.311	0.305	47.3	5	523	<.001

Table 10.10 Contribution of predictors on resilience

Model coefficients—CYRM TOTAL				
Predictor	Estimate	SE	*t*	*p*
Intercept	29.61	2.849	10.39	<.001
Teacher Support	1.88	0.714	2.63	0.009
Peer connectedness	3.48	0.886	3.93	<.001
School connectedness	1.78	0.950	1.88	0.061
Rule clarity	1.68	0.860	1.95	0.052
Reporting and seeking help	1.10	0.711	1.54	0.123

Table 10.11 Regression analysis result on the predictive power of wellbeing based on the dimensions of school climate

Model Fit Measures							
				Overall Model Test			
Model	R	R2	Adjusted R2	F	df1	df2	*p*
1	0.602	0.362	0.356	59.4	5	523	<.001

Table 10.12 Contribution of predictors on wellbeing

Model coefficients—wellbeing				
Predictor	Estimate	SE	*t*	*p*
Intercept	13.448	2.094	6.42	<.001
Peer_Connectedness	3.787	0.658	5.76	<.001
School_Connectedness	0.891	0.697	1.28	0.202
Rule_clarity	1.043	0.631	1.65	0.099
Reporting and seeking for Help	1.390	0.522	2.66	0.008
Teacher support	1.200	0.519	2.31	0.021

This path signifies the indirect effect of school climate on resilience through wellbeing, indicating a significant positive effect ($\beta = 0.204$, $z = 7.47$, $p < .001$). This suggests that school climate significantly impacts resilience indirectly by influencing wellbeing, while wellbeing itself impacts resilience, as well as the perceived school climate (there is also a direct effect of school climate on resilience) (see Table 10.13 and Fig. 10.3).

Table 10.13 Indirect and total effects of school climate to resilience, mediated by wellbeing

95% C.I. (a)								
Type	Effect	Estimate	SE	Lower	Upper	β	*z*	*p*
Indirect	SchClim ⇒ Wellb ⇒ Resil	3.585	0.4798	2.645	4.525	0.204	7.47	< .001
Component	SchClim ⇒ Wellb	7.880	0.4719	6.955	8.805	0.588	16.70	< .001
	Wellb ⇒ Resil	0.455	0.0544	0.348	0.562	0.347	8.36	< .001
Direct	SchClim ⇒ Resil	6.392	0.7302	4.961	7.823	0.364	8.75	< .001
Total	SchClim ⇒ Resil	9.977	0.6293	8.744	11.210	0.568	15.85	< .001

Note Confidence intervals computed with method: Standard (Delta method)
Note Betas are completely standardized effect sizes

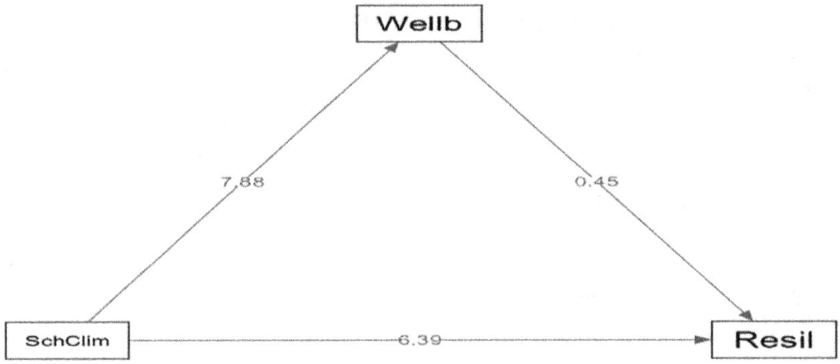

Fig. 10.3 Statistical diagram for mediation model: Mediation role of wellbeing between school climate and resilience

10.5.1.10 Discussion. Interpretation of Results

The overall objective of this research was to study the extent to which school climate influences two of the variables that are closely related to school success: resilience and wellbeing.

The first hypothesis tested the differences that occur in students from different grade levels in their perceptions of the aspects of school climate examined: teacher support, peer connectedness, school connectedness, rule clarity, reporting and seeking for help. The analysis showed that primary school students score higher on the dimensions of perceived teacher support, school connectedness, than their peers in higher grades (middle and high school). The information obtained is closely related to the results identified in the literature that capture the fact that in primary education, the relationship between students and teacher is closer because the teacher teaches most subjects and he/she spends most of the time with the students at school (Suldo et al., 2012). The same study showed that experiencing a high level of support from the teacher results in a significant increase in school engagement. Thus, the link between the two dimensions on which significant differences were found can be observed: teacher support and school connectedness. Also in terms of perceived teacher support, secondary school pupils also reported a higher level than high school pupils. The result obtained may be influenced by the fact that with advancement to higher educational levels, usually the size of the school also increases and the number of teachers is larger, the relationship between students and teachers becomes colder (Bru et al., 2010). However, in terms of their perception of reporting and seeking for help in the school environment and peer connectedness, no statistically significant differences were found between the categories analyzed. In the case of reporting and seeking for help in the school environment, the lack of differences between students in different grades can be explained by the influence of the practices that support these actions, as they are applicable to the whole school, not by grades. However, a particular role in encouraging reporting to and seeking help from school authorities is, according to studies, played by pupils' positive perceptions of teachers' actions during conflict (Aceves et al., 2010). Similarly, the difference in the rules clarity can be justified only between primary and secondary school pupils, as the rules are the same for all children, but at the beginning of school they are more frequently brought to attention with the aim of learning them, whereas in higher grades, it is often counted on the fact that they are already known by the pupils (Dockett & Perry, 2002).

The third hypothesis explored the relationship between students' perceptions of school climate and their level of resilience and wellbeing, as well. The analysis looked at each dimension of school climate in relation to resilience and wellbeing. The hypothesis was confirmed, identifying a directly proportional relationship across all five dimensions analyzed with resilience and with wellbeing. First, a positive relationship was confirmed between resilience and students' perceptions of teacher support, with a medium effect size. This is captured in the literature, with a close relationship with a teacher shown to be a very strong protective factor for student resilience (Conner et al., 2014). Second, a directly proportional relationship has been shown between student resilience and their peers' connectedness, with the effect being medium. In other words, the better connection students report with their peers, the higher their level of resilience. One possible explanation may be the positive influence that peer relationships have on their hope that they can successfully cope with academic challenges (Frisby et al., 2020). Also, the impact of this dimension on resilience has been shown to have a stronger effect than their relationship with their teachers (Gowing, 2019). Third, the analysis also included the established relationship between school connectedness and resilience. The results showed that as school connectedness increases, so does students' resilience. This relationship can be based on the positive effects that school connectedness has: reducing rates of violence, moderating the effect that exposure to violence has on students' behaviors, and increasing students' wellbeing (Foster et al., 2017). On the fourth dimension, rules clarity, a positive relationship is also identified between this and resilience, with a medium effect size. This result is also reinforced by the theoretical model of resilience in the educational environment, at the level of which one of the six components of the variable is the clear establishment of rules and boundaries in the school institution (Henderson, 2013). Between the last dimension analyzed, reporting and seeking for help and resilience, there is also evidence of a directly proportional relationship, with a medium magnitude of correlation. This relationship can be explained by the mechanisms of reporting and seeking for help positively influencing students' wellbeing and negatively influencing mental health problems (Aldridge & McChesney, 2018). According to the Positive Education there is a strong relationship between school environment and student's wellbeing.

Hypothesis 4 tested the extent to which students' perceptions of school climate dimensions can predict their level of resilience. Results show that 31% of the variance in resilience is explained by these school climate dimensions. Among them, teacher support and the clarity of rules in the school environment make a significant contribution. This influence may be due to the protective role that a close relationship with both a teacher and a peer has on resilience, and the support they can give children in overcoming adverse situations (Conner et al., 2014). In relation to the other dimensions included in the analysis, their role as predictors can also be justified by the theoretical model of resilience developed by Henderson (2013), who shows that actions such as "conveying to students a sense of caring and support, setting and communicating high expectations, providing opportunities for meaningful involvement in school activities, fostering prosocial bonding, developing a set of clearly established boundaries and rules, and developing life skills" are specific to the school climate dimensions analyzed.

The fifth hypothesis investigated whether students' perceptions of school climate can predict their wellbeing. The hypothesis was confirmed, showing that 36% of the variance in wellbeing is explained by these dimensions of school climate. Of the five aspects examined, teacher support, peer connectedness, and reporting and seeking for help make a significant contribution. Similar results are presented by Lester and Cross (2015) showing that school climate factors of feeling safe at school, feeling connected to school, and peer support are all protective of mental and emotional wellbeing over the transition period between primary and secondary school while connectedness to teachers is protective of emotional wellbeing.

Hypothesis 6 tested the mediator role of wellbeing in the relationship between perceived school climate and students' resilience. This result is consonant with other studies results. Lombardi et al. (2019) showed that improving school climate can improve students' engagement in school activities, but only when it modifies their wellbeing experience, not directly as the effect of school climate on engagement is mediated by wellbeing experience. So there is a mediator role of wellbeing between school climate and school engagement. School climate is directly related to students' wellbeing (Aldridge et al., 2016) as our study indicated.

Strengths and Limitations

The topic of this research refers to the relationships that are established between the dimensions of school climate, resilience, and wellbeing. Considering that the number of studies addressing this topic is low and that it has not been analyzed with reference to the Romanian educational system, educational institutions in Romania and the children who attend them, this short study provides valuable information on the dimensions of school climate where improvements should be made in order to positively influence students' life quality through the relationships established between them, resilience, and wellbeing. Another strength derives from the size of the sample studied, which provides an opportunity to generalize the results obtained on a larger scale. The inclusion of students belonging to all three levels of education, and the testing of differences between them, outlines important information that new educational policies should take into account, representing another strength of the present research.

The use of self-reporting as the sole method of data collection is one of the limitations of the study because errors often occur due to subjects' expectations, social desirability, even if confidentiality and anonymity are guaranteed.

10.5.2 Study on Teachers' Wellbeing in Romania

10.5.2.1 Aim and Objectives of the Research

This study aims to identify the relationship between perceived stress, resilience and teachers' wellbeing, how stress influences teachers' wellbeing and resilience, and the role of teachers' wellbeing in mediating the relationship between stress and resilience.

The research objectives are:

- assessment of the stress level and the level of teachers' wellbeing;
- studying the relationship between stress and teachers' wellbeing;
- identify differences by demographic variables (gender, background, length of teaching experience) in teachers' wellbeing
- identify differences by demographic variables (gender, seniority) in teachers' perceived stress
- identify differences in perceived stress, resilience, and wellbeing of teachers according to whether they attend training (counselling and emotional education)
- testing the mediating role of teachers' wellbeing in the context of the relationship between perceived stress and teacher resilience

10.5.2.2 Research Variables

- Independent variables: gender, age, seniority, training courses (counselling, emotional education);
- Dependent variables: perceived stress, teacher wellbeing, resilience.

10.5.2.3 Research Hypotheses

Hypothesis 1: Stress negatively correlates with teacher‘s wellbeing and resilience.
Hypothesis 2: There are differences in perceived stress, wellbeing, and resilience by gender.
Hypothesis 3: There are differences in perceived stress, wellbeing, and resilience according to seniority.
Hypothesis 4: There are differences in perceived stress, wellbeing, and resilience depending on the completion of counselling training courses.
Hypothesis 5: There are differences in perceived stress, wellbeing, and resilience depending on whether emotional literacy training is taken.
Hypothesis 6: Wellbeing mediates the relationship between perceived stress and teacher resilience.

This research is a quantitative cross-sectional study, investigating the correlations established between stress-wellbeing-resilience, following the application of online questionnaires by the University "Stefan cel Mare" of Suceava. Data analysis was carried out using Jamovi and SPSS 28 software.

10.5.2.4 Research Sample

The statistical population consists of 2948 preschool, primary, secondary, and high school teachers from rural and urban areas, aged between 19 and 69 years, with an average age of 38 years old (SD = 10.4) and an average length of service in the education system of 14 years (SD = 10.69), selected arbitrarily from the North East Region (47.9% are from urban areas, 52.1% are from rural areas, 25% are men and 75% are women).

The proposed research collected data to analyze correlations between variables in order to test the research hypotheses.

Questionnaires were completed in Google forms, online. Please note that the data was collected in 2020, 2021, 2022 by the students of the master program. The questionnaire was accompanied by informed consent and participants signed and agreed to participate in the study.

10.5.2.5 Instruments

The Psychological Wellbeing Scale developed by Carol Ryff measures wellbeing on six dimensions: *autonomy, environmental mastery, personal growth, positive relationships with others, purpose in life, self-acceptance. It has 42 items.* (Alpha Cronbach—0.872).

The Perceived Stress Scale (Cohen et al., 1983) contains 10 items (Alpha Cronbach—0.920).

The Connor Davidson scale for measuring resilience contains 10 items (Alpha Cronbach—0.900).

10.5.2.6 Data Analysis Strategy

Data processing of the questionnaires was carried out using the statistical analysis software Jamovi and SPSS, after they were entered.

10.5.2.7 Results

Descriptive statistics for study variables.

Descriptive analysis of the scores recorded for each of the study variables (stress, wellbeing, resilience) is presented in Table 10.14.

Hypothesis 1: a. Stress correlates negatively with teacher wellbeing.

Table 10.14 Descriptive statistics for study variables

	N	Missing	Mean	Median	SD
Perceived-stress	2947	3	26.5	27.0	6.02
Resilience	2947	3	40.5	41.0	5.93
WellBeing	2948	2	193.5	198.0	25.57

Analyzing the Pearson correlation between teachers' stress and their wellbeing, a negative correlation can be found between the two variables ($r = -0.451$, $N = 2947$, $p < 0.001$), which means that teachers who have a high level of stress have a low level of wellbeing. Stress correlates negatively with teacher resilience (see Table 10.15). Analyzing the Pearson correlation between teachers' stress and their resilience, a negative correlation can be found between the two variables ($r = -0.419$, $N = 2947$, $p < 0.001$), which means that teachers who have a high level of stress have a low level of resilience.

Hypothesis 2: There are differences in perceived stress, wellbeing, and resilience by gender.

To examine whether there are gender differences in teachers' perceived stress levels, wellbeing, and resilience, the independent samples *t*-test was used (see Table 10.16).

The results indicate that there is a significant difference between the level of stress perceived by women ($N = 2210$, $M = 27.0$, SD = 5.91) and the level of stress perceived by men ($N = 737$, $M = 24.8$, SD = 6.04): [$t(2945) = -8.959$, $p < .001$] (Fig. 10.4). Regarding wellbeing there is a significant difference (Fig. 10.5) between women and men, in the sense that women experience a higher level of wellbeing than

Table 10.15 Correlation matrix for study variables (***$p < 0.001$)

	Stress	Resil	WellB
Stress	–		
Resilience	−0.419***	–	
WellBeing	−0.451***	0.530***	–

Table 10.16 *T*-test for independent samples (in terms of gender)

		Statistics	df	p	Mean difference	SE difference		Effect Size
Wellbeing	Student's t	−2.992[a]	2946	0.003	−3.248	1.086	Cohen's d	−0.1272
Stress	Student's t	−8.959	2945	<.001	−2.264	0.253	Cohen's d	−0.3811
Resilience	Student's t	0.900	2945	0.368	0.227	0.252	Cohen's d	0.0383

men. When it comes about resilience, there is no statistically significant difference between women and men.

Hypothesis 3: There are differences in perceived stress, wellbeing, and resilience according to seniority.

Using *t*-test to compare means for independent samples (see Table 10.17), we got findings showing that the teachers with higher experience have lower levels of stress and higher wellbeing and resilience in comparison with teachers having less teaching experience.

Hypothesis 4: There are differences in perceived stress, wellbeing, and resilience depending on the completion of counselling training courses.

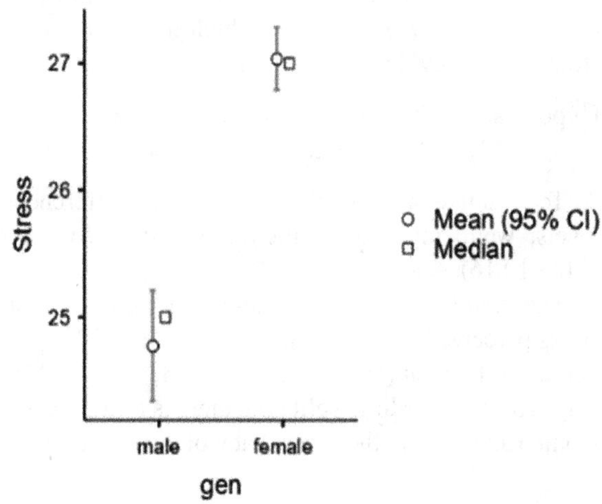

Fig. 10.4 Perceived stress differences in terms of gender

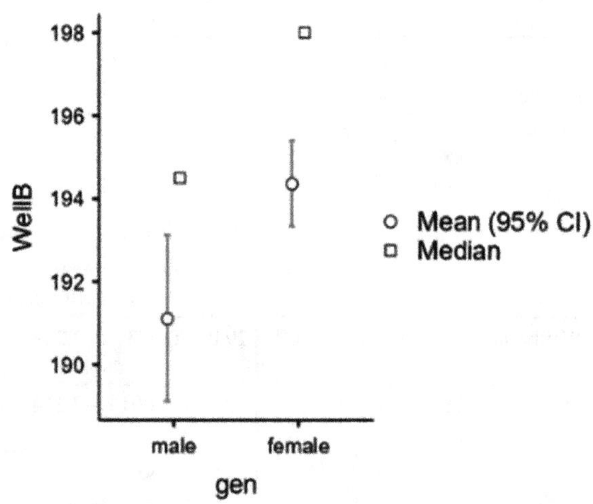

Fig. 10.5 Wellbeing differences in terms of gender

Table 10.17 *T*-test for independent samples (in terms seniority)

	Seniority	*N*	Mean	Std. Deviation	*T*-test
Perceived stress	> = 14 yrs	1318	25.3012	5.76728	$t(2745) = -9.504$
	<14 yrs	1429	27.4563	6.08958	
Resilience	> = 14 yrs	1318	41.0577	5.65830	$t(2745) = 4.814$
	<14 yrs	1429	39.9734	6.10901	
Wellbeing	> = 14 yrs	1318	198.3414	23.20328	$t(2745) = 9.609$
	<14 yrs	1429	189.0826	26.96562	

Using the *t*-test for independent samples (see Table 10.18), we find that there are significant differences between teachers who have taken counselling courses and those who have not, in that the former show higher levels of wellbeing and resilience and lower levels of stress than the latter. For comparing means of wellbeing, we used the Welch's *t*-test which does not assume equal variances, making it suitable for situations where Levene's test is significant.

We could easily see that teachers who attended a course related to school counseling have higher level of wellbeing and resilience and lower levels of stress in comparison with those who did not pursue any course in counseling. The results indicate a significant difference of stress (Fig. 10.6) $t(2945) = -4.55$, $p < 0.001$ between teachers who have followed counselling courses ($N = 2039$, $M = 26.01$, $SD = 5.96$) and those who have not followed such courses ($N = 908$, $M = 27.2$, $SD = 6.08$). In terms of resilience (Fig. 10.7), there were significant differences ($t(2945) = 4.83$. $p < 0.001$) between teachers who took counselling courses ($N = 2039$, $M = 40.9$, $SD = 5.83$) compared to those who did not take such courses ($N = 908$, $M = 39.7$, $SD = 6.10$). Analyzing the differences in wellbeing (Fig. 10.8) we find that there is a significant difference ($t(2945) = 5.28$, $p < 0.001$) between those who took counselling courses ($N = 2039$, $M = 195.2$, $SD = 25.01$) compared to those who did not ($N = 908$, $M = 189.8$, $SD = 26.44$).

Hypothesis 5: There are differences in perceived stress, wellbeing, and resilience depending on the completion of emotional education training courses.

Table 10.18 *T*-test for independent samples (in terms of attendance a counselling course

		Statistics	df	*p*	Mean difference	SE difference		Effect size
Stress	Student's t	−4.55	2945	<.001	−1.09	0.239	Cohen's d	−0.182
Resilience	Student's t	4.83	2945	<.001	1.14	0.236	Cohen's d	0.193
WellBeing	Welch's t	5.17	1656	<.001	5.37	1.04	Cohen's d	0.208

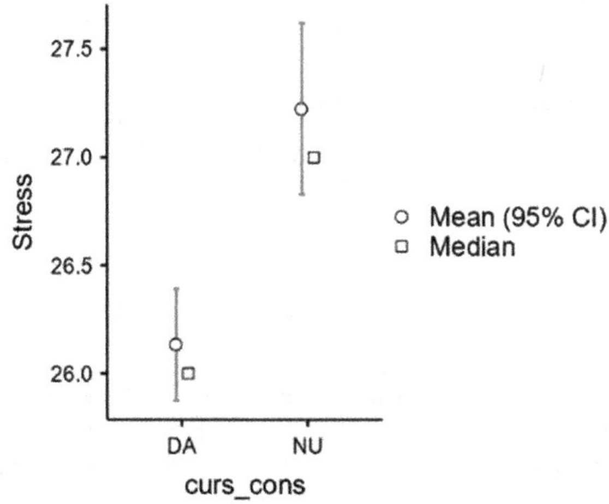

Fig. 10.6 Stress differences in terms of participating in counseling courses (DA-yes, NU-no)

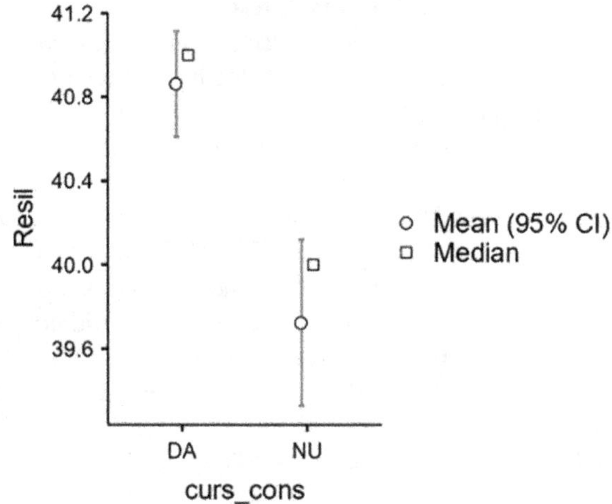

Fig. 10.7 Resilience differences in terms of participating in counseling courses

Using the *t*-test for independent samples, we find that there are significant differences between teachers who have taken counselling courses and those who have not, in that the former show higher levels of wellbeing and resilience and lower levels of stress compared to the latter (Table 10.19).

We could easily see that teachers who attended a course related to emotional education have higher level of resilience and lower levels of stress in comparison with those who did not pursued any course in counseling. The results indicate no significance related to wellbeing (Fig. 10.11) between the group of teachers who attended an emotional education course and the group who did not attend such a course. The results indicate a significant difference of stress (Fig. 10.9) $t(2945) = -3.06$, $p < 0.001$ between the teachers who attended emotional education courses (N = 1578, M = 26.2, SD = 6.04) and those who did not attend such courses ($N =$

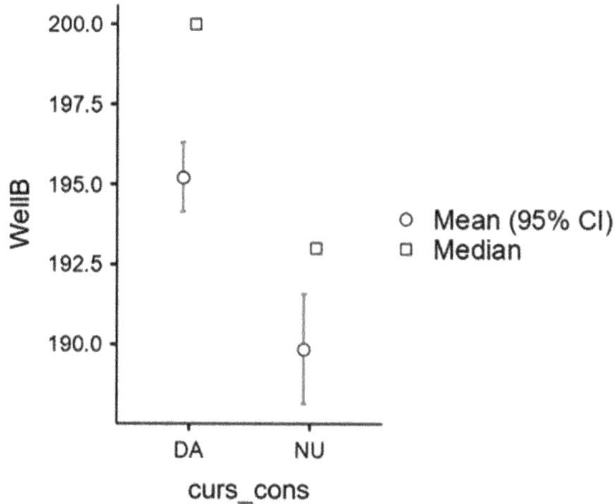

Fig. 10.8 Wellbeing (WellB) differences in terms of participating in counseling courses (DA-yes, NU-no)

Table 10.19 *T*-test for independent samples (in terms of attendance an emotional education course)

		Statistics	df	*p*	Mean difference	SE difference		Effect size
Stress	Student's t	−3.06	2945	0.002	−0.679	0.222	Cohen's d	−0.1129
Resilience	Student's t	4.33	2945	< .001	0.947	0.219	Cohen's d	0.1600
WellBeing	Student's t	1.32	2945	0.186	1.251	0.944	Cohen's d	0.0489

1369, $M = 26.8$, SD = 5.99). In terms of resilience (Fig. 10.10), there were significant differences ($t(2945) = 4.33$. $p < 0.001$) between teachers who took emotional education courses ($N = 1578$, $M = 41$, SD = 5.82) compared to those who did not take such courses ($N = 1369$, $M = 40$, SD = 6.02).

Hypothesis 6: Wellbeing mediates the relationship between perceived stress and teacher resilience.

We did a statistical analysis in JAMOVI testing the hypothesis that wellbeing mediates the relationship between perceived stress and teachers' resilience.

The findings indicate a significant negative indirect effect of stress on resilience mediated by wellbeing, significant negative direct effects of stress on resilience, and a significant positive effect of wellbeing on resilience. The statistical significance of these effects is marked by *p*-values less than.001, indicating strong evidence against the null hypothesis in all cases (see Table 10.20). This demonstrates the importance of wellbeing in buffering the negative impacts of stress on resilience among teachers (Fig. 10.12).

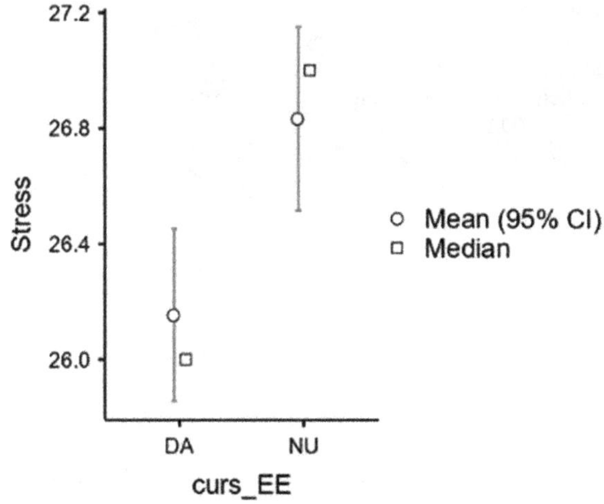

Fig. 10.9 Stress differences in terms of attendance at emotional education courses (curs_EE) (DA-yes, NU-no)

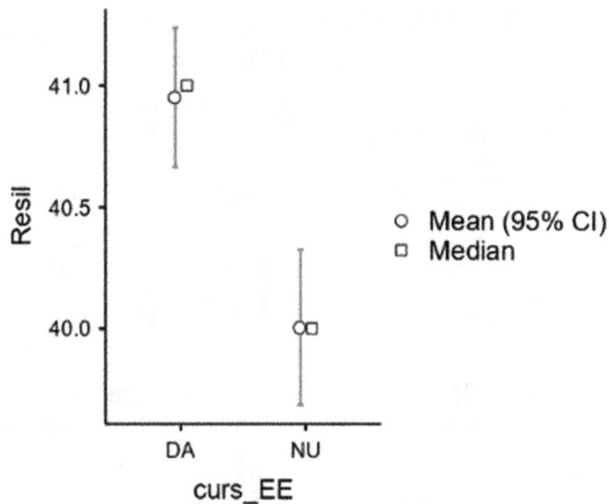

Fig. 10.10 Resilience differences in terms of attendance at emotional education courses (curs_EE) (DA-yes, NU-no)

This underlines the critical role of promoting wellbeing within educational settings to enhance teachers' resilience against stress. The findings are based on robust statistical evidence, providing a strong foundation for interventions aimed at improving teacher wellbeing and resilience.

10.5.2.8 Discussions

The present research aimed to investigate teachers' perceived stress and wellbeing, the relationships between stress and wellbeing, stress and resilience and how teachers' wellbeing mediates the relationship between perceived stress and resilience.

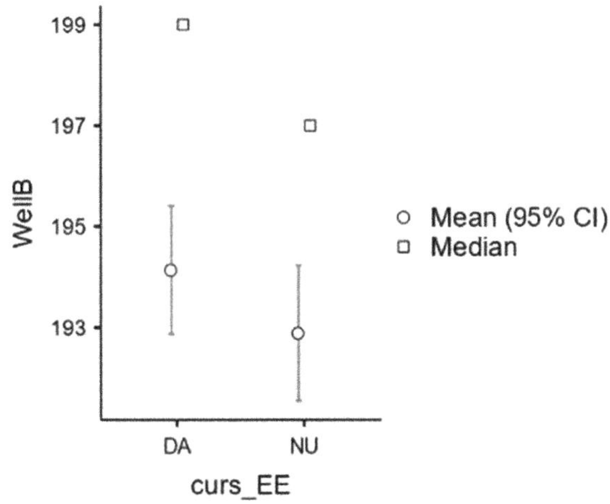

Fig. 10.11 Wellbeing differences in terms of attendance at emotional education courses (DA-yes, NU-no)

Table 10.20 Indirect and total effects for the mediation model: wellbeing as mediator between perceived stress and resilience

	95% C.I. (a)							
Type	Effect	Estimate	SE	Lower	Upper	β	z	p
Indirect	Stress ⇒ WellB ⇒ Resil	−0.1900	0.01025	−0.2101	−0.170	−0.193	−18.5	< .001
Component	Stress ⇒ WellB	−1.9148	0.06984	−2.0517	−1.778	−0.451	−27.4	<.001
	WellB ⇒ Resil	0.0993	0.00394	0.0915	0.107	0.428	25.2	<.001
Direct	Stress ⇒ Resil	−0.2232	0.01676	−0.2560	−0.190	−0.226	−13.3	<.001
Total	Stress ⇒ Resil	−0.4132	0.01649	−0.4455	−0.381	−0.419	−25.1	<.001

Teachers' perceived stress correlates negatively with wellbeing and resilience, a result that is consistent with previous research. Stress directly affects teachers' wellbeing, and school managers should pay attention to teachers' workloads in order to reduce them, create a safe, pleasant working environment, and regulate stressors at school (Liao et al., 2023; Woods et al., 2023). Female teachers predominate in the education system and experience higher levels of stress than male teachers (Liao et al., 2023). High levels of stress no longer had a large impact on wellbeing in teachers with high levels of coping (Woods et al., 2023).

The positive correlations between the research variables wellbeing and resilience lead to the idea that teachers have a positive attitude toward themselves and others, are able to have harmonious relationships with others, are resilient, are able to cope

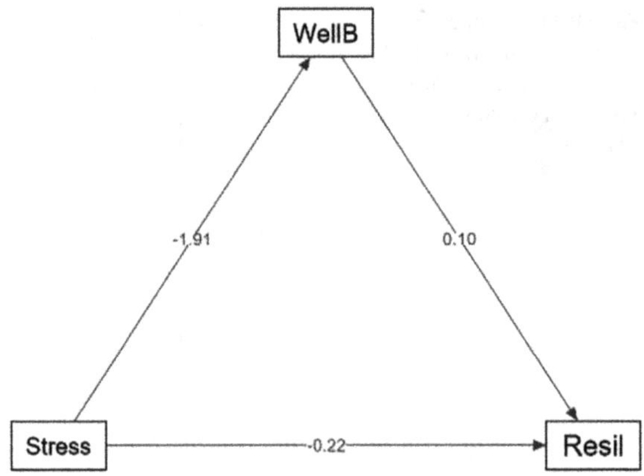

Fig. 10.12 Statistical diagram for mediation model

with external pressures, make effective use of their inner capacities and opportunities, have a purpose in life, continuously improve their skills, realize their own potential, so that they do not let external factors influence their work with students and teaching. These results are in line with the results of Pretsch et al. (2012), who found significant positive correlations between teacher resilience and wellbeing as well as job satisfaction, emphasizing that resilience might be particularly important for the wellbeing of teachers.

Research in the literature indicates that teachers experience high levels of stress but high levels of wellbeing, and that the teaching profession also brings satisfaction.

In a study conducted in Romania in 2017, the relationship between burnout-efficacy-wellbeing was analyzed and they concluded, as in our study, that personal achievement correlated positively with wellbeing dimensions, while emotional exhaustion and depersonalization correlated negatively with wellbeing dimensions (Bentea, 2017).

Given that the study participants recorded high stress, high wellbeing values, we might consider that teachers' wellbeing reduces perceived stress (Brasfield et al., 2019).

The *t*-test showed that there were gender differences in perceived stress levels, and wellbeing in teachers as shown in a study in Greece where women have higher levels of stress because they have more tasks in society (Galanakis & Alamani, 2020). Teacher counselling is needed to prevent stress, to avoid burnout, and to reach a higher level of wellbeing. There is also a need for both initial training in emotional competences and ongoing training through free training courses, both personal development for teachers and continuing professional development.

Related to the work experiences, there are few studies to underline this impact on teachers' wellbeing, stress, or resilience. Our results could imply the necessity of future research explicitly examining these relationships across different seniority levels for providing valuable insights for developing targeted support programs for teachers at various stages of their careers. According to our results, it is important to focus on the young teachers within their early career, to support their wellbeing and to diminish stress.

In terms of teachers' participation in specialized courses in counselling and emotional education, our study has shown that taking these courses can make a difference to wellbeing, stress, and resilience, in that it supports higher levels of resilience and wellbeing and lower levels of perceived stress. Similar results reported by Isidori et al. (2023) explore the synergy between counseling and resilience pedagogy, emphasizing the critical role of fostering resilience and professional counseling in addressing educators' challenges. This holistic approach promotes wellbeing through emotional support, coping strategies, and adaptability, underscoring the importance of such programs in creating a supportive educational environment (Isidori et al, 2023). Isidori et al, 2023, propose a practical framework for schools and policymakers to develop and implement targeted interventions to promote teacher wellbeing.

Recent studies have underscored the complex interplay among stress, wellbeing, and resilience in the teaching profession, highlighting wellbeing's crucial role in moderating these interactions. Research conducted by El-Sayed (2022) and Cho et al. (2021) supports the notion that wellbeing serves as a protective factor, mitigating the effects of stress on resilience and facilitating more effective coping strategies and mental strength among educators. This evidence points to the significant impact of enhancing teacher wellbeing, which not only improves individual health but also boosts job performance and resilience. The consensus among these studies is clear: wellbeing is indispensable in teacher support initiatives. Educational systems are encouraged to focus on wellbeing to bolster their employees' resilience, leading to a more nurturing and productive educational setting. Accordingly, a comprehensive strategy for teacher wellbeing is advocated, emphasizing psychological resilience, stress reduction, and the promotion of a positive work identity.

10.5.2.9 Conclusions

Our research highlights the strong positive correlations between teachers' wellbeing and resilience, and the negative correlations between perceived stress and wellbeing, and perceived stress and resilience. We found that teachers' stress and wellbeing differed in terms of gender and that women had higher levels of both wellbeing and stress. There are also differences in terms of work experience (seniority) and we found that less experienced teachers have higher levels of perceived stress and lower levels of wellbeing and resilience than their more experienced colleagues. We are looking at the differences that participation in counselling and emotional education training makes. We found that teachers who attended such programs experienced lower levels of perceived stress and higher levels of resilience. Those who attended counselling courses had higher levels of wellbeing compared to colleagues who did not attend any training. Our study also underscores the benefits of counselling and emotional education training in reducing stress and enhancing resilience and wellbeing. The findings advocate for incorporating such training into educational policies to foster long-term wellbeing and resilience in schools. Another important finding for our study is the mediating role of wellbeing in the relationship between perceived stress and resilience in teachers. This means that wellbeing acts as a strong buffer against perceived stress and reduces its impact on teachers' resilience.

All these findings have implications for educational policy, at school level and at regional or national level. It would be important to introduce more training courses in counselling or emotional education in order to create the conditions for cultivating wellbeing in the long term. At the same time, improving wellbeing could contribute to increasing resilience within Romanian schools. School managers and policy-makers should consider introducing courses on promoting wellbeing and increasing resilience as part of in-service training for teachers.

10.6 Conclusions. Theoretical and Practical Implications

We outline a comprehensive relationship between different theoretical models of wellbeing and the educational interventions, policies, and programs implemented in the Romanian education system to support students and teachers. It is in line with the school wellbeing model (Konu & Rimpelä, 2002), the PERMA and PERMA-H models proposed by Seligman (2011) and further developed by Kern (2022), and the concepts of resilience as described by Grotberg (1995a, 1995b). Our view (Table 10.21) aligns Romanian educational policies with each of these components, showing how policies support the development of wellbeing according to the integrated model of school wellbeing and resilience (proposed by the author), which includes the lines derived from Konu's model of school wellbeing, combined with elements of PERMA-H (Kern, 2022) and the three main pillars of resilience as defined by Edith Grotberg (1995a, 1995b).

It concludes that school wellbeing and resilience could be promoted through a variety of tools based on educational and social policies. These could include programs to enhance coping skills, social support, and mental health resources. All the Romanian initiatives presented in this chapter were aimed at improving the well-being of students and teachers. They could be seen as providing strong opportunities for health and achievement, ensuring financial support, nutrition, learning materials, and after-school programs to help students succeed. In the same vein, policies such as the National Curriculum, Elective Curriculum and "Together we take courage" aim to promote positive relationships between students, teachers, and the school community. These programs promote social and emotional learning, collaboration and community engagement and provide a good framework for promoting wellbeing and resilience. Curricula and European programs such as PROMEHS, SEEVAL, RodaWell, and FLOURISH are mentioned as explicitly promoting self-awareness, emotional awareness, positive emotions, engagement, emotional wellbeing, and a sense of meaning and purpose in students.

Our framework illustrates a multifaceted approach to student and teacher well-being in the Romanian education system, aligned with internationally recognized

Table 10.21 Descriptors of the integrated model of school wellbeing and resilience within Romanian schools

School wellbeing (Konu)	Models of subjective wellbeing—PERMA, PERMA-H (Kern, 2022; Seligman, 2011)	Resilience (Grotberg, 1995a, 1995b)	Romanian educational measures, policies, programs for students and teachers that meet the indicators proposed by theoretical models
Having	Health Achievements	I have	Law 198/2023; ARACIP, 2021; EURO200; Hot meal; School Supplies; After School; CRED; PNRAS; ROSE; CJRAE; PROF
Loving	Positive relationships	I can	National Curriculum; Elective Curriculum; Together we take courage; Early Education Curriculum
Being	Positive emotions Engagement Meaning	I am	National Curriculum; Elective Curriculum; Early Education Curriculum; European programs (PROMEHS, SEEVAL, RodaWell, FLOURISH)
Health	Health		Law 198/2023; ARACIP, 2021; Together we take courage;

models of subjective wellbeing and resilience. Each policy, measure, project, or program is designed to contribute to one or more aspects of wellbeing and resilience, demonstrating a holistic view of education that goes beyond academic achievement to include emotional, social, and physical health.

10.7 Competing Interests

The author has no conflicts of interest to declare that are relevant to the content of this chapter.

10.8 Ethical Approval

This study was performed in line with the principles of the Declaration of Helsinki. Approval was granted by the Ethics Committee of "Stefan cel Mare" University of Suceava (No. 111/30.01.2023).

For the study involving children, informed consent was obtained from their parents. Informed consent was obtained from teachers who participated in the study.

References

Aceves, M. J., Hinshaw, S. P., Mendoza-Denton, R., & Page-Gould, E. (2010). Seek help from teachers or fight back? Student perceptions of teachers' actions during conflicts and responses to peer victimization. *Journal of Youth and Adolescence, 39*(6), 658–669. https://doi.org/10.1007/s10964-009-9441-9

Aldridge, J. M., & Ala'I, K. (2013). Assessing students' views of school climate: Developing and validating the What's Happening In This School? (WHITS) questionnaire. *Improving Schools, 16*(1), 47–66. https://doi.org/10.1177/1365480212473680

Aldridge, J. M., Fraser, B. J., Fozdar, F., Ala'i, K., Earnest, J., & Afari, E. (2016). Students' perceptions of school climate as determinants of wellbeing, resilience, and identity. *Improving Schools, 19*(1), 5–26. https://doi.org/10.1177/1365480215612616

Aldridge, J. M., & McChesney, K. (2018). The relationships between school climate and adolescent mental health and wellbeing: A systematic literature review. *International Journal of Educational Research, 88*, 121–145. https://doi.org/10.1016/j.ijer.2018.01.012

ARACIP. (2021). *Ghiduri pentru aplicarea unitară a standardelor de evaluare. Volumul 2, Evaluarea internă şi externă a stării de bine*. Bucureşti.

Annex to Government Decision No. 994/2020. https://oportunitati-ue.gov.ro/program/programul-national-rechizite-scolare/#obiectivul-general-al-programului

Bentea, C. C. (2017). *Teacher self-efficacy, teacher burnout and psychological wellbeing*. European Proceedings of Social and Behavioural Sciences.

Botnariuc, P. F., Mironov, C., & Ţibu, S. L. (2023). Romanian teachers' needs and training pilot programme to implement SEE in a whole school approach. *Revista Romaneasca Pentru Educatie Multidimensionala, 15*(1), 331–351. https://doi.org/10.18662/rrem/15.1/699

Bota, O. (2013). Job satisfaction of teachers. *Procedia—Social and Behavioral Sciences, 83*, 634–638. https://doi.org/10.1016/J.SBSPRO.2013.06.120

Brasfield, M. W., Lancaster, C., & Xu, Y. J. (2019). Wellness as a mitigating factor for teacher burnout. *Journal of Education, 199*(3), 166–178.

Bru, E., Stornes, T., Munthe, E., & Thuen, E. (2010). Students' perceptions of teacher support across the transition from primary to secondary school. *Scandinavian Journal of Educational Research, 54*(6), 519–533. https://doi.org/10.1080/00313831.2010.522842

Cefai, C., Camilleri, L., Bartolo, P., Grazzani, I., Cavioni, V., Conte, E., Ornaghi, V., Agliati, A., Gandellini, S., Tatalovic Vorkapic, S., Poulou, M., Martinsone, B., Stokenberga, I., Simões, C., Santos, M., & Colomeischi, A. A. (2022). The effectiveness of a school-based universal mental health programme in six European countries. *Frontiers in Psychology, 13*, Article 925614. https://doi.org/10.3389/fpsyg.2022.925614

Cho, I.-K., Lee, J., Kim, K., Lee, J., Lee, S., Yoo, S., Suh, S., & Chung, S. (2021). Schoolteachers' resilience does—But self-efficacy does not—mediate the influence of stress and anxiety due to the COVID-19 pandemic on depression and subjective wellbeing. *Frontiers in Psychiatry, 12*, Article 756195. https://doi.org/10.3389/fpsyt.2021.756195

Cohen, S., Kamarck, T., & Mermelstein, R. (1983). A global measure of perceived stress. *Journal of Health and Social Behavior, 24*(4), 385–396.

Colomeischi, A. A. (2014). Emotional life as influence on work satisfaction. *Procedia—Social and Behavioral Sciences, 159*, 350–354. https://doi.org/10.1016/j.sbspro.2014.12.386

Colomeischi, A. A., Ursu, A., Bogdan, I., Ionescu-Corbu, A., Bondor, R., & Conte, E. (2022). Social and emotional learning and internalizing problems among adolescents: The mediating role of resilience. *Children, 9*(9), 1326. https://doi.org/10.3390/children9091326

Colomeischi, A. A., & Ursu, A. (2023). How does perceived stress relate to life satisfaction in pre-university teachers? The mediating role of wellbeing. *Revista Românească pentru Educație Multidimensională, 15*(3), 44–54. https://doi.org/10.18662/rrem/15.3/752

Conner, J. O., Miles, S. B., & Pope, D. C. (2014). How many teachers does it take to support a student?: Examining the relationship between teacher support and adverse health outcomes in high-performing pressure-cooker high schools. *The High School Journal, 98*(1), 22–42.

Decision No. 631 of 11 May 2022.

Decision no. 566/2022 approving the Methodology for the organization and functioning of nurseries and other early childhood education units, Official Gazette, Part I no. 437 dated May 4, 2022.

Dockett, S., & Perry, B. (2002). Smoothing the way: What makes a successful school transition program? *Education Links, 65*(1), 6–10.

Durlak, J. A., Domitrovich, C. E., Weissberg, R. P., & Gullotta, T. P. (2015). Social and emotional learning: Past, present, and future. In J. A. Durlak, C. E. Domitrovich, R. P. Weissberg, & T. P. Gullotta (Eds.), *Handbook of social and emotional learning: research and practice* (pp. 3–19). Guilford Press.

El-Sayed, N. (2022). The role of psychological resilience in reducing psychological stress among teachers. *Journal of Education and Health Promotion, 11*(1), 290. https://doi.org/10.4103/jehp.jehp_1835_21

Foster, C. E., Horwitz, A., Thomas, A., Opperman, K., Gipson, P., Burnside, A., Stone, D. M., & King, C. A. (2017). Connectedness to family, school, peers, and community in socially vulnerable adolescents. *Children and Youth Services Review, 81*, 321–331. https://doi.org/10.1016/j.childyouth.2017.08.011

Frisby, B. N., Hosek, A. M., & Beck, A. C. (2020). The role of classroom relationships as sources of academic resilience and hope. *Communication Quarterly, 68*(3), 289–305. https://doi.org/10.1080/01463373.2020.1779099

Galanakis, M., & Alamani, E. (2020). How gender and working conditions affect occupational stress and job satisfaction of general education's preschool and elementary teachers in greek public schools. *Psychology, 11*(2), 364–372.

Gowing, A. (2019). Peer-peer relationships: A key factor in enhancing school connectedness and belonging. *Educational and Child Psychology, 36*(2), 64–77. https://doi.org/10.53841/bpsecp.2019

Grotberg, E. H. (1995). *The international resilience project: Promoting resilience in children.* https://eric.ed.gov/?id=ED383424

Grotberg, E. H. (1995). *A guide to promoting resilience in children: Strengthening the human spirit* (Vol. 8). Bernard van leer foundation.

Henderson, N. (2013). Havens of resilience. *Educational Leadership, 71*(1), 22–27.

Henderson, N., & Milstein, M. M. (2003). *Resiliency in schools: Making it happen for students and educators.* Corwin press.

https://www.edu.ro/sites/default/files/_fi%C8%99iere/Legislatie/2023/OME_3783_2023.pdf

https://www.edu.ro/sites/default/files/_fi%C8%99iere/Legislatie/2023/OM_5181_2023.pdf (Euro200)

https://eurydice.eacea.ec.europa.eu/ro/national-education-systems/romania/romania

Ignat, A., & Clipa, O. (2012). Teachers' satisfaction with life, job satisfaction and their emotional intelligence. *Procedia—Social and Behavioral Sciences, 33*, 498–502. https://doi.org/10.1016/J.SBSPRO.2012.01.171

Ionescu, M. (coord.) (2010). Repere fundamentale în învãtarea si dezvoltarea timpurie a copilului de la nastere la 7 ani. Bucuresti. Ed. Vanemonde. ISBN 978-973-1733-16-6.

Isidori, E., Leonova, I., Abele, A., Caione, G., Zakharova, L., & Sandor, I. (2023). Teacher wellbeing: Between counseling and resilience pedagogy. *Educația 21 Journal* (25), Article 37. https://doi.org/10.24193/ED21.2023.25.37

Jefferies, P., McGarrigle, L., & Ungar, M. (2019). The CYRM-R: A Rasch-validated revision of the child and youth resilience measure. *Journal of Evidence-Based Social Work, 16*(1), 70–92.

Kern, M. L. (2022). A useful model for focusing on wellbeing in schools. In *Handbook of positive psychology in schools: Supporting process and practice* (p. 12). Routledge.

Konu, A., & Rimpelä, M. (2002). Wellbeing in schools: A conceptual model. *Health Promotion International, 17*(1), 79–87.

Law no. 126/2002 for the approval of Government Ordinance no. 33/2001 regarding the granting of school supplies for the school year 2001–2002, Official Gazette, Part I no. 198 on March 25, 2002.

Legea învăţământului preuniversitar 198/2023. Monitorul Oficial al României nr. 613/5.07.2023.(Law on Pre-university Education, 198/2023, Official Gazette of Romania, no. 613/5.07.2023).

Lester, L., & Cross, D. (2015). The relationship between school climate and mental and emotional wellbeing over the transition from primary to secondary school. *Psych Wellbeing, 5*, 9. https://doi.org/10.1186/s13612-015-0037-8

Liddle, I., & Carter, G. F. (2015). Emotional and psychological wellbeing in children: The development and validation of the Stirling Children's Wellbeing Scale. *Educational Psychology in Practice, 31*(2), 174–185.

Liao, J., Wang, X.-Q., & Wang, X. (2023). The effect of work stress on the wellbeing of primary and secondary school teachers in china. *International Journal of Environmental Research and Public Health, 20*(2), 1154. https://doi.org/10.3390/ijerph20021154

Lombardi, E., Traficante, D., Bettoni, R., Offredi, I., Giorgetti, M., & Vernice, M. (2019). The impact of school climate on wellbeing experience and school engagement: A study with high-school students. *Frontiers in Psychology, 10*. https://doi.org/10.3389/fpsyg.2019.02482

Methodological letter for the school year 2023–2024, No. 31,815/25.10.2023, GENERAL DIRECTORATE OF PRE-UNIVERSITY EDUCATION.

Methodological guidelines in Counseling and Guidance for successful transition from 8th grade to 9th grade, SUBJECT: COUNSELING AND GUIDANCE, IN 9TH GRADE IN THE SCHOOL YEAR 2021–2022, Bucharest, 2021.

Ministerul Educaţiei. (2023). *Raport privind starea învăţământului preuniversitar din România 2022–2023*. Bucureşti [Report on the state of pre-university education in Romania 2022–2023]. Bucharest.

Ministry of National Education, ORDER no. 4.694 of August 2, 2019, OFFICIAL MONITOR no. 686 of August 20, 2019. CURRICULUM FOR EARLY EDUCATION, (2019) Annex to M.E.N. 4.694/2.08.2019.

Nedelcu, A., Ulrich-Hyngum, C., Ciolan, L., & Ţibu, F. (2018). Educaţie cu stare de bine. După o reţetă româno-daneză. https://rodawell.fpse.unibuc.ro/wp-content/uploads/2019/04/RODAWELL.pdf

Obrad, C. (2020). Constraints and consequences of online teaching. *Sustainability*. https://doi.org/10.3390/su12176982

Obrad, C., & Circa, C. (2021). *Determinants of work engagement among teachers in the context of teleworking*. www.amfiteatrueconomic.ro. https://doi.org/10.24818/ea/2021/58/718

Order of the Minister of Education and Research No. 5287 / 09.10.2006. Annex to the order of the Minister of Education and Research No. 5287/09.10.2006, MINISTRY OF EDUCATION AND RESEARCH NATIONAL COUNCIL FOR CURRICULUM, School Programs for the Curriculum Area Counseling and Guidance, GRADES IX–XII.

Order of the Minister No. 5286/09.10.2006. School Curriculum for the Curriculum Area Counseling and Guidance GRADES I–IV GRADES V–VIII Approved by the Minister's Order No. 5286/09.10.2006.

Ortan, F., Simuţ, C., & Simut, R. (2021). Self-efficacy, job satisfaction and teacher wellbeing in the K-12 educational system. *International Journal of Environmental Research and Public Health, 18*. https://doi.org/10.3390/ijerph182312763

Pretsch, J., Flunger, B., & Schmitt, M. (2012). Resilience predicts wellbeing in teachers but not in non-teaching employees. *Social Psychology of Education, 15*, 321–336. https://doi.org/10.1007/s11218-012-9180-8

Rusu, P., & Colomeischi, A. (2020). Positivity ratio and wellbeing among teachers. The mediating role of work engagement. *Frontiers in Psychology, 11*. https://doi.org/10.3389/fpsyg.2020.01608

Seligman, M. E. P. (2011). *Flourish: A visionary new understanding of happiness and wellbeing*. Free Press.

Suldo, S. M., McMahan, M. M., Chappel, A. M., & Loker, T. (2012). Relationships between perceived school climate and adolescent mental health across genders. *School Mental Health, 4*(2), 69–80. https://doi.org/10.1007/s12310-012-9073-1

Woods, S., Sebastian, J., Herman, K., Hyang, F., Reinke, W., & Thomspon, A. (2023). The relationship between teacher stress and job satisfaction as moderated by coping. *Psychology in the Schools, 60*(7), 2237–2256. https://doi.org/10.1002/pits.22857

Zoller, K., & Bacskai, K. (2020). Teacher work and job satisfaction among Romanian lower secondary teachers. *Central European Journal of Educational Research, 2*(2), 93–100. https://doi.org/10.37441/CEJER/2020/2/2/7918

Chapter 11
Research of the Problem Concerning Preserving Psychological Health of Students During the War

Inna Kovalchuk, Maria Oliinyk, and Olena Homoniuk

Currently, the problem of preserving the psychological health of student youth raises an increased interest, as it is one of the conditions for the formation of professional self-awareness, identity and effective professional activity of the future specialist, especially under martial law.

The term "mental health" became relevant due to the report of the World Health Organization in 1979 on the topic "Mental health and psychosocial development of children" (Progress report of the World Health Organization for 1979). WHO experts tried to draw the attention of the world public to the protection of childhood and the need to ensure conditions that prevent deviations from the norm; the unity of mental, somatic, physical and social health and their mutual influence was especially emphasized.

The considerable attention, in WHO materials, was paid to family and school education, which can significantly influence the psychosocial development of children (Bevzenko, 2008).

According to the definition of WHO, mental health is a state of wellbeing when a person can realize his/her personal potential, resolve ordinary life stressful situations, work productively and efficiently, and contribute to the life of society (The World Health Report, 1998).

I. Kovalchuk · M. Oliinyk
Yuriy Fedkovych Chernivtsi National University, Chernivtsi, Ukraine
e-mail: i.kovalchuk@chnu.edu.ua

O. Homoniuk
Jan Kochanwski Unversity, Kielce, Poland
e-mail: elena_gomonyuk29@ukr.net

M. Oliinyk (✉)
Khmelnytski National University, Khmelnitskyi, Ukraine
e-mail: mariia.oliinyk@ujk.edu.pl; m.oliynyk@chnu.edu.ua

A. A. Colomeischi (ed.), *Wellbeing in Schools of Southeastern Europe*, Human Well-Being Research and Policy Making,
https://doi.org/10.1007/978-3-032-10525-7_11

The World Health Organization defined the following mental health criteria: "A person must have awareness and a sense of continuity, permanence and identity of his/her physical and mental "I"; a sense of constancy and identity of experiences in similar situations; self-criticism, criticism to mental activity and its results; correspondence of mental reactions (their adequacy) to strength and frequency of environmental influences, social circumstances and situations; the ability to self-management in accordance with social norms, rules and laws; the opportunity to plan and realize your own life; the ability to change your own behaviour depending on changes in life situations and circumstances" (Mental Health Declaration for Europe, 2005).

Due to the importance of the mental health issue of the nation, Ukraine, together with other progressive states, signed the European Declaration on the Protection of Mental Health (2005) and the European Social Charter. It states that "psychological health and mental wellbeing are the most important prerequisites for a high quality of life and productive activities of individuals, families, local communities and nations as a whole, as they allow people to perceive their lives as full and meaningful" (European Social Charter, 1996).

According to these documents, Ukraine has moved from the concept of treating mental illnesses to the concept of preserving and strengthening the mental health of the population, and since 2012 it increased to a thorough assessment of vulnerabilities and risks for the population various segments' mental wellbeing.

Ukraine also supports the Convention on the Protection of Human Rights and Fundamental Freedoms of 1950 in issues of the population mental health, ratified by the Law of Ukraine 1997; the European Concept of Human Rights №. 475/97-BP (2010), the Convention on the Rights of the Child, Ratified by the Resolution of the Verkhovna Rada of the Ukrainian SSR №. 789-XII (1991), the Convention on the Rights of Persons with Disabilities, Ratified by the Law of Ukraine (2009); the Resolution of the UN General Assembly "Transforming Our World: Agenda in the Field of Sustainable Development for the Period up to 2030" (2015).

Consideration of important aspects of these documents formed the basis for the development of the Concept of Mental Health Care Development in Ukraine for the period until 2030 (Mental Health System Transformation in Ukraine: Improving Mental Health Services & Bringing Mental Health Care in Line with International Standards, 2018).

Modern theoretical, experimental and applied approaches in psychology characterize mental health as a state of wellbeing in which a person can realize his/her own potential, cope with ordinary life stresses, work productively and efficiently, and also make a significant contribution to the life of the community. According to M. Mirov, the main function of mental health is the maintenance of an active dynamic balance between a person and the surrounding environment in situations that require personal resources mobilization (Mirov, 2020).

The study of scientific sources proves various approaches to the definition of the concept "mental health". This fact confirms its understanding as an integrated process.

Thus, in modern psychiatry, the definition of the concept "mental health" according to the formulation of T. Dmytryeva and B. Polozhey is widespread. Scientists consider it as a state of the individual psyche, which is characterized by the integrity and coherence of all mental functions of the organism, which provide a sense of subjective mental comfort, the ability to purposeful meaningful activity and optimal performance of social functions, adequate to universal human values and ethno-cultural features of the group to which individual belongs (Dmytryeva & Polozhey, 1994).

In philosophy, the problem of mental health is considered at the intersection of natural and social sciences. Thus, philosophy examines the place of mental health and mental pathology in the system of human relations to the world, to people and to themself.

Under mental health disorder, philosophy recognizes the inconsistency of biological, social and subjective being. Human is triadic in nature, i.e. spirit, soul, body. These parts cannot be separated (Dmytriiuk & Schastna, 2003).

Solving the problem of preserving human health in the modern world philosophy involves a change in worldview, i.e. a transition from the biosocial model of health dominant in society, which considers human health as adaptation to the surrounding biosocial environment, to the biosocial one, which is aimed at the comprehensive realization of spiritual and creative potential of the individual (Yashchyshan, 2011).

Researcher O. Dmitrieva fairly considers the categories "health" and "disease" to be the most important and offers the following definition: "Health should be realised as optimal mental, physiological, reproductive, and social activity of the organism, and disease as a condition that interferes with mental, physiological, reproductive and social activities of an individual" (Kostyuk & Kostiuk, 2018).

We share the approach of D. Kostyuk and V. Kostyuk, who, after analysing a pile of literature on the problem, identified the following key ideas of mental health research, i.e. mental health can be considered as equivalent to spiritual health; analysis of mental health actualizes the problem of normality and pathology in the mental health of an individual; the basis of a person's mental health is the character of the manifestation of the human in a person (Potapchuk, 2004).

The pedagogical approach to the concept of mental health can be characterized by five specific features as follows: anthropology (requires consideration of mental and spiritual components of health); integrity (referring to all knowledge about a human); personally oriented (the individual should be considered as an object and subject of activity in relation to his/her health, although these concepts are usually separated) and pedagogical nature (in the process of education and upbringing, a person masters the culture of a healthy lifestyle) orientation; humanism (health is considered as the main value of human life) (Yashchyshyna, 2011).

According to Ye. Potapchuk, "the mental health of an individual is a stable mental state of a person, which is a consequence of the balance or harmony of the external form and internal content" (Potapchuk, 2004).

We share the scientists' opinion that mental health can be equivalent to spiritual health.

In recent years, there has been an increasing proposal to consider the spiritual sphere of a person as the fourth dimension of health.

The native ethnopsychologist S. Boltivets (2000), in his work on the problem of the psychology of the Ukrainian ethnic group, draws attention to the dominance of the spiritual factor in the psychology of the Ukrainian people. The issue of the human soul health was considered by the Scythian philosopher Anaharz Prydnipryanskyi, Ukrainian philosophers and educators Feofan Prokopovych, Hryhoriy Skovoroda (Boltivets, 2000).

Researchers reveal the development of ideas regarding the problem of spiritual health in Ukrainian anthropological culture, which is defined by two religious worldviews—paganism and Christianity.

The ideas development concerning the spiritual health issue in the Ukrainian humanistic culture, which is determined by two religious worldviews as paganism and Christianity, is revealed by researchers.

E. Potapchuk, in his research, assumes the opinion that spiritual health is most likely a component of mental health, and not a separate component of general health (Potapchuk, 2004).

Based on the conclusion of V. Frankl, mental health is possible only when there is a certain tension between a person and the content from the outside, which a person needs to understand and implement (Frankl, 1992). According to the author's existential-psychological concept, a person in any condition, in any situation, strives for the content, validity and meaningfulness of their life.

According to V. Frankl's theory, there are three possibilities to achieve the meaning of life and get satisfaction from it: to perform any task or create anything; to expect something or to love someone; to overcome a difficult dramatic situation that cannot be changed. The researcher claims that a person is not filled with a desire for power or a desire for pleasure, but, first of all, with a desire for the meaning of life. Motivated by this desire, a person makes every effort to find the sense and realize it, as well as to meet and love another human being. Both these factors enable a person to experience happiness and satisfaction (Frankl, 1992).

The internal complexity and ambiguity of the phenomenon of psychological health are described in the concept of S. Freud's successor, E. Erikson. The scientist correlates personality characteristics with age, presenting them as several forms of identity that have already passed their main path of development, forms that still belong to it and shapes that exist in the stage of formation (Huzenko, 2007).

We believe that the basis of a person's mental health is the character of the manifestation of the human in a person. Such representatives of the humanist school drew attention to this as A. Maslou, K. Rogers. According to well-known scientists, the basis of psychological health is a person's desire to become and remain himself/herself, despite all the difficulties of life (Maslou, 2002).

However, A. Maslou saw great danger in equating mental health with an individual's ability to adapt to reality and considered an important manifestation of mental health to be the individual's ability to rise above the environment, to be independent from it (Maslou, 2002).

The Polish psychologist K. Dombrowski believes that the ability to always adapt to new conditions indicates moral and emotional immaturity, behind this ability lies the absence of a hierarchy of values and such a life position that does not contain the elements necessary for personality development (Befany, 2004).

The well-known foreign psychologist K. Rogers also considered self-actualization to be the highest level of a person's mental health development, but not as a final result, but as a constant movement the direction of an individual's own development. He claimed that a person has a natural, innate desire for health K. Rogers called a "fully functioning" person a person who realizes their potential and is characterized by such features as: openness to experience, an existential lifestyle, self-confidence, empirical freedom and creativity.

Psychological health is the basis of complete human development. The very concept of psychological health, introduced into scientific circulation by A. Kichuk, was included into the basic content of mental health as its part for a long time, due to which the experience of psychopathology was used in relation to a healthy person psyche. However, modern science distinguishes the spheres of mental and psychological health, i.e. psychological changes are reversible, their timely diagnosis and professional correction helps a person to develop self-regulation abilities that will enable him/her to overcome internal problems on his/her own before these issues become irreversible (Kichuk, 2019).

The modern development of psychology allowed researchers not only to separate the concepts of "mental health" and "psychological health", but also to mark the phenomenological field in which the concept of "health" is represented in its psychological aspects' totality.

The problem of psychological health of an individual was revealed through the relationship with various psychological phenomena, namely: the connection between mood and health; the psychological health criteria of participants in the educational process; peculiarities of students' mental health; the role of protective mechanisms of the individual and their significance for mental health; the assessment criteria and factors of psychological health formation; the problem of psychological health in the context of a healthy lifestyle, etc.

A significant contribution to the psychological health issue was made by foreign scientists of the twentieth century who have world recognition and authority in psychology. An important place among the studies is the analysis of mental disorders of the population under the influence of military conflicts that take place in various regions of the world, which is reflected in a number of foreign studies (Yashchyshyna, 2011).

The study of the psychological consequences of Russia's large-scale war against Ukraine has only just begun and is reflected in the scientific works of many Ukrainian authors.

Currently, there is also an approach to identifying the concepts of mental and psychological health. In particular, this can be traced in the scientific works of I. Haletska. The researcher singles out the most important component of a person's mental health, i.e. psychological health as a subsystem of mental health, which performs the main regulatory function in relation to maintaining balance in the health system as a whole, being the realisation of the socialization consequences and a factor in the effectiveness of the entire process and individual development at the same time. The author proposes to distinguish two levels in the structure of mental health; they are structural and procedural mental health (characteristics of processes and properties of the cognitive and emotional-volitional spheres) and psychological health, which covers semantic aspects of mental health, peculiarities of "I" and human noogenic sphere, beliefs, identity, as well as the spiritual sphere (Haletska, 2005).

Mental health is a multidimensional phenomenon containing various components, therefore, in scientific sources, the concept of "mental health" is identified with such concepts as "mental health", "spiritual health", "psychological health" and "personal health".

In our opinion, these concepts are identical to the term "mental health", because they reflect the same concept, i.e. "mental health". Therefore, there is no reason to use these concepts further.

Mental health is ensured at different but interdependent levels of functioning, i.e. biological, psychological and social.

Health at the biological level implies a dynamic balance of all internal organs and systems functions, their adequate response to environmental influences.

Health at the psychological level is related to an individual's personality.

Mental health can be affected by the dominance of character traits that are negative in nature, as well as the absence or insufficiency of morality, the wrong choice of value orientations, etc. The transition from the mental to the social level is very notional.

Mental properties of an individual do not exist outside the system of social relations in which it is included. A person is considered at this level, first of all, as a social being. Mental health is influenced by various social relationships, and the consequences of these influences can be both positive and negative. Only people with a healthy psyche feel like active participants in the social system. Existing educational neglect and unfavourable environmental conditions are often the cause of various forms of inadequate and unhealthy human behaviour in the society.

At the same time, in modern psychology there is an approach according to which the problem of mental health of an individual cannot be reduced to the analysis of the generalized concept of a specific sample, but it is advisable to consider it at the individual personal level.

Thus, V. Petkov distinguishes three levels of mental health, and they are as follows: the first level is the level of psychophysiological health; the second is individual and psychological; the third, highest level is personal and meaningful. Each of these levels has its own patterns of internal, neurophysiological organization of mental activity acts and its own criteria, patterns of passage. The first level is directly related to hereditary and biological characteristics, the second and third depend on the social conditions of education and upbringing (Petkov, 2015).

The basis of psychological health, according to O. Zavhorodnia, is the ability to integrate contradictions between external and internal reality, which is possible only if the ability to conscious self-regulation is formed, the rational-volitional sphere is developed, which creates a basis for social adaptation, without suppressing emotional spheres.

Mental health, being multilevel, can be disrupted at some levels while others remain relatively intact (Zavhorodnia & Kurhanska, 2008).

Researcher O. Kalitiyevska, relying on the proposed mental health model of B. Bratus, offers her understanding of personality functioning as the level of psychophysiological regulation; the level of socio-adaptive regulation; the level of semantic regulation; and the existential level, which influences the lower levels of personal activity. It is at the fourth level, notes Y. Yashchyshyna, that the individual makes an autonomous choice, shows not adaptive, but supra-situational activity, being the subject of changes in his/her life (Yashchyshyna, 2011).

Therefore, the authors came to the conclusion that mental health is not a diagnosis, but a means of human existence in the world, it is evidence of maturity, integrity of personal self-regulation mechanisms.

We believe that in the conditions of war, the mental health of students is threatened by the following factors as the instability of the emotional wellbeing of the individual, which is caused by threats of military bombings, the instability of the social environment where is the student (friends, relatives have died; good acquaintances have been called to participate in military operations, migration of the female population); the need to master new social patterns of behaviour in conditions of unstable electricity supply and fear of the future.

Considering these factors, we share the opinion that the study of students' mental health is an interdisciplinary problem and should attract the attention of scientists from medicine, psychology, pedagogy, economics, ecology and law. Therefore, the effectiveness of studying the mental health of students will depend on the coordinated interaction of specialists from all fields.

R. Sirko, in his study of the mental health of pupils and student youth, confirms that the state of mental health of a young person is determined by numerous personal and behavioural characteristics, a synthesis of social and biologically determined features of the psyche, which determine the peculiarities of communication, satisfaction with various aspects of family or educational relations (Sirko, 2002).

Studying the problem of mental health of students, D. Mirov notes that psychological health is a higher level of manifestation of mental health. According to the author, it is determined by the value-meaning content of personality development (Mirov, 2020).

Researcher A. Kichuk examines psychological health from the perspective of the reverse personality theory. The theory proposes the concept of motivational diversity. According to this concept, psychological health depends on the completeness of emotional and behavioural manifestations, i.e. it is manifested in a wide range of psychological states, in various emotional registers, and the experience of motivational diversity. Therefore, the conditions for healthy social development of the individual are the changes, inconsistency and instability, which serve as a defining characteristic of the contemporary postmodern world (Kichuk, 2019).

Among the studies of the psychological consequences in the aggressive war of Russia against Ukraine, there exists the problem of studying the essence and structure of the mental health of teachers in the conditions of war, its negative and positive expressions, the classification of the main problems related to the severity of the components of mental health, the determination of the resources necessary for its support and preservation.

The Department of Psychodiagnostics and Medical Psychology of Taras Shevchenko National University of Kyiv deals with the problems of health psychology.

The main areas of research of the department's scientists are the study of psychosomatic, personal and socio-psychological aspects of life, which are regulators of human mental health, the problem of maintaining the psychosomatic health of people of different age periods, the technology of counselling psychosomatic patients, etc.

Leading scientists of the Kostyuk Institute of Psychology of the Academy of Sciences of Ukraine also have modern scientific achievements in the study of health psychology. Scientists are engaged in the study of a range of problems related to the improvement of a person's mental health, the psychology of an individual healthy lifestyle. Researcher N. Kolotii offers a portrait of a mentally healthy personality. It is spontaneous, creative, cheerful, cheerful, communicative, with developed cognitive qualities, intuition, who is constantly developing, quickly adapts to changes, can be in a situation of uncertainty, without losing faith in a better future (Kolotii, 2003).

We are also impressed by the scientist's approach to the analysis of a person's mental health as a system of interconnected components. We believe that it can be adapted to understand the students' mental health. The components of mental health are axiological, instrumental and activity-motivational.

We understand the axiological component of a student's mental health as a student's perception of his/her intrinsic value, respect for youth, the ratio of his/her own self-esteem for value by other people. This gives an individual the opportunity to accept himself/herself and other people, to travel, to learn about culture and traditions. Possession of reflection, which allows you to coordinate behaviour with other people, serves as a means of self-improvement, promotes the free expression of feelings, without harming other people. When considering the influence of value orientations on the professional formation of a student's personality, a holistic system referring ideas about motivational and value-orientation spheres of professional activity has been developed in psychology.

It is advisable to analyse the instrumental component through the prism of professional activity orientation.

According to Zhavnerchyk O.V., professional activity involves the following structural elements: professional vocation, that is an aspiration (tendency) to a certain profession, which is based on knowledge of its purpose; professional intentions that is a conscious attitude to a certain type of professional activity; value orientations in professional activity grounds developed by society and accepted by an individual for evaluating the purpose of his/her work, choosing a system of spiritual values, rules of professional ethics; motives of professional activity are internal motivations that determine the direction of a person's activity in his professional behaviour as a whole and lead him/her to various aspects of professional activity; professional pursuits are the desire to achieve a result, a certain level of professional competence, which is determined by the person himself/herself, knowing the previous achievements; professional expectations are the expectations about one's possible successes. The activity-motivational component reveals a person's expressed feeling for self-improvement, which serves as the internal engine of the individual's vital activities (Zhavnerchyk, 2020).

At the same time, the identified components of mental health (positive attitude towards oneself and attitude towards other people, personal reflection and the need for self-development) are interrelated, or more precisely, they interact dynamically. For the development of positive rather than neurotic reflection, a person needs to have a positive attitude towards himself or herself. In turn, a person's self-development affects a change in attitude towards oneself. And personal reflection is a mechanism of self-development. Accordingly, it can be concluded that the attitude towards oneself, reflection and self-development interact between each other and are in constant cooperation.

From the definition of "human health" notion proposed by M. Honcharenko, in his valeological dictionary, it follows that the main characteristic of a healthy person is the ability to perfect self-regulation (Honcharenko, 1999). Self-regulation is interpreted as a special level of programming activity based on prediction processes; purposeful change of both individual psychophysiological functions and the neuropsychological state as a whole, as well as the character and method of action.

Therefore, a person's attitude towards himself/herself, reflection and self-development in the structure of a student's mental health are in constant interaction. Thus, neurotic manifestations of one of them inevitably affect other components of mental health.

Analysing mental health, it is necessary to take into account the issue of norm and pathology in mental health. We would like to emphasise the idea that the analysis of mental health exacerbates the problem of standard and pathology in the individual mental state.

Researcher Ye. Potapchuk emphasizes that determining the norm of mental health of an individual should be carried out in accordance with the age periods of its development. Therefore, in our opinion, it is necessary to talk about such types of norms of mental health as the norm of mental health of an individual at the stage of its formation; the standard of mental health of an individual at the stage of his/her development; the standard of mental health of a mature personality (self-actualization) (Potapchuk, 2004).

Given the potential complexity of the studied phenomenon, the problem of mental health criteria requires careful study and analysis. Despite the fact that scientists identify criteria for mental health, the issue of assessing its condition is still not resolved. None of the criteria can be unambiguously interpreted, since mental health is an integrative system that must be considered not only as a holistic phenomenon, but also taking into account the subjective objectivity of the situation and environment.

According to A. Adler's theory, psychological health criteria are directly related to how successfully a person is able to solve basic life tasks, i.e. work, make friends and love (Adler, 2015). Therefore, in assessing health, most researchers point out two main criteria as social (as a measure of ability to work, social activity, and a person's active attitude to the world) and personal (as a person's life strategy and the degree of self-regulation and life circumstances).

The analysis of scientific sources shows that the issue of mental health criteria was considered by M. Andros. The researcher considers the criteria of health to be the level of maturity of the cognitive, emotional and volitional sphere of the individual, planning and achieving a certain life goal, the level of adequacy of self-esteem and relationships in the microsocial environment of self-acceptance as an individual (Andros, 1998).

Ukrainian scientists emphasize the socio-moral orientation of the individual and emphasize that mental health involves the correspondence (inconsistency) of subjective images with the objects of reality and the nature of reactions, which are external stimuli, the content of life events; age-appropriate level of maturity of the emotional, volitional and cognitive spheres of the personality; adaptability in microsocial relations; the ability to self-control behaviour, intelligent planning of life goals and support of activity in their achievement (Kolotii, 2003; Petkov, 2015; Pyliahina, 2020).

We can see similar ideas in the scientific works of S. Boltivets, who considers individuality, activity, socialization, energy potential and self-regulation to be the main factors in mental health (Boltivets, 2000).

Researcher emphasize that mental health is characterized by the following signs as adaptive orientation of mental activity and behaviour, adequacy of age and environmental influence (Pyliahina, 2020).

Internal self-regulation of mental health is indicated by S. Maksymenko (Maksymenko, 2002). According to the scientist, the key criteria of positive mental health are the attitude to the "I"; growth, development and self-actualization of the personality; integration of the personality, autonomy; adequacy of perception of reality; skill and competence in relation to the environment (Maksymenko, 2002). We are impressed by the classification of mental health criteria presented by Yashchyshyna Yu. who divided the existing criteria according to their correspondence with the types of mental manifestation in the personality (processes, states, properties) (Yashchyshyna, 2011). As a result of this work, among the mental processes she singled out the maximum approximation of subjective images to the reality objects that are reflected (adequacy of mental reflection); adequacy of self-perception; the ability to concentrate attention on the subject; retention of information in memory; the ability to logically process information; critical thinking; creativity (ability to be creative, ability to use intelligence); discipline of the mind (management of the thinking process).

Regarding mental condition, it includes emotional stability (self-control); maturity of feelings according to age; management of negative emotions; free, natural expression of feelings and emotions; the capacity for joy; preservation of general (optimal) wellbeing.

Among the personality traits we can highlight the following: optimism; concentration (absence of vanity); poise; morality (honesty); adequate level of harassment; sense of duty; self-belief; inoffensiveness (the ability to get rid of hidden images); indolence; independence; immediacy (naturalness); sense of humour; goodwill; self-respect; adequate self-esteem; self-control; freedom; energy, activeness; purposefulness.

It is noteworthy that among the criteria of individual mental health, the degree of its integration, harmony, balance, as well as such components of its focus as spirituality (kindness, justice, etc.), focus on self-development and enrichment of the personality are of particular importance.

Researcher O. Honcharenko believes that the issue of health assessment criteria is key in the problem of mental health. At the same time, she notes that among the various signs, the mental balance criterion deserves special attention. With its help, it is possible to judge the character of a person's mental sphere, namely cognitive, emotional and volitional. Only in a mentally healthy, i.e. balanced person, we observe manifestations of relative stability of behaviour and adequacy to its external conditions; high individual adaptability of the organism to the usual fluctuations of the external environment; the ability to maintain the usual comfortable wellbeing, morphological and functional preservation of organs and systems (Honcharenko, 1999). The psychologist points out that the set of criteria for the main manifestations of a healthy psyche, which are most often cited in the literature, can be divided by types of mental manifestation (mental states, processes, properties, degree of self-regulation, etc.). The scientist singles out the following criteria for mental health:

- personality traits: optimism, concentration (lack of fussiness), balance, ethics (honesty, conscientiousness, tact, etc.), adequate level of demands (harassment), sense of duty, self-confidence, invulnerability to insults (ability to get rid of insults), diligence, independence, directness (naturalness), responsibility, sense of humour, benevolence, tolerance, self-respect, self-control;
- mental states: emotional stability (self-control); maturity of feelings, according to age; possession of negative emotions (fear, anger, greed, envy, etc.); free natural expression of feelings and emotions; the ability to rejoice; preservation of optimal feeling;
- mental processes: maximum approximation of subjective images to the objects of reality that reflect (adequacy of mental reflection); adequate self-perception; the ability to logically process information; critical thinking; creativity (ability to be creative, ability to use authority); self-knowledge; mind discipline (thought management); special importance is given to the degree of integration, its harmony, consolidation, balance, as well as such components of its focus as: spirituality (knowledge, striving for truth), the priority of humanistic values (goodness, justice, love, beauty, etc.), orientation to self-development, enrichment of your personality; self-management that is a healthy personality characterized by a strong purposefulness (gaining the meaning of life), will, energy, activity, self-control, adequate self-esteem; the social health of an individual is reflected in the following characteristics, i.e. adequate perception of social reality, interest in the surrounding world, adaptation (balance) to the physical and social environment; focus on public affairs, consumer culture, altruism, empathy, responsibility to others, selflessness, democracy in behaviour.

Researcher N. Honcharenko singled out six criteria of psychological health, namely a positive attitude towards one's own personality; spiritual growth and self-actualization; integrated personality; autonomy, self-sufficiency; adequacy of reality perception; competence in overcoming the demands of the surrounding world (Honcharenko, 1999).

The scientist N.Yarema, researching the problem of psychological health, cites a more extensive system of criteria, in particular: self-interest and public interest, self-management (self-control) and high frustration resistance, acceptance of uncertainty and flexibility, which is expressed in the plasticity of thinking, openness to changes, "scientific" thinking and focus on creative plans, self-acceptance, ability to take risks, long-term hedonism, neo-utopianism and responsibility for someone's emotional worries.

At the same time, it is important that foreign psychology takes into account ideas about the manifestation of mental health criteria depending on the conditions dictated by culture, or ideas about the influence on the manifestation of individual social characteristics (Yarema, 2015).

Representatives of health psychology interpret this notion as wellbeing in the broadest sense. Wellbeing is a multifactorial construct that represents a complex interrelationship of cultural, social, psychological, physical, economic and spiritual factors. This complex product is the result of the influence of genetic predisposition, environment and individual development characteristics.

Summarizing the above-mentioned opinions, we can emphasize that many criteria are repeated in a large number. It shows that they are not coincidental, but are interrelated and can be traced in the diagnosis of specialists' mental health in various fields of life.

Analysing the above criteria, we see that they are also related to the person's self (self-acceptance, individuality, activity, harmony, spirituality, self-analysis, self-regulation, self-actualization and others). This group of criteria reflects the personal qualities of a person, which are interconnected with the criteria that reflect the adequate social behaviour of a person, his/her relations with the environment and interaction with other people (socialization, social maturity, transfer of social roles, norms, values to his/her internal world, etc.).

In the conditions of Russia's war against Ukraine, the concept of criteria acquires special importance and demands its rethinking in the context of the new social situation. The life uncertainty, the unknown future, the plans absence or destruction and prospects led to growing emotional stress, increased anxiety, the appearance of fears, obsessive negative thoughts and constant experiences, which greatly affect the state of psychological balance of the individual, his psychological health.

It is worth substantiating the significance of the specified criterion, namely the acceptance of uncertainty, through the characteristics of the manifestations of two opposite personal traits, i.e. tolerance and intolerance to uncertainty.

Tolerance to uncertainty is a multilevel and multidimensional personal construct that reflects the cognitive aspect that characterizes the tendency to perceive the situation, the affective aspect which includes the emotional reaction to uncertainty and the conative aspect which demonstrates individual behavioural features of self-regulation in complex conditions that are associated with the uncertainty of the semantic foundations of individual's own existence.

Thus, a person intolerant to uncertainty shows a tendency to rigid categorization and making clearly opposite judgments, a desire to make hasty and unbalanced decisions, avoidance of obscure, unclear, incomprehensible situations and an emotional reaction to them, perception of uncertainty as a threat and rejection of everything new. As a result, in conditions of uncertainty, an intolerant individual undergoes a significant destabilization of psychological health. Therefore, awareness of a drastic change in the situation and the impossibility of influencing certain life events is an extremely important step that will help to maintain the psychological health of each person.

Tolerance for uncertainty, which is also considered as a person's ability to find the meaning of life in difficult conditions, will help to accept uncertainty and navigate in the existing life situation. An uncertainty tolerant person demonstrates such capabilities as:

- the ability to make decisions, to solve problems in situations where it is difficult to predict all possible consequences and in conditions of a significant lack of facts regarding the current situation;
- the ability to resist the lack of logic in incoming information;
- the ability to perceive new, unfamiliar and risky situations as stimulating;
- the ability to organize oneself and apply an effective social and psychological attitude, which involves the activation of affective, cognitive and behavioural components in a difficult situation;
- the ability to feel and produce positive emotions in ambiguous situations by perceiving them not as a threat, but as a certain challenge;
- willingness to adapt to an uncertain situation and use the available opportunities.

Therefore, acceptance of uncertainty and developed tolerance for uncertainty help the individual to avoid despair, not to give up, to activate and enlist all available individual resources for self-help and self-maintenance of psychological health.

In our opinion, such a criterion of psychological health as frustration tolerance of an individual also deserves special attention. The ability of the individual to resist the unfavourable and complex challenges of the modern world, to adapt to the environment in war conditions, actualizes the mentioned quality of the individual more than ever.

The problem of frustration tolerance is actively studied and developed in modern science. Interpreting this concept, scientists are unanimous in understanding that it is the ability of an individual to overcome difficulties, the ability to adequately assess a frustrating situation and predict a way out of it, the limit of the mental stress permissible level, exceeding which causes destructive changes in a person's psyche and behaviour.

We are convinced, the definition proposed by N. Chyzhenko deserves attention, which considers this phenomenon as a mental quality of an individual that allows to adequately endure frustrating situations, while demonstrating constructive behaviour on the way to overcoming frustration barriers.

According to the researcher, awareness of negative frustrating influences, adjustment to solving urgent life tasks and manifestation of optimism allow maintaining mental balance. A decrease in sensitivity to the influence of adverse factors depends on the level of frustration tolerance formation, which allows supporting the psychological health of the individual.

Considering frustration tolerance as mental stability, the researcher emphasizes that it is "the ability of an individual to resist external manifestations that bring a person out of a state of neuropsychological imbalance, and to independently return to a state of mental equilibrium" (Chyzhenko, 2006).

According to A. Husiev, frustration tolerance operates in the cognitive, emotional and behavioural spheres and allows an individual to withstand crisis manifestations that are associated with the uncertainty of his/her own existence (Husiev, 2007).

Based on the analysis of the studied sources, it can be determined that frustration tolerance is an integrative characteristic of the personality, the main components of which are stability, endurance in the attitude towards frustraters, motivation to overcome obstacles, life optimism, cognitive evaluation based on reflection and critical thinking processes, which involve the ability to predict successful overcoming of frustraters.

Regarding the criteria of psychological health, Ukrainian researchers note that there are a significant number of such criteria, the most relevant of which are personality traits, social and psychological adaptation, indicators of creative achievements (Yashchyshyna, 2011).

The criteria of mental and psychological health are common, but they are not absolutely identical, which indicates the affinity and simultaneous difference in the concepts of mental and psychological health, and confirms the expediency of differentiating these categories.

Mental health criteria are basic for assessing the normal functioning of the psyche and the level of the individual adaptation.

According to A. Ellis's concept, the criteria of mental health are the student's interest in himself/herself and in social events; ability to self-education; emotional (frustration) stability; flexible thinking; acceptance of uncertainty; the presence of plans for the future, the ability to take risks, hedonism and responsibility for the emotional state.

Thus, as we found out, researchers, describing the criteria of mental health, assign the main role to mental balance and the related harmony of the organization of the psyche and its adaptive capabilities, the adequacy of the subjective perception of objects, phenomena and circumstances, the correspondence of mental reactions the intensity of external irritants, the orderliness and causality of mental phenomena, critical self-evaluation and assessment of circumstances, the ability to adequately change behaviour in accordance with changes in the environment and its organization in accordance with accepted moral and ethical norms, a sense of attachment and responsibility in relation to close people, the ability to develop and implement the life plan.

The concept of "mental health criteria" requires clarification of the essence of such concept as "indicators".

At the end of the nineteenth century provisions on the main indicators of mental health were formulated. Its content emphasizes their relationship and interdependence with moral, mental, and physical health (Yashchyshyna, 2011). Based on the conducted studies, the researcher identified two levels of mental health—high and low. As the author fairly believes, groups with a high level of mental health are characterized by self-sufficiency, emotional stability, satisfaction with educational activities, the absence of emphasis and psychopathological manifestations; groups with a low level of mental health involves dissatisfaction with the social microenvironment, low ability to self-regulate, tendency to conflict, aggressiveness. But this constructive thought, unfortunately, did not receive further development either in domestic or foreign science, and now there is an opportunity to evaluate and adopt it by Ukrainian philosophers, teachers, psychologists, cultural scientists and other representatives of humanitarian disciplines.

It should be noted that identifying indicators of mental health of an individual is an important and difficult task, as it requires taking into account a complex personal characteristic of an individual, from the peculiarities of cognitive processes to the manifestation of mental properties, etc. In this regard, military researchers note that the boundary between a healthy and mentally ill person is quite conditional and only a specialist doctor has the right to determine it definitively.

The complexity of this task also lies in the fact that all these characteristics are too dependent on the influence of many social and psychological factors.

First of all, we are talking about their dependence on the influence of changes associated with a person's age, the general state of his/her health, relationships with the environment, etc. It is obvious that the indicators of mental health of a young man and an elderly person will be different. In addition, there is a need to pay attention to the requirements for indicators put forward by the specifics of professional activity.

Classics of psychology point to such indicators of mental health as: an individual's ability to self-development and the ability to realize actual needs.

Researcher O. L. Turynina singled out the following indicators of psychological health as the presence of deep moral convictions, readiness to overcome life's trials, the ability to adequately use one's own mental resources, personal initiative and a positive vector of attitude towards life (Turynina, 2017).

Indicators of students' mental health are their activity, cheerfulness, observation, adaptability to the conditions of educational activities in a higher education institution, low anxiety, emotional stability, ability to perceive and analyse information.

Researching mental health, I Pryb points to the peculiarities of the individual level of health, which is characterized by the integrity and coherence of all mental functions of the body, and the social level of mental health, in turn, indicates the level of mental health of the population (Pryb, 2016).

In foreign psychology, in addition to the individual level of health, six levels of health in the world community are also considered.

The first level is individual (health of an individual); the second is the level of health of a certain group of people (the person's immediate environment); the third is the level of health of formally defined organizations in society with which the vast majority of people interact and which affect the health of employees; the fourth is the level of health of the community, which is determined mainly by territorial characteristics or by ethnic, professional characteristics, political or religious beliefs, etc.; the fifth is the level of the country; and the last, the sixth is the level of the whole world (Tanella et al., 1998).

This structuring of health levels should emphasize the world community understanding of the connection between individual and public health, which determines the interdependence of all levels.

Based on the existing research on the mental health of students, we will determine the levels of mental health: high (creative), medium (adaptive), low (maladaptive).

Observations of the student sample make it possible state that students with a creative level of mental health and an average level of adaptive mental health prevail in Ukrainian higher education institutions.

The creative level characterizes people with stable adaptation to the environment, the existence of a strength reserve to overcome stressful situations and an active creative attitude to reality, the presence of a creative position. Such people do not need psychological help.

The medium level (adaptive) includes people who are generally adapted to society, but have slightly increased anxiety. This group of students can be classified as a risk group, as they do not have a reserve of psychological health and can be included in group work of a preventive and developmental focus.

A low level is maladaptive. It can include students with a violation of the balance in the assimilation and accommodation processes and use either assimilative or accommodative means to resolve the internal conflict.

The assimilative style of behaviour is characterized, first of all, by a person's desire to adapt to external circumstances to the detriment of his/her desires and capabilities. Its unconstructiveness is manifested in the rigidity and attempts of a person to fully comply with the wishes of others. There are few people with a low level of health among students.

The authors of the psychology textbook emphasize that a person needs psychological help and support to the greatest extent in his/her youth. Scientists draw attention to the fact that radical changes in personality development give rise to a large number of psychological problems, and they are adaptation, professional formation, interpersonal communication and family problems.

The mental health of students of higher education institutions depends on pedagogical and psychological factors. Pedagogical factors include learning conditions; accommodation; organization of educational activities; lack of individual approach by teachers; workload; etc.

Psychological factors include an individual's inability to control his/her own emotional states; low level of resistance to stressful situations; tendency to conflicts; insecurity of the individual in himself/herself; low self-esteem; insufficient sociability; incredulity.

Among students, changes in mental health are caused by external stress factors namely, changes in living conditions and self-esteem of the individual. Scientists claim that self-esteem plays a mediating role in reflecting life changes through increased sense of competence and experiencing stress.

Scientists point out that everything that a person lives by, that makes him/her happy in life, is connected with the future he/she seeks. This life perspective is a consequence of goal setting, i.e. one of the main properties of human consciousness, which consists in determining the goals of activity, behaviour and ways and means of achieving them (Moskalets, 2004). However, the destruction, loss of ideals, value orientations, which illuminate the individual's life perspective, are the determining worldview basis for the emergence of mental disharmony of the individual.

At the same time, according to the researchers, the socio-psychological maladaptation of the individual is expressed in the so-called behavioural reactions, in particular, in the reaction of emotional imbalance, in the pessimistic situational reaction, in the reaction of negative balance, in the situational reaction of demobilization, opposition and disorganization (Moskalets, 2004).

Each of these reactions has a negative effect on the mental health of the individual. Therefore, we will consider them in more detail.

The reaction of emotional imbalance is characterized by a distinct experience of a negatively coloured range of emotions (low mood, emotional discomfort, general dissatisfaction). This means a narrowing of the circle of communication and social contacts. With a rather deep reaction, fatigue increases and the mental protection effectiveness gradually decreases.

A pessimistic situational reaction is manifested, first of all, in changes in the worldview, the establishment of a gloomy, pessimistic worldview, judgments and assessments, in the restructuring of the value orientations system.

Inherent in such a worldview, the steady decrease in the level of optimism makes it difficult to plan for the future and gives rise to gloomy forecasts of troubles, which are seen as blows of fate that are useless to counteract.

The reaction of the negative balance is the weighing of reasons and the determination of the existence perspectives are limited due to incurable somatic diseases, old age and physical infirmity.

The situational reaction of demobilization is characterized by the most drastic destructive changes in the sphere of personal communication. A person avoids inclusion in any spheres of activity, except for the most necessary, mandatory, socially controlled.

Activity productivity is low, which increases mental discomfort, frustrating experiences, alienation and isolation of the individual.

The situational reaction of the opposition is characterized by an extra-punitive (total negativism) position with a steady increase in aggressiveness, an increase in harshness, categoricalness and unappealable negative assessments of other people and their activities.

The situational reaction of disorganization, its main component is anxiety, from which somatic-vegetative disorders originate as hypertensive and vascular-vegetative crises, drowsiness or insomnia. Dysthymic experiences of indecision, fatigue, loneliness, abandonment, alienation, isolation, helplessness, sadness, yearnings, depression, mental pain, etc., prevail in the formation of these reactions.

The literature analysis on the problems of students' mental health made it possible to consider it on an individual basis (taking into account age-related socio-psychological formations, gender characteristics, place of residence, the influence of the microsocial environment during the study at a higher education institution, features of the value-meaning sphere and characterological features of the subject, individual characteristics of self-regulation) and on the social (availability of a reference group, status, satisfaction with relationships in the family, group, degree of overload, stressful situations during training, social conditions, etc.).

Therefore, psychological health disorders depend on how the team perceives the individual, in which he works or studies, on personal success in the activity he performs. As a result, the disturbance of psychological balance experienced by students, teachers or employees in stressful situations is a disturbance of the emotional sphere, anxiety, aggressiveness, fears, etc.

The view of Czech rescarchers K. Blaga and M. Shebek, regarding the problem of intra-personal disharmony, is valuable in the course of research.

According to scientists, it is necessary to define this phenomenon, first of all, based on the understanding of the "I system" of the individual (fundamental acmeology is a science of the twenty-first century, 2019). So, the mature, developed "I system" is limited and combined with the so-called global I. Global "I" is the centre of personality. Its components are sincere processes, states, feelings, desires, goals. In addition, in the "I system" in addition to the global "I", there is a "hierarchical structure of axes of self-image and self-understanding". This structure contains such axes as: I am, I want, I have, ideal self, conscience, social role, who I will be, etc. Researchers believe that intra-personal disharmony occurs when there is a disintegration of the global "I" or any hierarchical structure of axes is broken.

Analysing the essence of students' mental health as a holistic phenomenon, we can talk about the following issues as the level of maturity of the cognitive, mental sphere of the individual; the level of maturity of the emotional and volitional sphere of the individual; planning and achieving life goals and aims of specific activities; the level of adequacy of self-esteem and self-acceptance as an individual; the level of adequacy of relations in the microsocial environment.

In terms of mental development, studentship is a period of intense human socialization, development of higher mental functions, formation of the entire intellectual system and personality as a whole. If we consider studentship, taking into account only biological age, then it should be attributed to the period of youth as a transitional stage of human development between childhood and adulthood. Therefore, in foreign psychology, this period is associated with the growing up process.

The psychological content of youth is closely related to the development of self-awareness, solving tasks of professional self-determination and entry into adulthood. In early youth, cognitive and professional interests are formed, and the need for work, the ability to build life plans, social activity, the independence of the individual, the choice of a life path are asserted. In youth, a person asserts himself/herself in the chosen business and finds professional skill, and it is also during this period that professional training is completed, and, therefore, the student period.

In age psychology, it is emphasized that in youth, a person is maximally capable of working, withstands the greatest physical and mental stress and is most capable of mastering complex methods of intellectual activity.

The problem of the student's emotional and value attitude towards himself/herself and his/her health is significant for modern psychology.

For a long time, there was a ban on selfishness in our culture, when loving others is virtuous and loving oneself is sinful. And these two meanings: self-love and love for others were opposed for a long time, when "the interests of everyone are subordinated to the interests of all" and "public opinion is higher than personal opinion". "If it is virtuous to love one's neighbour as a human being, then my love for myself should be virtuous, not vicious, since I am also a human being".

The idea expressed in the biblical commandment "love your neighbour as yourself" implies that respect for one's own integrity and uniqueness, self-love and understanding of inner self are inseparable from respect, love and understanding of another person.

A number of authors claim that only a high level of self-acceptance determines a positive attitude towards others.

Self-love, according to T. Tytarenko, acts as a kind of integral personal formation, which at the same time expresses the driving force of the "I", its active side, but not closed "in itself" and "for itself", but as a way of correlating the individual with the social world, others by people self-love as an indicator, criterion of interaction with the world plays an important role in the development of the value and moral sphere of the individual. This is one of the effective sources of increasing (decreasing) motivation, acquiring (losing) the meaning of life (Tytarenko & Dvornyk., 2022).

Mental health of students depends on a number of factors, and they are negative stressful situations, inability to maintain adequate relationships with others, conflicts, insufficient rest, social and living conditions, material situation, external stimuli (noise, etc.).

Preserving mental health is incompatible with the use of any psychoactive substances. Nicotine addiction is the most widespread mental disorder, which does not help to get rid of stress, but, on the contrary, increases its level, which contributes to the development of severe mental disorders. And since psychological health is definitely connected with mental health, since the latter creates a basis for psychological health, then one should pay attention to those factors that negatively affect a person, and be able to calmly approach the solution of adverse situations for preservation of a person's mental and psychological health.

The stress caused by the war has a negative effect on the effectiveness of activities and the mental health of students. Stress leads to an increase in the number of diseases of stress aetiology and, as a result, impaired work capacity, difficulty in adapting to new types and forms of learning, the development of reduced work capacity and the development of various forms of personal discomfort (the phenomenon of work alienation, desocialization, professional and personal deformation).

The main factors of the educational environment affecting the mental health of students in wartime conditions are as follows, physical conditions of study, i.e. the influence of the features of the room and household noises on the psyche of students. Unfavourable placement of the educational institution in relation to household sources and military noises contributes to the overstrain of the nervous system of students, causes excessive irritation, prevents the creation of a working atmosphere, negatively affects work capacity, assimilation of educational material and leads to the development of a stress reaction due to chronic stress on the psyche of students.

The peculiarities of the structure and climate of the educational institution also have a noticeable impact on the state of students' health. If students do not have the opportunity to take part in organizing their own life activities in the educational institution, an inadequate distance is established between the administration and student groups, and this contributes to an increase in the level of anxiety, a decrease in the level of self-esteem and tolerance to stress.

In the conditions of the educational process in Ukrainian higher education institutions, when analysing the problem of student stress, it is advisable also to take into account the state of mental health of the teacher as a full-fledged participant in educational interaction.

Such scientists as S. Dubyna, D., Khapchenkova and S. Bondarenko emphasize that the stress factor is an accompanying factor for teaching activities. Professional stress is associated with experiencing mental tension in conditions of high responsibility for decision-making, N. Sydorchuk truly notes (Dubyna et al., 2018).

Working under conditions of professional stress caused by military anxieties and professional tasks is a serious test of the teacher and student's physical and mental health, a test of the quality of professional interaction.

The professional activities of teachers and students are influenced by the following factors.

Firstly, it is the organization of the workplace; work overload; physical factors (temperature, noise, crowdedness); complexity of the performed activity; dissatisfaction with communication; concern about the consequences of possible mistakes; increased responsibility; etc.

Secondly, it is professional status, the problem of status; change of duties; transfer to another job; dissatisfaction with the prospect; etc.

Thirdly, it is remuneration for work, lack of clarity in remuneration; unequal pay, etc.

Fourthly, these are relationships at work as trouble with administration; conflicts with colleagues; unfavourable climate in the team; etc.

Fifthly, these are extra-organizational sources of stress as problems in the family; health problems; financial problems; problems of personal and organizational values (Sydorchuk & Tryhubchuk, 2018).

The peculiarities of the structure and climate of the student group play an important role in the student's mental health. Segmentation of student groups, misunderstandings due to the ambiguity of the goals by individual students and their status positions provoke the appearance of mental tension in the group. Desired role positions, the wish to belong to a certain reference group can change the motivation of students, provoke the appearance of an internal personal conflict, lower self-esteem and the formation of a stressful situation. Unsatisfactory position in the group provokes demonstrative forms of behaviour. Constant dissatisfaction with the position in the group contributes to the development of a stress reaction.

Low educational and methodological support also reduces the effectiveness of education and induces a negative attitude towards individual subjects and education in general, which leads to excessive neuropsychological stress.

In the period of acute socio-economic changes, another additional risk factor for maintaining mental health is strongly manifested, i.e. the social and professional uncertainty of the future specialist in society and the need to find a job, according to the level of education and professional training. Among the factors of mental health, it is advisable to pay attention to the students' attitudes and expectations related to future events.

In general, they can be divided into positive (optimistic) attitudes, manifested in the expectation of positive events, and negative (pessimistic), the manifestation of which is evidenced by the expectation of negative events. The former help to successfully overcome stress, as emotions experienced in difficult situations act as mechanisms for reinforcing activity. In the case of negative attitudes, emotions begin to show a destructive weakening effect.

Belief in low self-performance can lead to violations of cognitive processes in a stressful situation, for example, memory blockage and cognition in graduation exam situations for future specialists.

According to A. Bandura, the very perception of your own actions' effectiveness affects the course of mental, motivational and emotional processes, that is, it becomes an important regulatory mechanism for overcoming stress. The evaluation of the effectiveness of one's own actions in various situations showed the existence of a strong dependence on the content of situations and a minor influence of stable personal traits.

Comparing the concept of the effectiveness of one's own actions with the expectations theory, it should be emphasized that students' ideas about the effectiveness of their own actions do not always coincide with expectations regarding the consequences of their behaviour, especially in situations that do not depend or only partially depend on the subject himself/herself.

Here we need to mention one more factor that undoubtedly plays a significant role in the processes of effectively overcoming difficult situations. It is the so-called gratification crisis. The crisis of gratification is considered in health psychology as a phenomenon that can lead to a sharp increase in dissatisfaction with the results of one's activities, powerlessness, disappointment, frustration and a decrease in motivation for achievements.

The reason for its occurrence should be sought in the discrepancy between the effort invested and the reward received. The contradiction between somebody's contribution and the received reward leads to a decrease in wellbeing, the appearance of psychosomatic diseases, that is, it becomes the cause of the deterioration of the individual's mental health.

In studies of the student stress causes, it is often noted that one of them is insufficient identification with the student environment, perception of it as distant, sometimes even hostile. This is especially relevant for first-year students, who for the first time met new, different from school requirements.

The necessary assistance in overcoming this negative phenomenon can be found by the psychological service of the Higher Education Institution, providing various types of consultations and assistance in organizing educational activities.

One of the mechanisms of identification with the environment of activity is the sense of coherence described in A. Maslou's concept of mental health. According to the author's concept, it is connected with a positive assessment of the possibilities of solving a problem situation, the development of effective strategies for overcoming it and a positive life attitude.

The sense of coherence as a mechanism for overcoming stress, included in the process of identification with the environment, affects the positive expectations formation in the success of one's own activities, guarantees the rational use of one's capabilities and, thereby, contributes to the mental health preservation.

Researchers H.Dzvonyk and T.Savchenko single out six sources of stress when requirements and opportunities do not match, i.e. physical; social; personal; tasks peculiarities; structural features (individual or group activity); role features (possible initiative or subjugation) (Dzvonyk & Savchenko, 2011).

So, the generalization of the research of national and foreign scientists showed that the mental health of students is a complex, diverse phenomenon that manifests itself in mental and somatic reactions to stressful situations in the educational activities of an individual. It worsens emotional wellbeing and can negatively affect both physical and psychological health.

In the context of studying mental health disorders within students, there is a need to consider them in more detail. It is advisable to take into account the fact that during experiences of a social nature, there is a loss of satisfaction with the quality of relationships with fellow students, colleagues or higher leaders; decreased interest in those with whom it is necessary to communicate in status-role positions; dehumanization of relations, loss of benevolence, care and friendliness in situations of business communication; loss of interest in the environment; dissatisfaction with social and administrative support, feelings of alienation.

With experiences of a spiritual nature, dissatisfaction with self-realization is observed; experiencing the senselessness of spent efforts and hopelessness in the life plans implementation; loss of faith in one's own strength and potential; lowering the personal growth level; "loss of himself/herself".

During experiences of a physical nature, there is a loss of strength; ailments, insomnia, appetite disturbance; health deterioration.

With experiences of a material nature, there is a loss of enthusiasm and motivation for material earnings, a feeling of fatigue. In the case of psychological experiences, there is a loss of positive mood and emotional stability; decrease in self-esteem; a sense of desolation; lack of positive energy; loss of desires; dissatisfaction with one's mood and lack of cheerfulness; loss of mental balance (irritation, incontinence, fatigue, feelings of guilt, addiction, etc.); violations in the motivational and

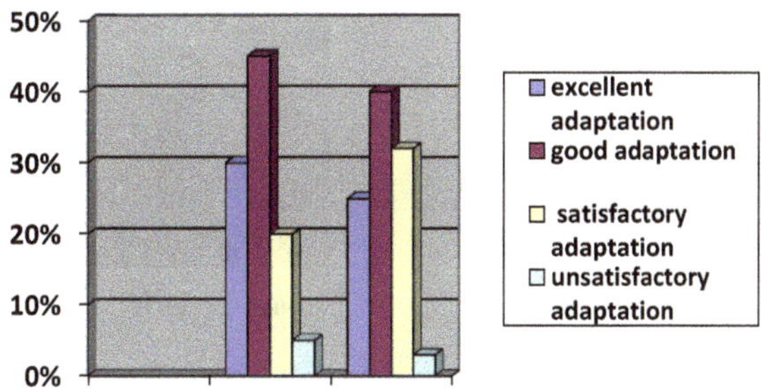

Fig. 11.1 Levels of students' adaptation of Ukrainian higher education institutions in war conditions

institutional sphere and in professional behaviour. As a result of this, there is mental (subjective), and in some cases, physical discomfort, a decrease or loss in activity and work capacity, a decrease in personal and social-psychological space (Dzvonyk & Savchenko, 2011).

In carrying out our own research, we sought to diagnose the mental health of students of Ukrainian higher education institutions, in particular, students of higher education at the bachelor's level of Yuriy Fedkovych Chernivtsi National University and Khmelnytskyi National University. For this purpose, diagnostic tests for adaptation, stress resistance, anxiety, emotional burnout and a questionnaire for self-assessment of the state of health were used.

The leading principles of diagnosis were defined: the principle of psychological research objectivity; the principle of multidimensional and multilevel existence of the researched subject; the principle of psychological phenomena in their development; the principle of creative self-activity; the principle of organizing formative and developing influences.

As for special principles, the following are highlighted by our conclusions, i.e. the professional competence principle; not harming those who participate in the research principle; the dispassion principle; the confidentiality principle; the voluntariness principle; etc.

We offered test materials for Ukrainian students in an electronic version as Google form.

To find out the peculiarities of students' adaptation to the educational environment, a questionnaire "Are you able to adapt quickly?" was used.

In 6 min, the students had to catch the pattern in the displayed numbers and letters. Answers completed without errors were counted. According to the test, which was passed by 150 people, the results shown in Fig. 11.1. were obtained.

As we can see from the figure, most of the respondents have good and excellent adaptation, and they are able to perform tasks that require stressing the emotional and volitional sphere. The indicator among boys is somewhat higher. We can explain this by the higher emotional threshold of boys compared to girls.

The chart illustrates within five per cent of students who have unsatisfactory adaptation. The conversation with them convinced us that these are people who have relatives in the war, they are sick, have the status of internally displaced persons or take care of sick relatives, that is, they are under the influence of strong emotional

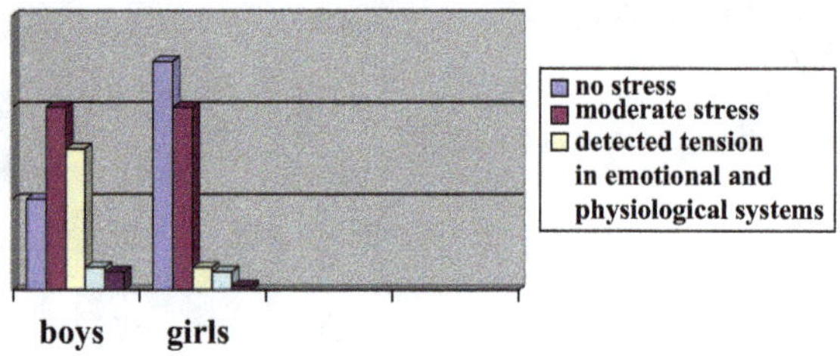

Fig. 11.2 Stress among students during the war

stimuli. Since their percentage on a sample of 150 people (100%) is insignificant, we can talk about the small influence of these students on the adaptation of other students.

To check the stress resistance of students in Ukrainian universities, we used the test of stress resistance according to V. Yu. Shcherbatykh (test for determining the level of stress). The test implementation created an opportunity to check the stress resistance of students based on intellectual, behavioural, emotional and physiological signs of stress. Figure 11.2 illustrates the results.

The diagram shows that almost half of the respondents' girls have no stress. Compared to boys, this indicator is higher.

We can explain the boys' stress by their passive participation in military operations on the territory of the state, a high level of involvement in volunteer activities and active discussion of military events.

At the same time, we have low percentages of depletion of adaptive energy reserves both among boys and girls.

Students who have illustrated this indicator need the intervention of a specialist, a qualified psychologist. Their condition requires a more detailed study, clarification of the condition causes, i.e. congenital or acquired, as well as corrective and rehabilitation assistance. In general, moderate stress prevails among the respondents. We can assume that this is influenced by frequent air alarms in the state.

Respondents generally rated their health as satisfactory. We chose the main criteria for self-assessment as physical condition on the border between norm and pathology; troubles in interpersonal relationships; unreasonable fears; violation of the harmony of creative abilities; and insufficient level of energy potential. Figure 11.3 graphically illustrates the responses.

Students are almost not bothered by unreasonable fears, but more than half of the respondents illustrate above-average indicators of problems in relationships with other people, which can be explained by the stress students are under and we note an insufficient energy potential level, which can be explained by the loss of body energy to ensure basic life activities. This is typical for people under chronic stress.

A special place in the diagnosis of mental health of students is occupied by the diagnosis of anxiety. The emotion of the "anxiety" type, performing signalling and evaluative functions in unfavourable situations for the individual, contributes to the development of psychological protection for the individual, which stimulates his/her search for a solution to the existing contradictions and therefore plays an important

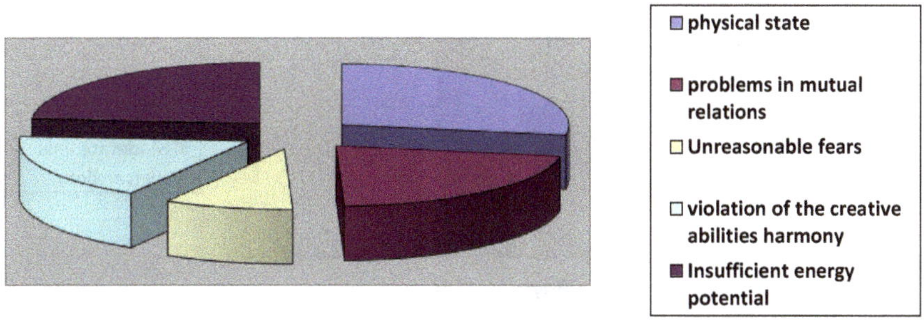

Fig. 11.3 Students' self-assessment of their health status

role in the dynamics of intra-personal disharmony. Despite the multifaceted and semantic uncertainty of the term "anxiety' in psychological research, it is most often used in two concepts: anxiety as a mental state and anxiety as a personality trait (anxiety).

In the first case, the term "anxiety" is used to describe an unpleasant emotional state characterized by subjective feelings of tension, anticipation of an unpleasant events development.

This condition arises in a situation of uncertain danger, threat.

In other case, anxiety as a trait, a personality trait, is characterized by a persistent tendency of a person to perceive a threat to his/her "I" in various situations and react to them by increasing the anxiety condition.

It should be noted that scientists have distinguished three groups of anxiety: personal, situational and pathological.

Personal anxiety is a stable and at the same time dynamic characteristic that reflects a person's tendency to perceive a wide range of situations and problems as threatening. It indicates increased inner restlessness and affects the peculiarities of perception and emotional-intellectual behaviour of a person.

Situational anxiety is peculiar temporary state that arises in unusual conditions and gives rise to such feelings as insecurity, fear and threat.

Pathological anxiety is a relatively stable and long-lasting state, the characteristic components of which are the depressing experience of vague fear and unpleasant anticipation of imminent danger. In addition to the signalling function, the alarm also performs the function of assessing the conflict situation. The assessment of a threatening situation leads to the launch of adaptive actions, protective mechanisms and other forms of adaptive activity, which have as their goal the elimination of the source of potential danger.

In the broadest sense, anxiety is a form of adaptation in a stressful situation; speaking about mentally healthy people, anxiety stimulates the emergence of defensive reactions to the situation. However, we note that the presence of low mood and the prevalence of negative emotions in a person can also be characterized by such a concept as depression, which has a wider meaning.

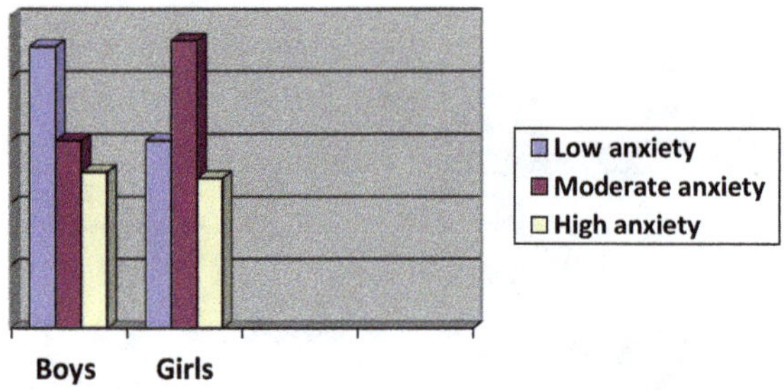

Fig. 11.4 Anxiety of students in Ukrainian higher education institutions

Students' anxiety was diagnosed using the Spielberger-Hanin test. The respondents were asked to read each of the given statements and cross out the corresponding number on the right depending on how the student feels at that particular moment. We calculated the indicator of situational (reactive) anxiety using the formula. The given results are presented in Fig. 11.4.

The figure illustrates the presence of high and moderate anxiety among students.

The obtained results were expected for our sample. We can explain the anxiety of students by the deterioration of the quality of life in connection with the war. But at the same time, they are not critical both among boys and girls.

The conducted survey convinced of the need to develop recommendations for improving the mental health of students in Ukrainian higher education institutions. We consider it expedient to pay attention to the following ways of its improvement:

1. Provision of adequate psycho-emotional space in student bomb shelters (reserve lighting, well-decorated walls of the shelter, availability of radios, televisions, Internet, places for rest and study).
2. Carrying out moments of psychological relief (tests, conversations based on situations, photos, humour) during lectures and seminars.
3. Creating and using animated presentations with the task of drawing a problem that worries.
4. Organising care for stray animals.
5. Optional meetings with priests show that religion and faith have a great potential to strengthen the mental health of an individual.
6. Work of groups in artistic creativity, psychological and medical care, volunteering.
7. In order to preserve the mental health of students in Ukrainian higher education institutions, it is advisable to take care of creating in the educational environment the recreation areas for students, cultivate moments of health during lectures, promote the psychological support of internally displaced students and conduct trainings.

Tests on the website "Anima" have proven themselves to be effective among psychologists. The project is aimed at helping internally displaced persons, military personnel and all those who are in conditions of increased stress. The tests are aimed at researching the neurobiological mechanisms of a person's mental state.

The study proved the urgency in the problem of preserving students' mental health. We summarized the approaches to defining this concept, analysed the difference between mental and psychological health of students, substantiated different approaches to defining criteria and indicators of mental health.

In our opinion, the nature of human mental health and its components should be considered as a systemic phenomenon, the essence of which can be understood through the study of existing concepts and views of scientists.

We share the opinion of scientists that mental health makes a person self-sufficient. Psychological health is associated with the concept of internal harmony of the individual, self-sufficient existence, and mental health is a state of mental wellbeing characterized by the absence of mental illnesses and medical conditions.

Empirical research has emphasized the expediency of strengthening work in the direction of preserving the mental health of students. For this purpose, we have proposed recommendations that require implementation in practice of work in Ukrainian higher education institutions.

Competing Interests The authors have no conflicts of interest to declare that are relevant to the content of this chapter.

List of References

Adler, A. (2015). The practice and theory of individual psychology: lektsyy po vvedenyiu v psykhoterapyiu dlia vrachei, psykholohov y uchytelei. Retrieved from: https://ia801504.us.archive.org/13/items/in.ernet.dli.2015.

Andros, M. (1998). Psykhichne zdorov'ia osobystosti: psykholohichne konsultuvannia kerivnykiv shkil [Mental health of the individual: Psychological counseling of school leaders.]. *Osvita i upravlinnia*. T. 2. №2, 63–69.

Befany, A. (2004). Psykhycheskoe zdorove kak proiavlenye lychnostnoi zrelosty."Psykholohiia osobystosti: dosvid mynuloho – pohliad u maibutnie" [Mental health as a manifestation of personal maturity. "Psychology of personality: Past experience—A look into the future"]. *Nauka i osvita*. № 6–7, 13–15.

Bevzenko, L. (2008). Styly zhyzny perekhodnoho obshchestva [Lifestyles of a transitional society]. K.: Instytut sotsiolohii NAN Ukrainy.

Boltivets, S. (2000). Pedahohichna psykhohihiiena. Teoriia ta metodyka [Pedagogical psychohygiene. Theory and methodology]: monohrafiia K.: Biuleten VAK Ukrainy, 302.

Convention on the Rights of the Child. (1991). Retrieved from: https://zakon.rada.gov.ua/

Convention on the Rights of Persons with. (2009). Retrieved from: https://zakon.rada.gov.ua/

Chyzhenko, N. (2006). Frustratsiina tolerantnist osobystosti yak afektyvnyi komponent optymizmu [Frustration tolerance as an affective component of optimism]. *Psykholohiia i osobystist*. № 2(10). Ch. 2, 146–155.

Dzvonyk, H., & Savchenko, T. (2011). Psykholohichni chynnyky vynyknennia profesiinoho stresu u menedzheriv [Psychological factors of professional stress in managers]. Materialy VII Miedzynarodowej naukowi-praktycznej konferencji "Europejska nauka XXI powieka 2011. (14), 62–72. Retrieved from https://lib.iitta.gov.ua/id/eprint/5385//

Dmytriiuk, N., & Schastna, K. (2003). Problemy psykhichnoho zdorov'ia molodi [Mental health problems of young people]. Imnforum siens for the future. Retrieved from https://www.inforum.in.ua/

Dmytryeva, T., & Polozhyi, B. (1994). Sotsyalnaia psykhyatryia: sovremennye predstavlenyia y perspektyvy razvytyia [Social psychiatry: Current concepts and prospects for development]. *Obozrenye psykhyatryy y medytsynskoi psykholohyy ym. V. M. Bekhtereva.* № 2.

Dubyna, S., Khapchenkova, D., & Bondarenko, S. (2018). Faktory, shcho vplyvaiut na studentsku uspishnist vyvchennia teoretychnoi dystsypliny [Factors influencing student performance in theoretical discipline]. K.

European Declaration on on the Protection of Mental Health. 12–15 Sichnia 2005 Roku. (2005). Khelsinki. Retrieved from https://apps.who.int/iris/handle/

European Social Charter. (1996). Retrieved from https://zakon.rada.gov.ua/laws/show/994_062#Text

Frankl, V. (1992). Man in search of meaning. Retrieved from https://psycnet.apa.org/record/1992-98457-000

Haletska, I. (2005). Metodolohichni problemy vyvchennia psykholohichnoho zdorovia [look at psychotherapy. Becoming human]. *Naukovi zapysky Instytutu psykholohii im. H. S. Kostiuka APN Ukrainy.* V. 26. / Maksymenko S. K., T. 1, 320–324.

Honcharenko, M. (1999). Valeolohycheskyi slovar [Valeological dictionary]. KhHU, 315.

Husiev, A. (2007). Do problemyformuvannia ta rozvytku tolerantnosti do nevyznachenosti [On the problem of formation and development of tolerance to uncertainty]. *Naukovyi chasopys Natsionalnoho pedahohichnoho universytetu imeni M. P. Drahomanova.* Ser. № 12. *Psykholohichni nauky.* K. № 17(41). Ch. 1, 101–113.

Huzenko, S. (2007). Zhyttievi kryzy v kontseptsiiakh [Life crises in the concepts of L. S. Vygotsky and E. G. Erikson.]. *Filosofiia. Psykholohiia. Pedahohika*: zbirnyk naukovykh prats. Ch. 1. № 2, 64–68.

Kichuk, A. (2019). Psykholohichnezdorovia osobystosti yak tsinnist i predmet suchasnoho psykholohichnoho znannia [Psychological health of the individual as a value and subject of modern psychological knowledge]. *Naukovyi visnyk Khersonskoho derzhavnoho universytetu. Seriia psykholohichni nauky.* V. 1, 36–40.

Kolotii, N. (2003). Psykholohichne zdorovia ta yoho otsinka v umovakh zahalnoosvitnoho navchalnoho zakladu [Psychological health and its assessment in a general education institution]: avtoref. dys. na zdobuttia nauk. stupenia kand. psykhol. nauk: spets. 19.00.07 Pedahohichna ta vikova psykholohiia. Kharkiv, 2003.

Kostiuk, D., & Kostiuk, V. (2018). Psykhichne ta psykholohichne zdorov'ia osobystosti: Poniattia, zmist ta kryterii [Mental and psychological health of a person: Concept, content and criteria]. *Visnyk Natsionalnoho Universytetu Oborony Ukrainy., 2*(50), 45–50.

Maksymenko, S. (2002). Psykhichne zdorovia ditei [Mental health of children]. *Psykholoh.* № 1 (1), 4–6.

Maslou, A. (2002). Toward a psychology of being. Retrieved from https://psycnet.apa.org/record/2005-06675-

Mental Health Declaration for Europe. (2005). Retrieved from https://iris.who.int/handle/10665/107625

Mental Health System Transformation in Ukraine: Improving Mental Health Services and Bringing Mental Health Care in Line with International Standards. (2018). Retrieved from https://moz.gov.ua/en/mental-health-system-transformation-in-ukraine-improving-mental-health-services-and-bringing-mental-health-care-in-line-with-intern

Mirov, D. (2020). Psykhichne zdorov'ia: poniattia ta struktura. Aktualni problemy osobystisnoho zrostannia [Mental health: Concept and structure. Actual problems of personal growth]. Retrieved from http://eprints.zu.edu.ua/29605/

Moskalets, V. (2004). V. Psykholohiia suitsydu [Psychology of suicide] (2004): posibnyk / K.: Akademvydav, 288.

Petkov, V. (2015). Anomalii rozvytku osobystosti yak psykholohichna problema [Personality development anomalies as a psychological problem]. *Visnyk Natsionalnoho universytetu oborony Ukrainy*. Retrieved from http://nbuv.gov.ua/

Potapchuk, Y. (2004). Sotsialno-psykholohichni osnovy zberezhennia psykhichnoho zdorov'ia viiskovosluzhbovtsiv [Social and psychological bases of preserving mental health of military personnel]: dys....dokt. psykh. nauk. 19.00.09.

Pryb, I. (2016). Osnovy sotsialnoi psykhiatrii i narkolohii [Social psychiatry and narcology. K.: IPK DSZU, 225.

Pyliahina, H. (2020). Medychna psykholohiia. T.2. Spetsialna medychna psykholohiia [Medical psychology. Special medical psychology]. K.: Novai knyhy.

Resolution 70/1 adopted by the United Nations General Assembly on "Transforming our world: The 2030 Agenda for Sustainable Development ". (2015). Retrieved from https://ips.ligazakon.net/

Sirko, R. (2002). Psykhichne zdorovia u starshomu yunatskomu vitsi yak predmet psykholohichnoho analizu [Mental health in older adolescence as a subject of psychological analysis]: dys... kand. psykhol. nauk: 19.00.01. L., 282.

Sydorchuk, N., & Tryhubchuk, M. (2018). Osoblyvosti profesiinoho zdorov'ia vykladacha zakladu vyshchoi osvity ta syndrom profesiinoho vyhorannia [Peculiarities of professional health of a teacher of a higher education institution and professional burnout syndrome.]. *Andrahohichnyi Visnyk: Nauk. Elektr. Zhurnal., 9*, 102–113.

Tanella, M., Dzhyrolamo, D., & Sartoryus, N. (1998). Annotyrovannaia byblyohrafyia psykhycheskoi epydemyolohyy [An annotated bibliography of psychiatric epidemiology]. K., 106.

The European Concept of Human Rights. (2010). Retrieved from: https://zakon.rada.gov.ua/

The Joint Action on Mental Health and Wellbeing. (2020). Retrieved from http://www.mentalhealthandwellbeing.eu/. he world health report 1998 Life in the 21st century (1998) Retrieved from https://santamaria.com.ua//

The World Health Report. (1998). Life in the 21st century: A vision for all (1998). Retrieved from https://apps.who.int/gb/archive/pdf_files/wha51/ea3.pdf

Turynina, O. L. (2017). Psykholohiia travmuiuchykh sytuatsii [Psychology of traumatic situations]: navch. posib. dlia stud. vyshch. navch. zakl. K.: DP "Vyd. dim "Personal".

Tytarenko, T., & Dvornyk, M. (2022). Yak dopomohty osobystosti v period perekhodu vid viiny do myru: sotsialno-psykholohichnyi suprovid [How to help a person during the transition from war to peace: social and psychological support]: praktychnyi posibnyk. Kropyvnytskyi: Imeks-LTD, 154.

Yarema, N. (2015). Psykholohichne zdorov'ia osobystosti [Psychological health of the individual]. *Yurydychna Psykholohiia., 2*, 106–113.

Yashchyshyna, Y. (2011). Sotsialni ta osobystisni chynnyky psykhichnoho zdorovia studentskoi molodi [Social and personal factors of mental health of students]. Dys. kand. psykh. nauk. 19.00.07- pedahohichna ta vikova psykholohiia. Luhansk.

Zavhorodnia, O., & Kurhanska, L. (2008). Psykholohichne zdorovia liudyny: teoretychni ta prykladni aspekty [Human psychological health: Theoretical and applied aspects]: monohrafiia. K: DP "Informatsiino-analitychne ahenstvo", 167.

Zhavnerchyk, O. (2020). Psykholohiia upravlinnia [Psychology of management]: Konspekt lektsii. ODEEKU.

Chapter 12
Conclusions. Building a Culture of Wellbeing in Education—Insights and Future Directions

Aurora Adina Colomeischi

This book intended to explore the concept and implementation of wellbeing in education, combining theoretical models with case studies from six South-Eastern European countries. By juxtaposing theory with field-based evidence, it provides a rich, multi-level understanding of how emotional, social, and psychological wellbeing is being integrated—or still needs to be—into national educational systems. This book set out to investigate how wellbeing in education is conceptualized, supported, and developed across Europe, with a special focus on the South-Eastern region. The theoretical part laid the groundwork for understanding how educational wellbeing is deeply interwoven with mental health promotion, family dynamics, school climate, and teacher resilience. Drawing on interdisciplinary literature and European policy analyses, these chapters provide a cohesive lens through which to frame subsequent empirical work.

The theoretical part pointed out important themes for deepen understanding of wellbeing as a priority not only at the policies level but also at the functional school levels.

As discussed in Chapter 2, wellbeing cannot be the sole responsibility of schools. European policy increasingly recognizes the need for integrated, intersectoral approaches, linking education with health, social protection, employment, and housing to reduce structural inequalities that affect children's wellbeing.

Chapter 3 highlighted that teacher wellbeing is not only a personal issue but a core component of school effectiveness. Teachers' resilience—shaped by working conditions, administrative support, and professional identity—profoundly influences both classroom climate and students' academic success.

A. A. Colomeischi (✉)
Faculty of Psychology and Sciences of Education, "Ştefan cel Mare" University of Suceava, Suceava, Romania
e-mail: adina.colomeischi@usm.ro

A. A. Colomeischi (ed.), *Wellbeing in Schools of Southeastern Europe*, Human Well-Being Research and Policy Making,
https://doi.org/10.1007/978-3-032-10525-7_12

Chapter 4 established that a positive, inclusive, and culturally responsive climate supports both mental health and learning outcomes, and school climate is a foundation for children wellbeing. It called for longitudinal and context-sensitive research to inform tailored interventions that respect local needs.

Chapter 5 emphasized that family stress and parental mental health are key predictors of student wellbeing. Parent-focused interventions—especially those enhancing co-parenting, stress management, and school engagement—are vital but under-researched in South-Eastern Europe.

These chapters collectively call for a paradigm shift: from treating wellbeing as an add-on or afterthought in education to embedding it as a core value, structural pillar, and right. The integration of models such as PERMA(-H), resilience theory, and systemic ecological frameworks underscores the need to move beyond fragmented initiatives toward holistic wellbeing systems.

Importantly, the book underscores that wellbeing is not a singular experience, but a relational, cultural, and systemic construct that plays out across personal, institutional, and societal levels.

The second part of the book focused on the analysis of wellbeing at school in different south-eastern European countries. Across the case studies, a shared recognition emerges: wellbeing is no longer a peripheral theme, but a central mission of modern education.

The chapter about Bulgaria emphasized systemic reform, stressing integrated policies and a "whole school" approach to enhance children's resilience and learning environments.

The chapter about Croatia underscored the importance of evidence-based SEL (social-emotional learning) programs and highlighted the PROMEHS curriculum as a promising model for sustainable teacher training and student wellbeing.

The chapter about Greece focused on teacher wellbeing, showcasing how supporting educators' emotional competencies directly improves student outcomes.

The chapter about Moldova offered a deep theoretical and structural model (Antoci & Mîslițchi) combining pedagogical, psychological, and social dimensions, with strong emphasis on teacher engagement and contextual challenges.

The chapter about Romania presented an integrated framework mapping educational policies and programs directly onto international wellbeing and resilience models—demonstrating strategic alignment with other theoretical models (PERMA-H, Konu, and Grotberg).

The chapter about Ukraine addressed wellbeing under conditions of extreme adversity, focusing on mental health and psychosocial support for students during war, which enriched the book with a humanitarian dimension of resilience.

While theory provided a vision, the case studies revealed the practical challenges of translating vision into sustained practice across diverse socio-political contexts.

Implications for policy, practice, and research should be drawn. Policymakers must acknowledge wellbeing as a measurable educational outcome, not merely a supportive condition. Based on European policies, coordinated national strategies can model how to embed wellbeing in curriculum, training, infrastructure, and legislation. The European countries benefit already by this focus on wellbeing at school provided by European educational policies, but Moldavia and Ukraine, as European acceding countries, could benefit as well in the future. Focusing on educators and practitioners, they need evidence-based training in SEL and trauma-informed practices, institutional cultures that promote both student and teacher wellbeing and collaborative frameworks that integrate schools with families and communities. Researchers are encouraged to conduct longitudinal studies on wellbeing interventions, to evaluate cross-national programs for cultural adaptability and impact and to investigate teacher wellbeing as a predictor of student wellbeing.

The variety of experiences presented in this volume confirms that wellbeing in education is a universal yet locally nuanced challenge. Investing in wellbeing today lays the foundation for a resilient, empathetic, and capable generation tomorrow. We urge educators, leaders, parents, and young people to collaborate in creating learning environments where every child is seen, supported, and inspired. It is our moral duty to care for the next generation because children only have one childhood, and we must ensure that school cultivates their full potential.

www.ingramcontent.com/pod-product-compliance
Lightning Source LLC
Chambersburg PA
CBHW052302310326
42230CB00003B/35
9783032105240